D1629852

TEXTBOOK OF ORTHOPAEDIC MEDICINE

2. Treatment by Manipulation, Massage and Injection

Also by James Cyriax

Textbook of Orthopaedic Medicine, Volume I
Diagnosis of Soft Tissue Lesions

Osteopathy and Manipulation
(1949: Crosby Lockwood)

The Slipped Disc
(1970: Gower Press)

Cervical Spondylosis
(1972: Butterworths)

Manipulation Past and Present
(1975: Heinemann)

TEXTBOOK OF
Orthopaedic
Medicine

VOLUME TWO

Treatment by Manipulation
Massage and Injection

JAMES CYRIAX MD (Cantab), MRCP (Lond)

*Honorary Consultant Physician in Orthopaedic Medicine,
St Thomas's Hospital, London; Visiting Professor in
Orthopaedic Medicine, Strong Memorial Hospital, University
of Rochester, New York, USA*

AND

GILLEAN RUSSELL MCSP

*Formerly Superintendent Physiotherapist, St Andrew's
Hospital, London, and Senior Physiotherapist, St Thomas's
Hospital, London*

Ninth Edition

Baillière Tindall · London

A BAILLIÈRE TINDALL book published by
Cassell & Collier Macmillan Publishers Ltd
35 Red Lion Square, London WC1R 4SG
and at Sydney, Auckland, Toronto, Johannesburg
an affiliate of
Macmillan Publishing Co. Inc.
New York

First published in 1944 as
Deep Massage and Manipulation

Eighth edition 1971
Revised and reprinted 1974
Ninth edition 1977
Reprinted 1977

ISBN 0 7020 0638 6

Spanish edition (Editorial Medica Panamericana, Buenos Aires) 1973
French edition (Masson et Cie, Editeurs, Paris) 1976
Italian edition (Editore Piccin, Padua) in preparation

Printed in Great Britain by
Cox & Wyman Ltd, London, Fakenham and Reading

Preface

Advances in orthopaedic medicine over the last thirty years have brought about many welcome changes in doctors' and physiotherapists' work. Gone is the justification for vague methods with widespread intention and little effect. Gone too are the days of infiltrating tender spots at random with a local anaesthetic solution or a suspension of hydrocortisone. Thanks to improved diagnosis, such blunderbuss measures are now being replaced by treatment directed to the lesion alone, referred pain and tenderness being ignored. Until the first edition of this textbook appeared twenty-seven years ago, the diagnostic problems posed by trouble in the radio-translucent moving parts appeared insoluble. The clinical method of selective tension set out in Volume I, supplemented when necessary by confirmation by diagnostic local anaesthesia, has since made it possible to single out a lesion with remarkable accuracy. Treatment must keep pace. As these diagnostic measures become ever more widely practised, so must the doctor's needle and the physiotherapist's finger be used with ever greater exactitude. It is, therefore, the aim of this book to foster precision in treatment, whatever form it may take.

Physiotherapists manipulate for a specific purpose and administer deep friction to an accurately localized lesion. Doctors also manipulate and give injections at a well-defined point within the structure at fault. To the description of manual methods was therefore added in the eighth edition equal consideration of standard injection techniques. For the first time, both aspects of one therapeutic problem are catered for—medical and physiotherapeutic—with the result that manipulation, traction, injections and deep friction are set out in one volume. For this reason, it is my hope that doctors and physiotherapists alike will consult it for the proper performance of their overlapping work.

Another feature of the book first introduced in the eighth edition is a summary of the physical signs identifying each disorder under consideration. This jogs the reader's memory and enables a fresh assessment to be made whenever necessary on the site of the trouble and on its response to treatment. This knowledge also helps the physiotherapist to make up her mind when great enough alteration in the signs has supervened to warrant reference back to the physician for further advice. Whenever effective methods of treatment are employed, the decision *not* to continue forms an important part of her responsibility. Lately the inclusion of physical signs

has carried a fresh advantage. It has been shown that hydrocortisone can
be driven through the skin into the deeper tissues by phonophoresis with
ultrasonic waves. This has opened a new field for the physiotherapist,
but it involves her in interpreting physical signs and directing her steroid
suspension with the same accuracy as is necessary for deep friction.

All the spinal manipulative methods described here were devised with
reference to the intervertebral disc. They do not depend on the osteopathic idea of restoring a full range of movement to a spinal joint, nor on
the chiropractic notion of the displaced vertebra. They have no autonomic
effects and can thus be used on normal healthy people. All physiotherapists should be familiar with them; and they will also wish to master the
deep friction techniques. All the injections can be carried out by any
medical man interested in an exact diagnosis and proper siting of a needle.
In short, this book contains a record of the standard tuition given by me
to the medical and physiotherapy students at St Thomas's Hospital until
my retirement at the end of 1969. I then went on teaching for another five
years at St Andrew's, London, where Gillean Russell, already my senior
physiotherapist at St Thomas's for five years, loyally accompanied me. I
cannot value too highly the support she gave me over that decade. She is
now in private practice.

Then the publishers pointed out that my advancing years placed the
future of this book in jeopardy, and called for an associate editor (to carry
on after my death, so I took it). I did not have far to seek. Gillean Russell
not only has an excellent grasp of the diagnosis and treatment of the
medical lesions of the moving parts, but she is also fully versed in the
manual techniques that they demand. To these talents she adds a third:
sensitive perception of English usage, a gift by which I lay great store. It
was therefore a great pleasure to me, and a great relief to my publishers,
when she agreed to step in to close the impending breach. Continuity of
knowledge is now secured for would-be physiotherapists as yet in their
cradles.

December 1976   JAMES CYRIAX

Contents

Teaching Facilities offered by the Author

1. Six-day course in orthopaedic medicine twice a year. Please write to Dr J. Cyriax, 32 Wimpole Street, London W1, whereupon a programme is sent, six months ahead, for acceptance or refusal.

2. Weekend courses for final-year physiotherapy students. These are held on a Saturday–Sunday basis, 10 a.m. till 6 p.m. each day. As often as we accumulate twenty applicants from various schools the course is given. Please write to Dr Cyriax's senior physiotherapist, 32 Wimpole Street, London W1.

3. A doctor or a physiotherapist can, by previous arrangement, sit in on my private consultations, but only one at a time.

4. Private tuition from my staff is available.

TAPED RECORDINGS

Copies of *audio-recordings* of lectures are available on cassette tapes at a cost of $35.00 each. Copies of *audio-visual tapings* of lecture demonstrations are also available at a cost of $80.00 each. These may be ordered from: Media Co-ordinator, Medical Center Media, Box 709, University of Rochester Medical Center, Rochester, New York 14642, U.S.A.

List of Illustrations

Part I
Principles and Technique of Manipulation and Massage

1
Logical Treatment

When I was a medical student I read and re-read Bertrand Russell's *Sceptical Essays*. He put forward convincing arguments in favour of reason as against mere custom as a basis for conduct and set out the radical changes that would follow the application of this logical code to ordinary daily life. I was much influenced and to this day have tried to follow his precepts, applying them to the best of my ability to my medical work. This endeavour has led me away from many traditional ideas, and towards a factual approach, sometimes with disturbing effect on others. Clearly, traditional orthodoxy cannot be challenged without upsetting the *status quo*, but work based on observation and reasoned deductions from it engenders interest and must finally gain acceptance. Now, thirty-two years after the first edition of this book appeared, the idea of treatment applied to the lesion is no longer a debated proposition. Even so, though the (so I should have thought) unarguable concepts put before the reader are simple, much of today's physiotherapy would be revolutionized if they were acted upon.

My work is based on three principles:

1. All pain arises from a lesion.
2. All treatment must reach the lesion.
3. All treatment must exert a beneficial effect on the lesion.

These three postulates seem unexceptionable enough to me, but they are violated daily, to the lasting detriment of doctors' and patients' views on physiotherapy. Acceptance would not alter in-patient treatment or orthopaedic work, for treatment is then clearly based on an accurate concept of the disorder present. For example, a patient with a fracture or after an orthopaedic operation would still need exercises; after thoracoplasty, posture would still require attention; general anaesthesia would still call for breathing exercises; bronchiectasis would still necessitate postural drainage.

Consider by contrast the fate of the out-patient with pain in the neck, trunk or limb in whom the radiograph shows nothing relevant. If something is out of place, does the physiotherapist attempt reduction? If a tendon or muscle is strained, does she apply deep friction to the affected point? If a ligament is sprained, is she expected digitally to maintain mobility at the tear? Unhappily, it is much more likely that she is asked to give heat and massage to the area of the pain, followed by exercises. Even when the diagnosis of, say, a displaced fragment of intervertebral disc has been reached, it is still unusual for the physiotherapist to be asked to try to put it back. When a muscle or tendon has been strained, further tension increases symptoms; now, too, exercises have no value. The heat that is so often ordered usually affects only the skin and superficial fascia. Such heat might help skin disease (though I doubt it); it certainly cannot affect tissues lying beyond these rays' reach. Penetrating heat rays exist and can increase blood supply along their route. Deep heat is useful in sepsis, bringing more leucocytes to the area and hastening resolution. But there are no bacteria to kill off in, say, lumbago, a stiff shoulder or a sprained knee. All that deep heat can do is to promote blood-flow and increase oedema—both of which are already excessive after trauma. Any reader would smile superciliously if he heard that in Asia the devils were driven out of a man's painful back by the application, let us say, of hot dung; but here today many doctors are not ashamed to order, and physiotherapists to give, infra-red rays in lumbago. What is the difference?

Clearly diffuse massage, whether given gently or deeply, has no part to play in soft-tissue lesions. Indeed, the obvious futility of this type of massage has led to the virtual abandonment of friction for all purposes. This is most unfortunate, since a number of lesions exist for which there is no alternative treatment, and a curable disorder becomes regarded as intractable for lack of trained personnel.

The employment of diffuse massage is based on the concept that it is beneficial to increase the circulation within the painful area. Increasing the circulation is advantageous only in septic conditions; but these, for other reasons, are not treated by radiant heat or massage. Supposing the local circulation were temporarily increased, in say, a tennis elbow, a sprained knee or lumbago, what possible benefit would accrue? Does increased circulation break down adhesions in a tendon, move a strained ligament or reduce an intra-articular displacement? Clearly not. It washes away, its advocates maintain, toxins and waste products. What toxins and waste products are these? A painful muscle or joint hurts the instant that strain falls on it, long before any waste products have begun to accumulate. Even if waste products were present, would it be sound policy to remove them as fast as they were formed, rather than to deal with the lesion responsible for their presence?

It is usual when the pathological concept of some syndrome changes to alter the treatment correspondingly. For example, in the olden days lumbago was thought to be due to muscular inflammation (Gowers, 1904), i.e. fibrositis, and treatment was given to, and did in fact affect, the muscles. Heat, massage, exercises—these did reach the muscles and the treatment was a logical extension of what was then believed. Nowadays the patient with lumbago is told that he has a slipped disc (Cyriax, 1945), implying that something is out of place. This is indeed true; but what is the treatment? Manipulative reduction? Not at all; the same heat, massage and exercises as he would have received at the turn of the century. Even today most people have to go outside the medical and physiotherapy professions to various shades of lay manipulators for rational therapy for spinal intra-articular displacements. A curious paradox results. It has now become obvious that these men, biased and untutored as they may be, have for all these years been giving what logic now shows to be the correct treatment for many spinal troubles, whereas under the best medical auspices the rational treatment—namely, manipulation—has been withheld. At St Thomas's Hospital, when we realized what lumbago really was, we thought out and tried out methods of treatment based on the new idea. We attempted direct action on the lesion, ignoring the unaffected muscles. Similarly, we no longer waste time giving quadriceps exercises to a recently sprained ligament at the knee; we treat the ligament itself, thus enabling the patient to use his knee so well that no wasting has time to come about. When contraction of a muscle pulls on a painful scar within itself or in a tendon, we try to get rid of the inflammation in the scar, or even the excess scar tissue itself.

This book represents an attempt to bring reason to bear on the problems of orthopaedic medicine as applied to non-specific painful disorders of the moving parts of the body. Due emphasis must be laid on the fact that the measures used are not dependent on the whim of any individual; it is the nature and position of the lesion that determine treatment. Throughout, the choice of method depends on the diagnosis. Accurate treatment follows as a logical result and requires a high degree of knowledge and skill.

Treatment of the type with which this book is concerned demands a great deal more from the physiotherapist than the routine switching on and off of lamps, massage over a wide area, and some desultory exercises. Each patient must be individually studied and the aim of treatment explained to him so that cooperation is gained. Minor variations in the anatomy of the part to be treated must be noted and the major variations in patients' capacity to bear pain must be taken into account. Patients must be questioned about any change in their symptoms at every attendance, and each session usually begins with an examination that reveals at once any alteration in the physical signs. It is by constant thoughtful handling of the moving parts of the body that the physiotherapist learns her craft.

Adequate manipulation demands knowledge of the range of movement at a joint and of the sensations imparted to the hand as each extreme is approached and the ability to estimate that tissue resistance has mounted to the point when the thrust should be applied. The different effects of different techniques must be appreciated, together with the capacity to choose the correct measure for different types of lesion. During treatment by deep friction great precision in siting of the patient and of the physiotherapist's hand is essential; throughout the session she keeps her mind on her finger-tip. This type of work involves her in much more concentration and care than most of her other work. There is nothing routine about it; each patient and each lesion must be assessed and given expert and individual attention. This extra knowledge and attitude is more trouble, but has the compensating virtue that the physiotherapist who cures a patient well and quickly feels justifiable pride in her own handiwork. Patients too are quick to appreciate genuine treatment and the atmosphere created is a reward in itself. It is by this means that all members of the physiotherapy profession—teachers and practitioners alike—should seek to reverse the justified scepticism with which doctors regard some of their work. The medical profession has a true regard for members of the physiotherapy profession and physicians and surgeons alike value their work on inpatients. But the doctor who hears that 'a bit of heat, some massage, a few exercises' is what a patient of his was given has some difficulty in reconciling such 'treatment' with what he saw carried out so effectively in the wards of his teaching-hospital. He begins to think of physiotherapy as a placebo, or valuable chiefly for its psychological effect: ideas that must be strongly resisted. There is no room for such damaging attitudes when treatment concentrated on the lesion is the order of the day.

It is by accurate treatment that doctors' interest will be retained and public esteem at present extended to lay manipulators brought back to the qualified physiotherapist to whom it rightly belongs. Deep friction and mobilization both figure in the Chartered Society of Physiotherapy's syllabus; manipulation is expressly excluded. Hence many students still qualify without appreciable grounding in the two most important ways of using their hands in treatment.

IMPENDING PITFALL

I see an awkward situation looming. Courses in manipulation have lately been given to graduate physiotherapists who had not been grounded in this work as students. This is indeed a step in the right direction, but it must be remembered that it is highly undesirable to teach manipulation in isolation from clinical medicine, merely as a series of techniques. It must be taught in conjunction with clinical examination and diagnosis, otherwise the manipulating physiotherapist becomes an indiscriminating technician. For thirty years all my students have been grounded in manipulation, it is true, but my emphasis throughout has been on the manner in which the clinical examination is conducted which alone enables a decision to be reached on whether this measure is indicated or not. It also enables the operator to decide what type of technique to employ, and to follow with proper understanding the significance of the relevant changes in physical signs as the session progresses.

Great attention must be paid to this aspect of tuition on manipulation, otherwise the qualified physiotherapist may sink to the level of the self-styled bonesetter. Many of these men treat everyone who crosses their threshold—suitable and unsuitable cases alike—by their particular brand of forced movement. Most of their clients need no manipulation at all, but neither patient nor bonesetter has the medical knowledge to realize that. It is true that these men get an occasional dramatic success which the patient broadcasts to all. But there are also a large number of avoidable failures which are not mentioned: a patient quite easy to put right, did they but know it, but not by manipulation.

A physiotherapist who has become disillusioned with routine measures may well start manipulating and obtain a sequence of good successes in her early series. Thus encouraged, she may begin to regard manipulation as a near-panacea, in the osteopathic and chiropractic way. Unless given a factual theoretical basis for assessing the need for this treatment, she may be led away by a burst of enthusiasm. This is a danger which can be simply countered by insisting on exact clinical localization of the lesion, i.e. examination before and during the session.

In students, this logical attitude is not difficult to inculcate and ensures that the physiotherapist maintains her proper status; for she possesses a firm theoretical foundation on which to base her work. It is no help to argue that the doctor makes the diagnosis and the physiotherapist merely carries it out. She is not just a technician, carrying out orders like an automaton; she uses her own judgement. For this reason, examination and diagnosis have always formed, in my view, the larger part of all instruction in manipulation. It is not whether the hand is held so or so that matters; it is the proper selection of cases based on an informed clinical examination, with which she must be fully conversant.

Here lies the hiatus to which I hope greater attention will be paid in future postgraduate courses.

2

Theory and Practice of Massage

Massage is given in many ways for many purposes. This book is concerned only with those manual techniques, frictional and manipulative, that reach the lesion and do good there. Superficial techniques applied at a distance from the lesion cannot be expected to help. Observation of the results of this sort of work—the only sort of work most doctors ever see—has led many medical men to regard massage as entirely worthless, at most as affording transitory palliation. Hence this book is devoted to putting forward a standard massage and manipulative technique in the assurance that it will achieve consistent results, and in the hope that it may eventually lead to general agreement on the indications for, and techniques of, manual methods.

Radiant Heat and Massage

If radiant heat were really beneficial, no patient should be asked to spend time and money on travelling to a hospital to receive such rays for a short period two or three times a week when he could easily receive similar irradiation at home in front of his own fire for many hours a day in comfort. Not only would it save the patient much inconvenience, but it would reserve hospital departments' time and space for more sensible purposes. In fact, of course, superficial heating does no good to deep-seated lesions; moreover the wasted expenditure is considerable, for Glanville has worked out that six treatments by radiant heat cost the National Health Service £5. Six aspirins would cost a penny. Yet, though logically indefensible, heat is often ordered, to the lasting discredit of physiotherapy.

Doctors and patients are impressed by results. Doctors must be convinced that, though diffuse massage is not beneficial, the results of adequate friction given to a definite spot are often dramatic and can surpass all other methods now known. Even more is this true of manipulation, for the prescription of heat and massage to disorders (e.g. lumbago) in fact requiring manipulation is a frequent and lamentable error that should in justice bring discredit on the prescriber only, not on the physiotherapist who carried out a doctor's request. But patients unfortunately tend to esteem or decry the operator on the basis of results. Hence the main effect of withholding logical treatment for many displacements, i.e. reduction, has been to play us straight into the hands of lay manipulators, and to transfer public esteem to various denominations of bonesetter. This is a situation that all who have the good name of physiotherapy at heart will wish to reverse.

TYPES OF MANUAL TREATMENT

1. Deep Effleurage

This technique serves to relieve congestion. Swelling is treated in many situations by upward stroking of sufficient depth to remove it. The chief indications for effleurage are oedema and traumatic periostitis.

Oedema

Whether the oedema appears as the result of an injury, of the removal of a plaster cast from the lower limb or of venous thrombosis or is of the type known as angioneurotic, effleurage is usually indicated for its diminution or removal. A crêpe bandage should be applied tightly at the end of each session and kept on until the next session. The massage should be given daily, sometimes more often. In the treatment of oedema due to heart failure, phlebitis, nephritis or lymphatic obstruction caused by carcinomatous invasion, massage is only a temporary palliative. The oedema about an infected area must not be treated by massage, and hereditary oedema of the leg (Milroy's disease) and oedema due to filaria (elephantiasis) are not benefited. The oedema that always occurs after an amputation, especially at the lower limb, should be treated not by massage but by continuous pressure bandaging, tightened several times a day.

Traumatic Periostitis

Since the periosteum is attached to a motionless structure—bone—the formation of adherent scars is harmless. Deep friction is, therefore, never required. The periosteum is painful because it is swollen, and no more need be done than to reduce the swelling by firm, but not painful, deep effleurage, given daily. If a subperiosteal haematoma is present, aspiration will much hasten the patient's recovery, since blood is absorbed very slowly thence.

2. Deep Friction

The most potent form of massage is deep friction. By this means, and by this means alone, massage can reach structures far below the surface of the body. Since the source of pain in patients for whom manual methods are required so often lies in muscle, tendon or ligament, whether as the result of injury or repeated strain, a penetrating technique is clearly essential if such tissues are to be affected. It is thus vital to every physiotherapist faced with the treatment of a variety of common disorders that she should be fully acquainted with this—the most remedial—type of massage.

When mobility is to be maintained at, or restored to, those moving parts which from their nature or position are apt to develop adhesions or scarring, deep friction is often the method of choice, either alone (as in the case of tendons) or in association with passive movements (for some ligamentous lesions) or with active movements without tension on the healing breach (for minor muscular ruptures). An important part of a physiotherapist's knowledge consists in choosing and applying whichever type of therapeutic movement is best adapted to the patient's disorder.

DEEP MASSAGE

The philosopher who sits in an armchair and considers the question of deep massage in the treatment of painful lesions is driven by apparent logic to the conclusion that it is never called for at all. Clearly, he says to himself, if a structure is already damaged, massage given with penetrating effect can only irritate it the more. Alternatively, massage so administered that it does not reach the lesion is obviously valueless. The essential fact about deep friction is as follows: it applies therapeutic movement over only a very small area. The movement is the more effective for being so concentrated. Indeed, greater movement may easily be imparted locally by the physiotherapist's finger than could ever have been obtained by any amount of the most strenuous exercises and it moves those very tissues on which manipulation has no effect. On account of its purely local action, deep friction must be applied to the exact site of the lesion; otherwise it is useless. Indeed, it is harmful, in so far as it hurts the patient without bringing him any eventual benefit.

Mode of Action of Deep Massage
A penetrating technique is required in the treatment by massage of deep-seated lesions. Given properly, deep friction has a dual effect. It induces (1) traumatic hyperaemia and (2) movement.

1. *Traumatic Hyperaemia*
Enhancement of the blood supply diminishes pain. Apparently it acts by increasing the speed of destruction of Lewis's P-substance, the factor responsible for the pain. Heat and counter-irritants soothe for the duration of their application, also as the result of a similar enhancement of blood-

flow. They have no lasting effect upon the type of lesion under discussion, because no other change than the circulatory is secured. Deep massage results in a more lasting hyperaemia and it appears to be in this way that the friction, though in itself painful, is found at the end of the session to have allayed the symptoms for a while. In other words, deep massage given to the lesion itself affords temporary analgesia, and during this period treatment can be given that pain would otherwise have prevented.

2. Movement

By moving the painful structure to and fro, it is freed from adhesions both actually present and in the process of formation. Clearly massage applied parallel to the length of a structure follows the course of the blood and lymph vessels, whereas transverse friction does not. Hence longitudinal frictions merely move blood and lymph along, whereas *transverse friction moves the tissue itself*. In most conditions, there is nothing wrong with the circulation, hence there is no advantage in trying to alter it. I regard the lasting benefit that so often follows massage in muscular, tendinous and ligamentous lesions as accruing from the application of therapeutic movement to the affected part.

Deep Massage for Muscular Lesions

The main function of muscle is to contract. As it does so it broadens. Hence full mobility in broadening out must be maintained or restored in muscles that have been the seat of inflammation, whether caused by one or by repeated strains. Resolution by fibrosis is occurring or has already occurred. The effect of deep transverse friction clearly consists in mobilizing the muscle, i.e. separating the adhesions between individual muscle fibres that are restricting movement. If passive restoration of full mobility of a muscle is followed by adequate active use, these adhesions do not re-form; cure results.

The principle governing the treatment of muscles during the acute or chronic stage is the same. The endeavour must be to prevent the continued adherence of unwanted young fibrous tissue in recent cases, or to rupture adherent scar tissue in long-standing cases. To stretch out a muscle does not widen the distance between its fibres; on the contrary, during stretching they lie more closely. Whereas, then, for the rupture of adherent scars about a joint forced movement is required, interfibrillary adhesions in muscle can be broken, not by stretching, but by forcibly broadening the muscle out. Particularly is this true of the fibres of attachment of muscle into bone, where the vicinity of stationary tissue restricts the mobility of adjacent muscle. *Thus, deep transverse frictions restore mobility to muscle in the same way as manipulation frees a joint. Indeed, the action of deep transverse friction may be summed up as affording a mobilization that passive stretching or active exercises cannot achieve.*

After the friction has restored a full range of painless broadening to the muscle belly, this added mobility must be maintained. To this end, the patient should perform a series of active contractions with the joint placed in a position that fully relaxes the affected muscle, i.e. the position that allows the greatest broadening. Strong resisted movements should be avoided until the scar has consolidated itself; otherwise, started too soon, they tend to strain the healing breach again. Athletes in particular must not return to full sport too early.

Deep Massage for Ligamentous Lesions

In recent cases, after any oedema that may be present has been removed by effleurage, the site of the minor tear in the ligament should receive some minutes' friction. The purpose is to disperse blood-clot or effusion here, to move the ligament to and fro over subjacent bone in imitation of its normal behaviour (thus maintaining its mobility) and to numb it enough to facilitate movement afterwards. The least strength of friction which achieves these results is called for. Hence, when friction is started during the first day or two after a sprain, the ligament need be moved only a few times. One minute's treatment thus suffices, since as yet there are no unwanted adhesions to break down. But it may well take ten to twenty minutes' effleurage and gentle friction to enable the patient to accept the one minute's valid treatment—actually moving the damaged tissue. When the lesion becomes less severe and tenderness is abating, friction maintained with increasing strength for five, ten, then fifteen minutes is called for.

When acute traumatic arthritis is present at a joint such as the knee, muscle spasm so limits movement at the joint that it is impossible to maintain the mobility of a ligament in the usual way, i.e. by moving the bones to and fro under it. In such a case the only physiotherapeutic alternative is to use the human finger to move the ligament to and fro over the bone in imitation of its normal behaviour. This is the very mobilization that transverse friction achieves, provided that it is given deeply enough to reach the injured fibres of the ligament.

In chronic cases deep friction is given to fibrous structures such as ligaments in preparation for manipulation. The friction thins out the scar tissue by which the fibrous structure is held abnormally adherent, and so numbs it that rupture by forcing becomes tolerable. However, in the case of the dorsal ligaments at the wrist, the coronary ligaments at the knee, the femoral extent of the medial collateral ligament at the knee and the sacrococcygeal ligament, the massage is itself the mobilizing agent and no forcing of movement follows.

Deep Massage for Tendinous Lesions

In acute and chronic teno-synovitis the way deep massage acts is somewhat different. On logical grounds it has been widely held that teno-synovitis, being as a result of overuse, should not be treated by further friction. Nevertheless this is the very condition in which massage achieves some of its quickest and most brilliant results. The phenomenon of crepitus proves that roughening of the gliding surfaces occurs. The fact that slitting up the sheath of the tendon at open operation is immediately curative shows that it was the movement between the close-fitting sheath and the tendon that set up the pain. Hence it would appear that manual rolling of the tendon sheath to and fro against the tendon serves to smooth the gliding surfaces off again. While the causative overuse was longitudinal friction, the curative is transverse.

In those tendons that lack a sheath, deep massage acts by breaking up scar tissue at the insertion of the tendon into bone or within its substance. Since no sheath exists, there is no reason to suppose that some slight roughening of the surface of the tendon would cause symptoms. Deep friction provides the only method whereby the physiotherapist can bring lasting relief in these cases. The alternative is local infiltration with hydro-cortisone, which disinflames the scar, but leaves this still in existence, Hydrocortisone, when it succeeds, is a quicker method of securing relief, but it is followed by a higher frequency of recurrence on account of the persistence of the scar.

Since the cause of teno-synovitis and tendinitis is overuse, no exercises follow. Splintage is quite unnecessary; the patient is merely told to avoid any exertion that hurts.

MASSAGE TO THE DERMATOME

This is a revival of a method of friction advocated by P. G. Hensler, a doctor in Kiel (Germany) who died in 1805. It was later carried on by E. D. A. Bartels in 1835, working in Berlin. He stated that 'deeply-lying organs corresponding to the area of skin to which friction is administered can thereby be stimulated in a beneficial manner'. But logic demands that massage can be given usefully only to lesions within reach of the human finger. This fact greatly restricts the number of conditions for which massage can reasonably be ordered. An ingenious scheme for restoring a wide scope to massage and making it appear suitable for a variety of deep-seated disorders has been elaborated inGermany. It is called 'Bindegewebs-massage' (connective tissue massage) and involves treating the dermatome belonging to the same segment as the diseased tissue. This concept brings all lesions back within the ambit of massage again. This doubtless well-meaning attempt to justify treatment given other than to the lesion is a retrograde step which must be resisted in the same way that chiropractors' equally clever idea that all disorders respond to spinal manipulation must be strongly countered.

MASSAGE WITH CREAMS

When deep friction is given, the physiotherapist's finger and the patient's skin must move as one. The application of any cream, ointment or powder, or even previous heat leading to local sweating, makes the skin slippery and must be avoided. But for centuries laymen's expectations have been periodically aroused that rubbing in this or that cream or liniment has a curative value. The effect postulated is local, not systemic as in mercurial inunction for syphilis. Naturally, it makes not the slightest difference to the deeper tissues what is or is not rubbed into the skin; for all agents that penetrate are absorbed by the blood in the cutaneous capillary system and removed. Counter-irritation results, of course, and the patient may feel a pleasant glow, but it is probable that, by drawing more of the available blood towards the skin, the flow through the underlying tissues becomes diminished for the time being. But minor ephemeral ischaemia is not likely to do good, since analgesic measures rely on an increase in the local circulation.

The uselessness of rubbing in any cream, liniment or embrocation, however convincingly advertised to the layman and, even more assiduously, to physiotherapists, is worth stressing. Thousands of pounds are wasted on these remedies by laymen and National Health Service alike. Such striking claims were made twenty years ago by Moss for a massage cream containing adrenaline that the Empire Rheumatism Council set up a sub-committee to investigate. It reported that whether adrenaline was present in the cream or not made no real difference to the result, and that none of the systemic effects of adrenaline was noted. The inherent unlikelihood of a superficial inunction having any effect, let alone a lasting effect, on deeply placed tissues is by no means obvious to laymen.

MUSCLE RELAXANTS

Contrary to general belief, muscle spasm about a joint is not painful. This is obvious at the distal parts of a limb, e.g. knee or wrist, where the muscles in spasm and the joints lie in different places. It is less obvious at the joints of the trunk or at the shoulder and hip, where the muscles overlie the joint. All that the muscle does is to contract, just as it would on voluntary movement at a normal joint, to prevent overstretching of a sensitive structure.

Muscle spasm is not constant; it springs into action at a certain point in the range to protect an arthritic joint or a sprained ligament. It also serves to approximate the edges of a partial muscular rupture. In these cases, the muscle spasm is largely beneficial. For example, when part of the meniscus is displaced at the knee, the hamstring muscles contract to prevent full extension of the joint, thus sparing ligamentous overstretching. This is advantageous and the treatment is not to relax the muscles but to reduce the displacement. Muscle spasm results from a lesion and is abolished when its cause ceases to operate.

It suits the advertisers' book to put forward the view that it is the muscles guarding the damaged tissue which set up the pain, not the lesion itself. In lumbago, they allege that the pain arises from muscle spasm, whereas anyone can see that the patient's back is fixed in slight flexion, not in the fully extended posture that would result from spasm of the erector spinae muscles. Moreover, some patients with lumbago deviate away from the painful side: an impossible position in muscle spasm. These arguments are ignored and muscle relaxants are advocated for a large variety of unsuitable conditions. When the lesion is excessive muscle tone, e.g. cramp or spasticity, such drugs can reasonably be prescribed, but they are contra-indicated in sprains, strains, arthritis or disc lesions, which should receive treatment directed to the lesion. The only exception is lumbago treated by rest in bed. Here, though of doubtful value, they are at any rate harmless and may enable the joint to move a little more during relief from weight-bearing.

3
Technique of Deep Friction

When massage is to be given to muscle, tendon, ligament or joint capsule, two principles must be observed. They are that the massage must be given (*a*) to the right spot and (*b*) in the most effective way. Clearly, only the place whence a pain springs requires treatment, but the referred pain so often present in the conditions sent to a Physiotherapy Department creates immediate difficulty, for the site of the pain and even of the tenderness does not then correspond with the site of the lesion. Since deep massage applies therapeutic movement only locally, it is by no means enough merely to apply friction somewhere close to a lesion. To give massage to a normal structure only a little to one side of the correct spot is quite valueless. There are many conditions unsuited to treatment by deep massage; these should not receive it. There exist other disorders calling for friction; this must then be given to the exact spot whence the pain originates, but it must be remembered that this does not necessarily lie within the area in which the patient *feels* the pain. Massage has acquired a bad name because it is so often applied to perfectly normal tissues, the site of referred pain and tenderness. In consequence, a most effective method of treatment, when applied correctly, is in danger of abandonment.

Once agreement has been reached on the truism that the actual site of the lesion alone requires treatment, the question naturally arises of how a penetrating effect is best imparted to massage. The principles are:

1. *The Right Spot must be found*
   The identification of the precise spot where the physiotherapist must apply her finger depends entirely on knowledge of anatomy. For example, at the shoulder, massage is often given to a stated part of a stated structure and no question arises of asking the patient if that spot is tender or not; at other sites the diagnostic movements may have singled out the tissue at fault, search for tenderness *along that structure* picking out the exact site of the lesion, whose boundaries are then accurately defined.

When asked to give massage to a named structure, the physiotherapist must decide which part of that structure is affected and give treatment directly to that spot only. This takes time, thought, knowledge and trouble, and she must not be hurried.

2. *The Physiotherapist's Fingers and the Patient's Skin must move as one*
Should movement take place between the patient's skin and the physiotherapist's fingers, then the friction is expended on the patient's skin.
When penetration is required, this can be secured only by rubbing the
patient's skin and subcutaneous fascia against his muscle, ligament or
tendon. The whole art of giving deep friction without damaging the
patient's skin depends on mastery of this technique. Vigorous friction
between the physiotherapist's finger and the patient's skin soon raises a
blister. When, on the other hand, the skin and superficial tissues are drawn
to and fro over the area to be treated, they stand the strain perfectly
well. The application of spirit before, during and after treatment helps to
dry the skin, as does a wisp of cotton wool between the operator's finger
and the area to be treated. Such precautions minimize the risk of friction
occurring between two moistened surfaces which can quickly result in a
blister. Some transient redness of the skin usually follows, but no more.
Occasionally, in fat patients, a little subcutaneous bruising may appear
a day or two after the massage; rarely a nodule may form in the adipose
layer. The patient is usually quite unconscious of either, and both soon
disappear. Sometimes it may be advisable to alter the area of skin receiving
pressure from time to time during one session. The finger may be applied
to the lesion after the skin has been drawn to one or other side. When
the choice has to be made, it is always preferable to be sure of reaching
the right spot than to spare the patient some hours' soreness of his skin. The
doctor must back the physiotherapist up should a patient complain. For
the patient to understand the position, it has only to be pointed out that
deep massage to a tender point cannot be painless.

3. *The Friction must be given* across *the Fibres composing the Affected
Structure*
Striated structures must receive massage given transversely. It is only
thus that each fibre is drawn away from its fellow and mobility restored to
muscle; it is thus that a ligament is made to reproduce its normal movement over bone; and it is thus that the surface of a tendon may be smoothed
off. The thicker and stronger the structure, the more must friction be
given to it strictly across the grain.

4. *The Friction must be given with Sufficient Sweep*
The amplitude of the to-and-fro movement of the physiotherapist's
fingers must be great enough to ensure that the frictional element is
paramount. Only thus can effective separation of each fibre from its fellow
be secured. The limiting factors are only the size of the area requiring
treatment and the elasticity of the overlying skin. In this connection it is

unfortunate that students are often taught to impart deep friction by a circular movement of the thumbs. When this method is used for deeply situated lesions no physiotherapist—however strong her hands—can avoid giving what amounts to pressure without enough friction. This should be avoided as it is painful and seldom curative.

It is a grave fault when, in giving massage, pressure replaces, instead of augments, friction. Thus, while it is true that adequate massage to an inflamed, and therefore tender, spot is bound to be painful, the fact that massage is painful is no guarantee that it is correctly given. *Unless the friction is given with a sufficient transverse sweep its curative value is lost.*

5. *The Friction must reach Deeply Enough*

The vigour with which deep massage is given is proportional to the toughness and distance from the surface of the tissue at fault. When, for example, the thick tendons at the shoulder require treatment, the limiting factor is the physiotherapist's strength. She cannot rub hard enough to do harm; her difficulty is to rub hard enough to do good. The friction must not start until she is pressing hard enough to feel her digit engaged against the edge of the tissue at fault.

The frictional element in deep massage is always paramount; pressure augments, but must never replace, friction. If this essential point is neglected a painful treatment results which has no curative value. During each session, physiotherapists unaccustomed to this sort of work do better to give a friction that really reaches the lesion for a few minutes at a time, pausing between whiles, than to rub gently, and hence in vain, for a longer period.

6. *The Patient must adopt a Suitable Position*

A position must be adopted that ensures the requisite degree of tension on, or relaxation of, the tissue to be treated. Some structures, notably the tendons about the shoulder, lie out of reach of a physiotherapist's finger unless the patient is first put into the position dictated by anatomical considerations.

7. *Muscles must be kept Relaxed while being given Friction*

Since it is the substance of a muscle rather than its surface that is affected, the massage must penetrate deeply. Hence the patient must keep his muscle relaxed throughout the administration of the massage. Since his instinct is to steel himself against the discomfort of the friction by contracting it, he has to be taught to avoid this reaction. Moreover, he must be placed in a position in which the part controlled by that muscle lies limply.

After-treatment—In order that the patient shall maintain the added range of painless broadening that the massage has afforded, he should be shown an exercise that contracts the muscle to the maximum. This must be achieved without putting appreciable strain on the damaged area. To this end, the joint is fixed in the position that fully relaxes the muscle, and he is then asked to carry out a number of maximal contractions; alternatively, faradism can be used. For example, if the knee or elbow is held fully flexed, full contraction of hamstrings or biceps can be carried out without straining the injured fibres. The more recent the injury, the more important it is not to pull on the fresh fibrous tissue in the healing breach. Exercises against resistance should be avoided until the scar has consolidated itself.

8. *Tendons with a Sheath must be kept Taut*

In teno-synovitis the roughening is confined to the outer surface of the tendon and the inner surface of its sheath. The friction is intended to smooth off the two gliding surfaces. To this end the tendon must be stretched so that it forms an immobile basis against which to move the sheath. Should the tendon remain lax, it and its sheath are rolled against adjacent structures and little good results.

POSITION OF PHYSIOTHERAPIST AND HER HANDS

The physiotherapist's best position for nearly all deep massage is to be seated by a low couch; her hands and forearms can then remain horizontal. She should place her hands in such a way that they rest naturally on the patient, ensuring that the movement about to take place shall be natural too. She should then adjust the position of her body so as to bring her upper limb into line with her hands. In general the digit, hand and forearm should form a straight line, being kept parallel to the movement imparted, the distal interphalangeal joint being slightly flexed. Much extension at the wrist or flexion at the metacarpophalangeal joint reduces the strength of the friction and forces the distal finger joint into full extension, painfully straining it.

If much deep friction is to be given in the course of a day, it is essential to use the hands alternately and to use now the fingers, now the thumb, for affecting the same place. Full ambidexterity is most useful. When part of a limb is to be treated, the physiotherapist's hand is best used in a grasping position, applying the index finger to the lesion; her other hand steadies the limb.

The work must be shared out among different muscles of the physiotherapist's limb. For example, if the finger or thumb is held firmly against the structure to be treated, and the friction is induced by a wrist, elbow, shoulder or trunk movement, two sets of muscles are in action and more power is achieved for less effort. No matter how strong the physiotherapist, she cannot give effective friction by alternate flexion and extension movements of the fingers or thumb for she is then pressing and moving with the same muscles. *The whole hand must move.*

Suitable Positions of the Physiotherapist's Hands
There are four main ways in which a physiotherapist may use her hands to the best advantage. They are:

1. *The Index crossed over the Middle Finger*
(Occasionally one thumb may be used instead of the crossed fingers.) This technique is well suited to linear areas, such as the attachment of a ribbon of tissue to bone: for example, the insertion of either patellar tendon or the fibular origin of the lateral ligament of the ankle. This is also the best way to affect a tendon at the ankle or each collateral ligament at the knee. This position of the fingers is also required when massage is given to a structure ensconced between two bones, e.g. the musculotendinous junction of the supraspinatus. One finger should be pressed on to the lesion and the friction imparted by rolling the finger to and fro over it. This movement is set up by alternating rotation of the forearm.

2. *The Middle Finger crossed over Index*
When a structure forming part of a limb is to be treated, the physiotherapist naturally grasps the limb, thus using her thumb for counterpressure. The fact of curving the fingers means that the index no longer reaches to the distal phalanx of the middle finger; hence the tip of the middle finger should reinforce the index on the nail.

3. *Two Finger-tips*
Depending on how the fibres of the structure to be massaged run in relation to the physiotherapist's hand, the index and middle finger-tips, or the middle and ring finger-tips, should be used. A length of tendon can be suitably dealt with in this way.

4. *The Opposed Fingers and Thumb*
This is the pinching position. The physiotherapist, having grasped the structure, applies friction by pulling her hand towards herself. The tendons at the shoulder, the coronary ligament at the knee, the biceps brachii muscle, and the tendo Achillis provide instances of this usage.

THE PHYSIOTHERAPIST'S WORKING DAY

Interval between Sessions

Gentle massage, especially for the treatment of oedema or of a recent injury, is best given daily, sometimes more often. Deep friction, however, can seldom be given more often than every other day, for the spot is too tender the next day to permit adequate treatment. The strength of the massage must not be abated if tenderness persists, but the interval between sessions should be prolonged. The proper moment to give the next treatment is when excess of tenderness has worn off, no matter how long this may take. The interval is usually from two to seven days. Patients should not be given a 'course' of so many treatments. They should be treated either until well or until no further improvement accrues. Alternatively, the method may be found useless after adequate trial; it should then be abandoned. It should be borne in mind that local tenderness due to deep friction often persists long after disappearance of pain due to the lesion. These symptoms—tenderness and pain—must be clearly distinguished, and *treatment must cease as soon as the pain has been relieved, irrespective of the persistence of tenderness*. All the physiotherapist need do is to test the affected structure clinically—if a ligament, by passive stretching; if a muscle or tendon, by the appropriate resisted movement. As soon as such testing elicits no pain, treatment ceases.

Number of Patients treated Daily

To do her work properly, the physiotherapist must not be rushed. Clinics exist at which thirty, forty, even fifty patients are treated during a seven-hour day. This implies giving less than a quarer of an hour's attention to each patient. Individual treatment cannot then fail to degenerate. Alternatively, the patient may attend for class-work of dubious advantage to him. Few indeed among the conditions commonly dealt with in a physiotherapy department yield to such 'treatment', and departments that practise this form of 'physiotherapy' defeat their own ends; for they lose, not save, time.

The fact is that in the long run patients are relieved much more quickly when clear instructions are given and the physiotherapist has enough time to implement them properly. The period allotted for each case must be sufficient not only for giving an adequate amount of manual treatment, followed when necessary by the appropriate exercises unhurriedly performed, but also for allowing the physiotherapist time to draw breath and collect herself, ask the patient a few relevant questions, re-examine the function of the tissue at fault, put him into the right posture comfortably, find the exact spot, and arrange her own position satisfactorily. Time thus spent is essential to the performance of good work. Striking results can be obtained by cutting down the number of patients treated daily until every physiotherapist has as much time as she wishes for each. Although a lesser number of daily treatments is given, the decrease becomes more than counter-balanced by the number of patients it is then possible to discharge.

At a mixed clinic the very most that a physiotherapist can be expected to deal with properly is twenty patients a day. If, as is quite usual, a considerable proportion suffer from lesions calling for deep massage or strenuous manipulation, somewhat fewer than this, say sixteen, is desirable. No physiotherapist, however strong and willing, can give manual treatment all day long; hence patients should be so spaced that two heavy cases do not follow each other.

Clinical Notes

The patient must always be treated by the same physiotherapist at each attendance, and she should keep his notes up date throughout. She should write down any change in his clinical state and any variation in her treatment. After a series of manipulations is completed, the result of each manoeuvre should be set out, so that, if the future brings a recurrence, the physiotherapist who then deals with him knows which technique proved most effective last time.

If a change of physiotherapist is necessary, the new physiotherapist should be present at the final treatment by her colleague, so that she knows exactly what is being done. This is particularly important when a joint is being stretched out or manipulative reduction is under way.

REFERRED PAIN AND 'FIBROSITIS'

During the first half of this century any pain in the trunk, especially on its posterior surface, was apt to be ascribed to 'fibrositis'. It was at that time an extremely common diagnosis in Britain, having been put forward by Sir William Gower in 1904 as the cause of lumbago and enthusiastically accepted for 44 years until it was debunked (Cyriax, 1948). In a different context fibrositis, i.e. inflammation of the fibrous tissue, is a perfectly genuine condition. For example, in a sprained ligament, a tennis elbow, rheumatoid arthritis or epidemic myalgia, fibrous tissue is certainly inflamed, but this was not what was implied by 'fibrositis' then.

'Fibrositis' was not accepted in the USA and Canada during those years. Just as this concept has become almost obsolete over here, it is beginning to appear in transatlantic books and articles. The reader may thus need a warning against this transposed revival and England must be on its guard against its introduction from abroad.

The notion of 'fibrositis' is based on palpation without adequate previous assessment of function (see Volume I). Its advocates suppose that tenderness of a muscle implies some lesion within it. In fact, a muscle lesion is shown to exist when the appropriate resisted movement is found to be painful. If a muscle contains an area of tenderness but resisted contraction of that muscle provokes no pain, then it is the site of referred tenderness. At the trunk this is a very frequent occurrence, the patient fingering the painful region and soon finding what is called a trigger point, a myalgic region, etc. There is no doubt that this is a genuine finding, but it represents a referred phenomenon. It is not caused by any lesion of the muscles, certainly not inflammation of the fibrous tissue. It is the result of pressure on the dura mater, with pain referred extrasegmentally, and is always accompanied by a small area of deep localized tenderness within the painful area. The patient finds this and avers that this is where his lesion lies. The patient is wrong, but his insistence may mislead both doctor and physiotherapist into treating that spot. One shudders to think of the hours of massage and the injections of first procaine and now hydrocortisone that have been applied to a referred symptom.

The mistaken attribution by the patient is simple to disprove. In the first place, when the allegedly inflamed muscle is tested, it is found to be strong and painless. In the second place, other movements unconnected with the muscle are found to set up the pain in the muscle. For example, in what used to be called 'scapular fibrositis' the movements of the cervical spine often hurt in the cervical area, whereas the scapular and arm movements do not hurt. Thirdly, the alleged area of inflammation can be moved from one muscle to another within a few seconds. In an alleged case of 'scapular fibrositis', manipulation of the neck during traction shifts the small fragment of disc and with it the tender spot. In this way the 'myalgic area' can be moved from, say, the infraspinatus to the supraspinatus, to the levator scapulae, or to the trapezius in the course of a few minutes, the patient confirming the shift. When painless movement has been restored to the neck in every direction, the peripatetic 'trigger spot' has disappeared.

Every time one of these spots is mistaken for the primary lesion, untold opportunities are afforded for a gratuitous advertisement for lay manipulation. I therefore hope indeed that this revival in the Western hemisphere will soon die out. I am old enough to remember the havoc caused to us, and the aid we unwittingly gave to laymen, as a result of this outworn concept. Let it not be revived.

LEGAL POSITION OF THE PHYSIOTHERAPIST

All effective methods of treatment are potentially dangerous, precisely because they have an effect. To a profession that has become accustomed to using harmless palliative measures this fact presents new difficulties. A technician has few problems, merely doing what is asked; but the physiotherapist who uses effective treatment shoulders unwonted responsibility. She should be proud of this situation, since it implies that she has reached the higher status that qualifies her to present an individual opinion and to undertake her duties at her own discretion.

In his paper on the legal aspect of a physiotherapist's duties, Baylis (1966) points out that, though she must not take on a case except at a doctor's (or dentist's) request, he is not legally responsible for any injury caused by her negligence. He is liable only if he unreasonably ordered the treatment that caused the damage. She might well be cited too if she knew that what was ordered was unsuitable, yet carried it out notwithstanding.

It follows that a physiotherapist is entitled to a mind of her own and, if she disagrees with a doctor's instructions, is under no compulsion to carry them out. If she considers that the diagnosis is mistaken, it is her duty to draw the doctor's attention to the facts on which her view is based. Should she fail to do so, for fear of offending the doctor, she would be legally responsible for any suffering caused by the diagnostic error. It follows that the physiotherapist has a right to know what diagnosis has been arrived at. If the doctor refuses this information, she is at liberty to give or not to give the treatment ordered, as she prefers. In my view, she is wise to refrain from treatment in an undiagnosed case, except by inert methods.

A difficult situation arises here. Many phrases are used between one doctor and another to their satisfaction, but are not precise enough to help a physiotherapist. She might well be asked to treat the 'rotator cuff syndrome'; it would then be up to her to decide which part of the supraspinatus, infraspinatus or subscapular tendon required deep friction. Or she might be asked to manipulate the neck for 'cervical spondylosis', of which readers of Volume I of this book will know that there are sixteen varieties. This blunderbuss term is also used by doctors, and covers similar but not identical disorders in which manipulation may be most beneficial, useless or, in a few instances, very dangerous.

The legal situation clearly demands that the physiotherapist, if she is to maintain a professional as opposed to a technician status (as I should wish), must be taught how to identify the tissue at fault in lesions of the moving parts. Only with this knowledge can she make sure of applying her treatment to the correct spot. When it comes to manipulation, whatever the doctor may order, it is the operator who has the final say on whether this treatment shall be performed or not. Moreover, it is only the operator who, as the extreme of range is approached, discerns the end-feel. This extremely informative sensation, which may indicate that a case which looked suitable clinically, in fact is not, is available to the manipulator for the first time at that moment. This finding cannot be predicted with certainty by any doctor, however experienced. It is, therefore, essential that the physiotherapist should be well versed in clinical examination and in the different sensations imparted to her hands, particularly when spinal lesions or arthritis at the shoulder are in question. Otherwise, she cannot form an opinion in advance on whether to manipulate or not, which manoeuvres to attempt or to avoid, nor can she re-examine after each passive movement to assess progress. She must know the indications and contra-indications, and how to look out for favourable and unfavourable signs. This is important and rewarding work, but it also involves the operator in care, thought and perception, with a due sense of responsibility to the patient and an awareness of legal pitfalls.

FEES IN PRIVATE PRACTICE

When radiant heat and massage are given, let us say, in a case of lumbago, or a patient with supraspinatus tendinitis is given heat and exercises, or a tennis elbow is given ionization or ultra-violet light, methods are being employed that have years of traditional sanction behind them. This does not alter the fact that such measures have no effect on the lesion present.

A physiotherapist in private practice may, however, base her work on quite a different principle. She may, when it is indicated, carry out manipulative reduction at the spinal joints, give deep massage to the supraspinatus tendon, stretch out the tendon in a tennis elbow. This sort of physiotherapy requires expert knowledge of a much higher order. Moreover, patients get well rapidly as the result of accurate employment of difficult manual techniques based on a precise understanding of applied anatomy.

In my view, the reward for physiotherapy of this high standard should be commensurate with the extra skill and endeavour involved and the enhanced effectiveness of treatment. Otherwise the earnings of the physiotherapist who gives exact treatment and thus cures her patient quickly will actually be less than those of her colleague who, relying on tradition, does not even attempt precise methods. It is thus my considered opinion that those who practise accurate measures deserve a fee at least double the usual one. This concept is incorporated in the Norwegian Health Service, where manipulation is paid for at twice the rate for ordinary physiotherapy.

THE IMAGE OF PHYSIOTHERAPY

Most people have little idea of what physiotherapy consists. Their concept alternates between a strong stern woman administering exercises and a kindly soul offering heat and soothing massage. Happily, neither of these images bears much relation to fact.

Doctors labour under different, but equally lamentable, misapprehensions. They, as students, see how useful the physiotherapist is in the wards. They see her avoiding postoperative venous and respiratory stasis, teaching patients to walk again, giving exercises after fractures and orthopaedic operations and affording neurological rehabilitation. After qualification, doctors realize that the sort of case admitted to the wards is now far out-numbered by, for example, stiff necks, painful shoulders, bad backs and sprained knees. These are treated in the out-patient department; thus the student may never see this work done. Doctors have no doubts, therefore, about the value of in-patient physiotherapy but are pardonably vague about those aspects of physiotherapy which they were never shown. Hence they are apt to play safe and to order placebo treatment (e.g. heat and exercises) when in fact quick success would have followed a physiotherapist giving the proper treatment. From this uncertainty arises the damaging idea that physiotherapy is often merely a second-rate form of psychotherapy and that lay manipulators are to be preferred.

All the physiotherapists who graduated from St Thomas's until 1969 were taught by me how to maintain or restore mobility at joints, ligaments, muscles and tendons, and in particular how to deal with spinal joints blocked by internal derangement.

If doctors' attention was drawn to the success of this aspect of physiotherapists' work, they would be happy to order accurate measures. The problem is that of education, mainly of doctors but also of the general public. The Chartered Society might well issue a pamphlet and publish memoranda in the medical press so that doctors know what physiotherapists can do, and the public what to expect. They can then insist that they get it.

'PHYSIOTHERAPY, PLEASE'

There are those who deprecate this request: I disagree. It should be regarded as an honour when a doctor uses this open phrase. He is saying 'this patient needs a physiotherapist's knowledge, and I rely on her to single out a lesion and give it effective treatment'. This is how a colleague, not a technician, is addressed. Such a request is far preferable to a routine prescription for 'heat and exercises', which forces her to give useless treatment against her better judgement.

The status of the physiotherapist depends on what doctors and patients find she can do. This depends in turn on two factors: her skill in assessing the nature of the lesion, and swift results of treatment. When a doctor finds he can count on her for accurate localization of the tissue at fault, he will be happy to delegate work to her. His simplest way of implying this trust is by 'physiotherapy, please'. When patients discover—and report to their doctors—that this prescription has led to rapid cure, the status of the physiotherapist is assured.

4
Indications For and Against
Deep Massage

INDICATIONS FOR DEEP FRICTION

Muscles, tendons and ligaments respond well.

Muscular Lesions
The function of a muscle belly is to contract. When it contracts it broadens. The action of deep friction after a muscle has suffered a minor rupture within itself is to move the muscle *in imitation of its normal behaviour,* thus restoring full painless broadening out.

Recent Trauma
No scar tissue has yet formed unwanted adherences; hence it is a question of maintaining the capacity of the muscle to broaden fully and to render such active contraction painless.

If immediate local anaesthesia is carried out, the massage starts the next day; if not, as soon as the patient is seen. The intention is to prevent scar tissue from matting the muscle fibres together, without interfering with the fibres consolidating themselves in the healing breach. Broadening out in the absence of tension is secured by transverse friction; the massage must reach the right spot but at first need not last long or be really vigorous. It should be followed by active movement of the damaged muscle; this maintains the added excursion towards broadening resulting from the massage. Passive stretching and resisted movements both strain the healing breach and are to be avoided. Indeed, resisted movements or active exertion carried out before healing is complete carry the risk of further rupture, particularly in the case of the hamstring muscles. After the massage, the limb is placed in the position that fully relaxes the affected muscle, whereupon contractions are started, either voluntary or induced by faradism. As a result, full active broadening is achieved without any strain falling on the uniting gap. Resisted movements should not be given until healing is complete.

Long-standing Scars

Scarring mats the fibres together and the range of broadening out of the belly during contraction is impaired. This must be restored passively and then maintained actively. To this end really deep massage is given for as long as possible (say twenty minutes) to the site of the scar. The transverse friction broadens the muscle out passively. This added range is now maintained by an exercise actively contracting the muscle to its fullest extent. Ordinary exercises are useless and exertion is best avoided until the patient is well. Resisted exercises do not increase mobility and are likewise valueless.

Lesions at the Musculo-tendinous Junction

At this situation, neither local anaesthesia nor a steroid infiltration is effective. The former is sometimes effective in minor tears in a muscle belly; the latter in a lesion at a tendon. At the musculo-tendinous junction, the proximity of rigid tendon prevents the restoration of mobility except by manual means. Hence the sort of strains that affect athletes and ballet dancers, especially at the leg, are often entirely incurable except by deep friction.

Tendinous Lesions

Tendons with a Sheath

Roughening of the synovial surfaces of a long tendon possessing a sheath is known as teno-synovitis. There are no adhesions; hence no movement is limited. Every time the tendon moves within its sheath pain is evoked; in the more severe cases, crepitus is palpable as the roughened surfaces slide against each other. In teno-vaginitis the primary impact is on the tendon sheath, but the gliding surface is affected too, identical symptoms resulting. Cure consists in smoothing the surfaces off again. This is simply obtained by rubbing the tendon sheath on the tendon, not up and down (this is often the cause) but transversely. During the massage, the tendon is kept stretched so as to provide an immobile base against which to move the tendon sheath circumferentially. Hence a lesion caused by longitudinal friction is cured by transverse friction. Exercises merely increase the causative trauma and are contra-indicated. The patient is warned to avoid such activities as hurt.

In the olden days, teno-synovitis was treated by splintage and heat, which was cumbersome, uncertain and took a very long time, even when it did prove effective. Nowadays, deep massage is given whether the condition is recent or long-standing, and it is immaterial whether crepitus is present or not. Alternative measures are injection of hydrocortisone or operative slitting up of the tendon sheath.

In bacterial teno-vaginitis (e.g. compound palmar ganglion) massage is, of course, harmful. Rheumatoid or gouty teno-vaginitis may affect the tendon sheaths at the wrist and ankle; nodules may also form on tendons as a complication of rheumatoid arthritis or xanthomatosis. None is susceptible to treatment by physiotherapy of any sort.

Tendons without a Sheath

This condition is known as tendinitis. A strain may tear some fibres in a short tendon (e.g. suprapinatus tendinitis, tennis elbow). A painful scar often forms in the substance of the tendon or at the teno-periosteal junction. Here self-perpetuating inflammation may result. As long as the scar remains inflamed—and this may last for years—every movement involving use of that muscle hurts.

Two treatments exist:

1. Steroid suspension, which converts an inflamed scar into one free from inflammation. However it leaves the scar in existence. It is quick and effective but the recurrence rate is about one in five.
2. Massage: deep friction would seem to get rid of the pain by breaking up the scar itself. This takes longer, but there is naturally little tendency to recurrence. It is my policy to start treatment by one or two infiltrations of the scar with hydrocortisone. If this fails, or the trouble recurs after a month or two of freedom, massage is substituted.

Ligamentous Lesions

Ligaments join two bones, allowing movement between them. Their mobility is at right-angles to their long fibres.

Recent Sprain

The immediate treatment of such ligaments as lie within fingers' reach consists in moving them by deep massage. In recent cases the friction eases pain and moves the ligament to and fro over bone *in therapeutic imitation of its normal behaviour*. The maintenance of mobility at a damaged ligament has its most spectacular results at the knee, where traumatic arthritis so limits movement as to prevent the bones being moved adequately under the ligament: this has to be passively moved over the bones instead. In these recent cases the friction need not last long nor be very vigorous, since the fibroblasts are young and very weakly attached. During the first few days, no endeavour is made to increase range at the joint passively; the massage without forcing has this effect. Later, movement at the sprained joint must be gently increased passively: the same movements are then repeated actively. In the case of the lower limb instruction in gait follows. Patients treated by friction to the point of a minor ligamentous rupture, followed by movements, get well very much more quickly than those treated by diathermy or diffuse massage and the same movements. The existence of bruising forms no bar to the immediate employment of massage; this will not cause recurrence of the haemorrhage.

Chronic Sprain

Chronic ligamentous sprain results from scars holding the ligament abnormally adherent to underlying bone. These result from healing during a period of insufficient movement, part of the ligament developing unwanted adhesion to bone. Owing to the reduced mobility of the ligament, vigorous use of the joint it spans resprains the ligament. Hence these adhesions must be ruptured by forced movement. This may be carried out under general or local anaesthesia or under massage analgesia. The virtue in massage to the site of a chronic ligamentous sprain is the movement imparted to the ligament and the consequent thinning out and disengagement of these adhesions. The numbing effect of the hyperaemia induced by the friction also comes into play and makes forced movement practicable through a larger range than would otherwise have been possible.

There are three exceptions to this rule. When adhesions have formed about the ligaments at the capitate bone at the wrist, at a coronary ligament at the knee, or at the anterior tibio-talar ligament at the ankle, manipulation is harmful and massage alone is the only successful treatment, however long the disorder has lasted.

CONTRA-INDICATIONS TO DEEP FRICTION

Massage should not be given in the treatment of the following conditions. (By 'massage' is meant such friction as actually reaches the structure named. Except in bacterial infection, gentle massage, being without effect on deep-seated lesions, is neither helpful nor is it harmful.) Massage should not be attempted, of course, when the structure at fault lies clearly beyond the reach of the physiotherapist's finger. For example, no useful purpose is served when a patient with osteoarthrosis of the hip-joint receives massage, whether gentle or deep, to his gluteal or quadriceps muscles. This is merely where the pain is felt, not where its source lies. In such a case friction is not so much contra-indicated as a waste of effort.

1. Inflammation due to Bacterial Action

No medical man would send such a case to a physiotherapist with a request for *active* treatment. Short-wave diathermy, which heats the part and thus increases the blood-flow through the inflamed tissue, provides the only effective physiotherapeutic measure when the lesion lies deeply. For superficial sepsis ultra-violet light may be required.

2. Traumatic Arthritis of the Elbow-joint

The proper treatment of an injury at the elbow which has resulted in traumatic arthritis is rest in flexion or intra-articular hydrocortisone. Massage and, more particularly, efforts to increase the range of extension at the elbow passively are useless; moreover, they are held to carry the risk of provoking myositis ossificans. Treating a sprained elbow joint actively lays the doctor and physiotherapist open to medico-legal difficulties.

3. Ossification or Calcification in Soft Structures

Extensive ossification of a ligament contra-indicates all active treatment, but the tiny areas of calcification that occur in ligament, tendon or capsule some time after a severe sprain may be ignored. At the knee, ossification in the tibial collateral ligament is rare and known as Stieda-Pelegrini's disease. The remote possibility of its occurrence should never be regarded as a contra-indication to active treatment of injuries to this ligament. Such treatment should be avoided only when the radiograph shows the typical shadow.

At the elbow, calcification in either of the collateral ligaments is sometimes seen, but, since the elbow is never treated actively for any articular sprain, this has little bearing on treatment. Calcification in a tendon, most often the supraspinatus, contra-indicates massage; it is useless but not actually harmful.

4. Bursitis

Inflammation of a bursa, from whatever cause, is made worse or at best is unaffected by massage. The treatment of bursitis is rest and infiltration with hydrocortisone; if it contains blood, aspiration; if it contains pus, evacuation. If these fail, excision may be required in some situations.

5. The Rheumatoid Types of Arthritis

Friction to the capsule of the joint is harmful in the acute, subacute and chronic stages of rheumatoid, gouty and villous arthritis and in the arthritis complicating psoriasis, lupus erythematosus, ankylosing spondylitis, Reiter's disease or ulcerative colitis. In most of these disorders, intra-articular injection of hydrocortisone is the treatment of choice. However in gout, phenylbutazone is indicated; in gonorrhoea, penicillin; but in non-specific urethritis no treatment exists as yet.

6. *Pressure on Nerves*

Theoretically it is just as unreasonable to give friction to a tendon as to a nerve sheath; for both are fibrous structures whose outer surface can suffer from excessive friction. Nevertheless, in practice deep massage to a tendon is as beneficial as it is harmful when applied to a nerve sheath. The cause of the pressure, e.g. a displaced disc, a cervical rib, a swollen tendon or too tight a ligament, should be dealt with.

MASSAGE TECHNIQUE

Doctors are regarding massage with increasing scepticism, as a mere placebo. This attitude is justified, since they have so few chances of seeing the results of massage properly administered. This opinion can be speedily reversed, and it is important that it should be, otherwise within a few more years the conditions curable by deep friction alone will be held intractable, not because they are difficult to relieve, but for lack of personnel trained to employ these techniques. It was therefore good news when in 1967 the Education Committee of the Chartered Society of Physiotherapy was asked to investigate the value of different ways of giving massage. This report, published two years later in their Journal, struck a welcome note on the negative side; it recommended the abandonment of beating, hacking, pounding and of abdominal massage as examination subjects. On the positive side, the report was disappointing since nowhere in it was considered *massage to a lesion*. No better reason for retaining other massage techniques was put forward than tradition and custom:

'From the extent to which massage is in use today it is obvious that it must continue to be taught and examined.' No hint was offered on what sort of massage might be regarded as beneficial, and throughout the entire report no mention is made of massage so given as to penetrate to and affect the lesion itself. The maintenance of mobility by digital means, i.e. deep localized friction to a stated part of a named tissue—the subject of one-third of this book—was ignored. Since this is the truly remedial and irreplaceable type of massage, often providing the only effective measure for disorders otherwise intractable, it is very disappointing that only vague methods with imprecise intent were dealt with.

A letter submitted for publication then drawing the Committee's attention to this hiatus in the report on their deliberations was not printed, but was rejected with the statement that its contents would be put before the Education Committee at its next meeting. Seven years have now elapsed and no addendum has appeared. Since the physiotherapy profession would benefit so greatly from the Committee's recognition of the remedial type of massage, a further meeting devoted to this subject merits urgent consideration. Another advantage would also accrue, for at this moment physiotherapists and laymen are competing in the manipulative field. Since accurate massage is almost unknown to these men, this mastery would put physiotherapists into a unique therapeutic position.

DISORDERS CURABLE ONLY BY DEEP FRICTION

The insoluble steroids have provided an effective alternative for many disorders previously curable only by massage (Cyriax & Troisier, 1952). There exist a number, listed below, that remain intractable except by deep transverse massage. There is a danger, now that massage is becoming a forgotten art in Europe and America, that these conditions will be considered intractable, not because the cure is unknown, but for lack of therapists able to apply the remedy.

Subclavius belly
Supraspinatus, musculo-tendinous junction
Biceps, long head
Biceps, lower musculo-tendinous junction
Brachialis, belly
Supinator, belly
Ligaments about carpal lunate bone
Adductors of thumb
Interosseous belly at hand
Interosseous tendon at finger
Intercostal muscle
Oblique muscles of abdomen
Psoas, lower musculo-tendinous junction
Quadriceps expansion at patella
Coronary ligament at knee
Biceps femoris, lower musculo-tendinous junction
Anterior tibial ⎫
Posterior tibial ⎬ musculo-tendinous junction
Peroneal ⎭
Posterior tibio-talar ligament
Anterior fascia of ankle joint
Interosseous belly at foot

5

Active Movement

So far as the treatment of deformity and the result of injury or overstrain are concerned, exercises fall into two main categories—namely, those for muscles and those for joints. Since the type of exercise required depends entirely on its *purpose*, clarity on this point is essential.

EXERCISES FOR MUSCLES

1. Active Exercises

These are used to prevent adhesions forming within or about a muscle. Thus they are called for equally after a few fibres have been torn within a muscle, as in the avoidance of adherence of muscle to bone, e.g. to the callus of a fracture of the femoral shaft. To send a patient back to exertion soon after minor damage to a muscle is mistaken policy; for he is apt either to hold the part stiffly (thus avoiding therapeutic movement) or to allow a series of excessive pulls on the healing breach, each leading to a relapse. Active movement of the muscle suffices for the formation of a supple scar that becomes painless quickly. Since it is full broadening of a muscle that is so important, exercise or faradism given soon after injury to a muscle belly must consist of active contraction of the affected muscle performed while the joint is held passively in the posture that fully relaxes that muscle. If this is done, a maximal active contraction can be performed without pulling on the breach strongly enough to lead to renewed rupture of the healing fibres. This is particularly important when the hamstring, quadriceps or calf muscles suffer minor rupture, since relapse is commonplace unless time has been given for a mobile scar to consolidate itself. Passive movements are, of course, valueless in the treatment of recent muscular injuries. Resisted exercises should be employed only when recovery is nearing completion.

2. Assisted Exercises

When a muscle is short and has to be stretched out, resisted exercises increase its tone and are therefore contra-indicated. Active exercises alone are ineffective, but active movements in the required direction strongly assisted by the physiotherapist are often successful. Alternatively, the patient's own body weight may be thus employed, e.g. in the treatment of an equinus deformity.

Assisted exercises are also useful in obtaining full excursion of the chest-wall; the assistance is then given by the physiotherapist's or patient's own hands. When, however, the patient is taught to raise his diaphragm to its fullest extent by drawing in his upper abdomen at the end of expiration, this is an example of one set of muscles giving assistance to another.

3. Resisted Exercises

These have the purpose of strengthening muscle. It should hardly be necessary to state again the obvious truth that massage and passive move-ments contribute nothing towards strengthening muscle. The power of a muscle depends entirely on how well and how often the patient uses it. Use against resistance, whether of the body weight, of an appliance, of the patient's other muscles, or given by the physiotherapist, is, of course, far more effective than mere unimpeded active movement. The atrophy of muscle that is an invariable consequence of arthritis, immobilization or disuse should be combated by resisted exercises. The optimum degree of resistance is that which the patient is just able to overcome; it should be applied evenly, elastically and maintained to the very end of the movement. Whether the resistance is applied by the physiotherapist, by means of springs and pulleys, by the strength of the patient's other limb or by his body weight is in theory immaterial. In practice much time and staff are saved, when a large number of patients are to receive similar treatment, if suitable apparatus is to hand. In the later stages of rehabilitation, gymnastic classes, occupational therapy, drill and organized games increase muscle power, control and physical fitness.

4. Active Movement under Local Anaesthesia

In the immediate treatment of any muscular injury, the unrestricted movement that local anaesthesia secures possesses great therapeutic value. Movement under local anaesthesia produces its most spectacular results in recent rupture of some fibres of the gastrocnemius muscle. The muscle is exercised while the patient sits, so as to avoid further strain on the healing fibres.

5. Exercises resisted within the Free Range

These are useful when the muscles about an arthritic joint require strengthening. The movement must be so resisted that the extreme of the possible range is never reached. This technique is valuable after operations on joints, in particular immediately after meniscectomy at the knee.

EXERCISES FOR JOINTS

Contrary to general belief, mobility is maintained at a joint just as well by passive as by active movement. Provided that the joint is moved, the agency is immaterial. It is the muscles about a joint, not the joint itself, that are influenced by the type of the movement.

1. Active Exercises

These are employed to retain mobility at a joint, at times slowly to increase range. Their cardinal use is to keep normal structures normal. Thus all the joints of an injured part not actually immobilized should be put through their full range of movement daily, preferably actively, and therapeutic occupations selected that bring the limb into effective play. The after-treatment of many reduced fractures and orthopaedic operations involves the performance of a suitably graded series of exercises. In such cases passive movements are usually valueless, the joint recovering at a fixed maximum rate that is attained only when the proper exercises are con-scientiously performed. In the case of the lower limb, exercises without weight-bearing precede those carried out standing up.

When injury to a nerve has led to muscular paralysis, the full range of movements at the joints served by the paralysed muscles must be preserved pending the return of conduction along the nerve. For this purpose the patient should be taught how to perform the requisite movements for himself; for example, by using other muscles of the same limb (e.g. climbing up a wall by means of the fingers in paralysis of the abductors of the shoulder), by assisting the movement with the other limb or by using gravity, a pulley or body weight. Such patients should be kept under periodic observation; clearly they do not require to attend hospital several times a week for passive movements for a palsy.

2. Passive, then Active Movements

These are used to increase the range of movement at a joint. Joints at which adhesions limit movement must, wherever possible, have the range increased until it is full in every direction. The proper technique for increasing movement at a joint is passive forcing followed by the patient's immediate repetition of the movement.

In the treatment of postural deformities of the spine the greatest possible correction should be attained passively, before giving the exercises that maintain it.

3. Static Contraction and Exercises so Resisted that no Movement occurs

These are employed when a diminished range of movement at a joint is desirable. A joint may be so disorganized that all movement is painful, and the patient unwilling for arthroplasty. This is often the position in advanced osteoarthrosis of the hip. An attempt to stabilize the joint by increasing the strength and tone of the muscles about it may be made by the use of faradism, static contractions or exercises so resisted that no movement takes place. Exercises are given for the same reason to the short flexor muscles of the foot in the treatment of strain of the mid-tarsal joint or plantar fascia. The increased strength of these muscles diminishes articular movement, thus relieving the fibrous structures of excessive stress.

4. Active Exercise with Passive Effect

When a patient who is standing is asked to squat, his knee becomes fully flexed. He performs an active movement, but it is not contraction of the hamstring muscles which brings about full flexion, but body weight, i.e. a passive agency. Indeed, no muscle exists which can fully flex the knee. Again, when a patient stands and bends his knee, keeping his heel on the ground, he stretches his soleus muscle. An active movement once more causes passive stretching.

EXERCISES AND DISC LESIONS

Exercises are often prescribed for disc lesions causing pain in the back or lower limb, the idea presumably being to strengthen the sacrospinalis muscles so that they can support the lumbar joints better. As normally given these exercises are harmful, moving the joint during compression. Stability at the lumbar joints is dependent on ligaments and the engagement of the lateral facets, not on muscle power. If displacement of the disc substance is present, moving the spinal joints increases pain and is both unkind and useless. If complete reduction has been effected, the patient, provided he never moves the joint again, will not be able to provoke another displacement. He must therefore learn to keep his lumbar joints motionless in a good position, i.e. in lordosis, by maintaining a constant postural tone. It is the duty of the physiotherapist to inculcate the idea of preventing movement at a weak joint liable to internal derangement by constant muscle guarding. This is *the* effective exercise for backache—and the one most seldom taught.

FARADISM VERSUS EXERCISES

In theory, faradism achieves no more than the patient can do for himself by voluntary action. There are, however, four situations in which electrical stimulation is very useful.

1. *Postoperative inhibition*—For the first few days after, say, a meniscus has been removed from the knee, the patient may find it very difficult to contract his quadriceps muscle adequately. Faradism then does it for him, until active control returns.

2. *Minor muscular ruptures*—When some violent exertion, usually during sport, tears some fibres in the quadriceps, hamstring or calf muscles, athletes report faster progress when treatment includes faradism. The function of muscle is to contract and it is then important that full broadening out of the muscle should be restored as soon as possible, without any strain falling on the healing breach. To this end, the joints are fixed in the position of full shortening of the muscle before the stimulation begins. This implies: for the quadriceps, sitting upright with the knee extended; for the hamstrings, lying prone with hip extended and knee held fully flexed; for the gastrocnemius, full flexion of the knee and plantiflexion of the foot.

3. *Weak feet*—Faradic foot baths often achieve more contraction of the short muscles of the sole than voluntary effort, especially in middle-aged women.

4. *Hysteria*—The patient may have the idea so fixed in his mind that a group of muscles is paralysed, that his attempts to move a limb fail. If now electrical stimulation is used to show him that they can be made to work, he may be persuaded. Faradism alone does not suffice; it must be followed at once by encouragement and repeated active exercise of the movements that he had found hitherto impossible. Often such symptoms are thus quickly removed, even without dealing with the underlying psychological fault.

6

Passive Movement

Today passive movement is under a cloud, but quite undeservedly so. Emphasis on active movement is justified in rehabilitation after reduction of fractures and orthopaedic operations, though even in these conditions passive movements have a restricted scope. In a number of common disorders, by contrast, passive movement plays a vital part in treatment. It must be realized that mobility at a joint is maintained or restored by movement *at that joint*; the agency is immaterial. Whether a movement is performed actively or passively has a profound influence on muscle tone and power, but the effect on the joint itself of movements of equal range is the same, whether they are carried out by the patient's own muscles or passively. There are several thousand lay manipulators in Britain today making an excellent living by performing simple passive movements that physiotherapists have so far failed to carry out. This situation is reversible as soon as physiotherapists come to accept passive movement as a normal method of treatment and part of their everyday work.

A number of movements exist that cannot be carried out actively; some others are voluntarily performed only with great difficulty owing to the mechanical disadvantage at which some muscles work (e.g. flexion at the knee). At many joints, therefore, it is almost or quite impossible for a patient actively to overcome limitation of movement. Moreover, after a fracture, an operation, or a sprain, discomfort and apprehension often combine to limit movement to a greater extent than is necessary for the protection of the damaged structure. Particularly in recent cases, therefore, passive movement is often called for in maintaining movement at a time when adequate active movement is beyond the patient's powers.

Three principles should be borne in mind:

1. Patients themselves should not be expected to break adhesions at their joints.
2. Patients themselves should not be expected to stretch out the capsule of a large joint.
3. Patients themselves should not be expected to reduce intra-articular displacements.

In each case the hope is vain; the movements required must be carried out passively by a skilled manipulator.

LEVERAGE

Naturally, the longer the lever, the less force the physiotherapist need use for manipulation. Thus, when the knee has to be forced towards flexion, the nearer the lower end of the tibia she places her hand, the more effective her pressure becomes. But she should not hold the foot, since control is diminished as soon as another joint is allowed to intervene unnecessarily between the joint to be manipulated and the physiotherapist's hand.

When rotation of the thorax on the pelvis is forced, the pelvic and thoracic levers are about the same length and each receives equal pressure. When, however, the femur is used to lengthen the pelvic lever, the hand on the knee has two or three times the force of the hand on the shoulder. Hence the physiotherapist distributes her weight so that most of it falls on the patient's thorax, and uses her arm muscles to move the long lever, thus securing the maximum torsion strain.

Useful levers exist all over the body. For rotation at the cervical joints, the occiput and maxilla provide suitable pressure points. The elbow bent to a right-angle provides the forearm as a lever for lateral rotation of the humerus at the shoulder, and the tibia is used in the same way when the knee is bent or the femur medially rotated. The dorsiflexed foot is used to rotate the tibia laterally at the knee. The longest lever is the fully abducted thigh added to the width of half the pelvis, employed for rotating the pelvis on the thoracic spine during traction.

TISSUE RESISTANCE

The intending manipulator must learn what each extreme of range at every joint in the body feels like. There are several different sensations imparted to his hand when an articular movement is carried as far as it will go.

1. *Bone-to-bone*, e.g. extension at the elbow or knee. The movement stops abruptly with the sensation of two hard surfaces engaging. Should this hard sensation obtrude itself in a direction which normally ends softly, the arthritis is unsuitable for forced movement.
2. *Leather*, e.g. rotation at the shoulder or hip, flexion at the wrist. The movement comes to a firm stop but can be pressed a little further by the use of some strength, with the sensation of stretching a scarcely elastic tissue like leather. If this extra amount of range can be obtained with little or no increase in pain, forcing movement is likely to be successful.
3. *Springy block*. There is no analogue to this sensation at any normal joint. It is caused by internal derangement and is best felt when the

meniscus is displaced at the knee. Extension no longer ends with the normal bone-to-bone feeling but with a soft sensation coupled with a springy recoil.

4. *Muscle spasm.* When gentle forcing evokes muscle spasm coming on with a sudden vibrant twang, the case should be investigated further and all passive movements avoided. The cause may be acute arthritis but fracture and secondary malignant deposits close to the joint also give rise to this abrupt sensation.

5. *Emptiness*, e.g. flexion at the elbow, hip or knee. There is no stop; the joint feels as if it would go further but unavoidable pressure against another part of the body prevents further movement, e.g. thigh against abdomen. If this sensation is felt before the extreme of movement is reached, the patient begging the examiner to desist from a movement that he can feel will perfectly well go further, serious disease may well be present, alternatively hysteria. Secondary deposits in the ilium, for example, or at the upper part of the femur limit hip flexion in this empty way. Great circumspection is thus called for when this sensation is evoked.

End-feel during Manipulation

Forcing must not start until tissue resistance has made itself apparent. The novice is apt to apply the manipulative thrust too soon, 'forcing' a movement that in fact exists already without forcing. The sensation of resistance starting tells the manipulator when to apply this force, but he does so only if it is the right sort of resistance. The twang of muscle spasm or the hard feeling of bone hitting bone warns him against any such attempt. It is, therefore, important to realize that the manipulator's hand, as the thrust is in process, performs two distinct functions: motor and sensory.

Motor

The hand applies the manipulative force at the last moment. Hence, the manipulation must not be thought of as a movement of large amplitude. If, say, the range of movement is 90°, the joint is taken through 89° and is then in position for the manipulation proper to start. Resistance is just becoming perceptible. At this point the manipulative thrust is begun and may well have a further amplitude of only one or two degrees. Proper control is quite unattainable if a wrench of 90° range is attempted.

Sensory

As the joint approaches full range, tissue resistance is felt. The manipulator is quick to distinguish the various sensations imparted to his hand, and to act on this information before the manipulative thrust is complete. Depending on the end-feel, he presses on or stops. Moreover, the decision on whether to repeat that manoeuvre or not, or to abandon the attempt altogether, depends in part on how final a stop the movement came to. The other factor is the result of the manipulation, i.e. a change in the degree or position of the pain, as reported by the patient, and in the physical signs, as determined by the manipulator.

PURPOSES OF PASSIVE MOVEMENT

Passive movements are best considered according to their purpose; the chief reasons for forcing movement at a joint are set out below. (Reduction of fractures, dislocations, and disorders such as a hernia fall outside the scope of this book.)

1. *To break Adhesions*

When minor ligamentous adhesions limit movement and cause pain, they should be manipulatively ruptured. The movement is performed in the direction that disengages the scar in the soft tissues from its abnormal adherences, but does not rupture the useful scar tissue present in the healed breach. Adhesions that have later to be ruptured by manipulation are particularly liable to form at the ankle and knee, when healing of an injured ligament is allowed to take place during insufficient movement.

The manipulation consists in taking the joint as far as it will comfortably go, and then, with a sharp jerk, pushing it further. The movement is sudden, controlled and firm; it hurts at the moment when it is done, but there is no afterpain to speak of.

Gross adhesions may result from prolonged immobilization following fractures. In such cases several manipulations under anaesthesia are often successful in restoring considerable range. The movement is a hard sustained push continued until, with tearing of fibrous tissue, the joint is felt to yield. The physiotherapist gives vigorous after-treatment.

Indication—A ligament is a local reinforcement of the capsule of a joint. Hence those movements that stretch an adherent ligament cause pain, the other movements that do not stretch it are of full range and painless. Thus the presence of adhesions about a ligament is signalled by a small (proportionate) amount of limitation of movement in one or two directions, coupled with a full range of movement in the other directions. Limitation of movement in every direction indicates arthritis and shows that forcing by a quick jerk is inapplicable.

Extent—Before mobilizing a joint it is essential to know its range of movement. For example, rotation in full flexion often has to be undertaken at the knee-joint, though it is a movement that the patient hardly ever uses and may not know to exist. This rule applies equally to planned manipulation as to the gentle movements given by the physiotherapist soon after injury. It is also important to be aware of ranges of movement that are not under voluntary control and therefore not reproducible actively, e.g. antero-posterior gliding at the carpus or knee.

After Anaesthesia—The importance of after-treatment cannot be over-stressed. Unless this is carried out fully and promptly the mobilization seldom does much good; for, in the absence of adequate movement after the adhesions have been ruptured, they quickly reform. The patient must have the range of movement that was obtained under anaesthesia repeated at the earliest possible moment afterwards—before he leaves the couch, and again not later than the following morning. Much insistance, help and encouragement must be given by the physiotherapist to achieve this important result, and in patients unable to bear pain well or in whom strong scars parted only after much forcing, great patience and persuasion may be required. Nevertheless, the after-treatment of mobilization is, if anything, more important and more difficult than the original forcing under anaesthesia. The physiotherapist should be present at the mobilization, and must report at once all cases in which she cannot afterwards reproduce the range obtained under anaesthesia.

The physiotherapist should see patients with lesions of any severity once daily for at least the first week. She should first ask the patient to demonstrate how much active range he has and then increase the range passively until the limit attained under anaesthesia is reached and, if possible, surpassed. This may be quite easy, or take some time. The patient is then asked to repeat these movements himself. Finally, he is shown exercises designed to maintain the range of movement of the joint in each direction, and asked to carry them out several times a day. It is often possible to devise exercises that, though actively performed, stretch a joint passively. For example, when a patient tries to squat, his body weight is flexing his knee and dorsiflexing his foot passively, and the movement has much more force behind it than that obtained by voluntary contraction of any muscle.

2. To Stretch the Capsule of a Joint

When the thick strong capsule of a joint needs to be stretched out, the quick movement that serves to break adhesions is inappropriate, for it merely hurts the patient and leads to further muscle resistance. To stretch out a tough structure, e.g. the capsule of the hip-joint, shoulder-joint or mid-tarsal joint, requires many repetitions of a long steady push maintained for as long as the patient can bear it, say a minute.

In the end, dense capsular adhesions do yield, but no increase in the range of movement can be expected after the first session or two. The result comes slowly; patient and physiotherapist must show forbearance and persistence respectively.

Since the treatment hurts, short-wave diathermy can be used to heat the joint before the manipulation begins. This diminishes the pain. Diathermy used in this way may well be termed the physiotherapist's analgesic. Heat, whether by short waves or microwaves, has a bad name because it is often ordered on its own or to be followed only by exercises. Having warmed the joint, it must then be stretched out while the blood-flow remains increased; otherwise nothing therapeutic has been achieved.

3. To Reduce an Intra-articular Displacement

This is a very common requirement, for all joints that contain intra-articular cartilage are apt to suffer from internal derangement. At others, small pieces of cartilage may become detached (with or without an osseous nucleus) and then displaced. This is a very common event at any spinal joint and at the knee; it also occurs less often at the elbow, jaw, and tarsal joints.

Traction is often a help and provides an example of one sort of passive movement increasing the effect of another. By separating the articular surfaces, the loose fragment is given room to move; pain is also diminished and the patient thus enabled to relax more easily. In general, a series of manipulations is tried in progression and continued until full reduction is secured or it becomes clear that the displaced fragment is irreducible. In contradistinction to the rupture of adhesions, the joint is not primarily moved in the direction in which movement is restricted. For example if trunk flexion is limited in lumbago, or knee extension is limited when the meniscus is out of place, the way to restore the movement is not at all by forcing the joint in the restricted direction—this is harmful—but by performing manoeuvres calculated to get the displaced fragment back into position, thus unblocking the joint. The methods are more subtle and less direct than those required for the simple rupture of an adhesion. A gentle start is made and the patient examined after each manoeuvre for subjective or objective change. This enables the physiotherapist to decide whether to go on or stop, and what to do next. It is interesting to note that, if forcing in one direction has resulted in full reduction, movement in the other directions becomes unblocked also. Hence in manipulation for an intra-articular displacement, but not for adhesions, forcing one way restores range in the other directions as well.

Once the loose fragment is fully in place, instruction must be given to the patient on the prevention of recurrence. The postures to avoid should be explained, and the question of retentive apparatus arises.

4. *To Stretch a Muscle*

A quick movement does not stretch out a muscle, whereas a strong sustained pull has this effect. A good example of this purpose is congenital torticollis resulting from contracture of the sterno-mastoid muscle. The muscle is stretched out by repeated manipulation and the baby's head fixed in the overcorrected position. In talipes equino-varus the calf muscles require similar treatment.

5. *To Stretch a Tendon*

When a painful scar exists at a teno-periosteal junction (as in the common variety of tennis elbow), a sharp jerk may widen the gap and allow the two surfaces, now separate, to heal individually. This treatment is indicated when only one of several tendons attached to the same area of bone is affected.

6. *To Reduce a Bony Subluxation*

This is not uncommon at the wrist. The direction of the displacement is determined and digital pressure during traction, or a gliding movement during traction, are performed according to circumstances. Subluxation at the carpus reducible by gliding is the only common disorder, but downward subluxation of the radius on the humerus (pulled elbow) occurs in children under eight years of age.

7. *To Correct a Deformity*

Sustained pressure without jerking is needed. In talipes equino-varus the varus deformity at the heel and the adduction and inversion of the forefoot must be corrected by the physiotherapist, who maintains a strong torsion strain. Traction is not required. Stiff joints in babies with arthrogryphosis are treated on similar lines.

Unstable fixation of a joint (fibrous ankylosis) in an unsatisfactory position may require correction by sustained traction in recumbency. Once a good position has been secured, fixation in plaster is usually necessary.

Plastic surgery can be used to overcome contractures of the soft parts limiting movement; as soon as possible after the operation, the physiotherapist begins to increase range in the desired direction.

8. *To Maintain Range at Joints whose Muscles are Paralysed*

Quite gentle movements are called for, usually soon after the occurrence of a hemiplegia or during convalescence from anterior poliomyelitis, peripheral nerve palsies and other disorders leading to muscular weakness.

9. *To Maintain or Restore Movement at a Joint soon after an Operation or an Injury*

Immediately after, say, a fracture of the surgical neck of the humerus, the patient's active movements do not suffice to maintain range at the shoulder-joint. Gentle, assisted, active movements are required after some fractures, some operations on bone and often, for example, in the treatment of a sprained ankle or shoulder.

The force with which gentle movements should be applied must strike a balance between an excess of vigour and an excess of gentleness. The movements must not be so forcible as to overstretch the fibrils normally attached within the healing area; nor must they be so gentle as to fail to disengage fibrils that are forming abnormal attachments. A safe rule is to push movements to the point of discomfort but not of pain. All the possible movements of the joint should be attempted passively, one by one, and a small but definite increase in the range of movement should be achieved each day. The patient then repeats these movements actively. *In fractures* two opposite requirements often conflict. The fracture must heal in the absence of movement so that dense adhesions may form and lead to bony union. On the other hand, any associated injury to soft parts must heal in the presence of enough movement to avoid adhesions. Sometimes, as in Colles's fracture, maintenance of reduction by splintage is the overriding consideration, in which case the associated sprain of the ulnar collateral ligament has for the moment to be disregarded. By contrast, in a fracture of the surgical neck of the humerus, it is the fracture that should be disregarded and the soft parts that receive immediate treatment.

10. *To Show a Patient what to do*

In spastic paresis or hysteria the patient may not have a clear idea of what is wanted or of his own capabilities.

The passive movement must be carried out with enough force to overcome gently the patient's muscular resistance and may have to be repeated a great number of times until the patient has learnt what to do.

11. *To Distract the Bone-ends*

Traction is a method of treatment that requires separate mention; for it is clearly a passive movement, but not one included within the concept of the passive forcing termed 'manipulation'.

TRACTION

This can be used as an adjuvant to manipulation or as a treatment in itself.

Adjuvant Traction

Clearly an attempt to reduce an intra-articular displacement is much more likely to succeed if the bone-ends are brought apart as far as possible; the loose fragment is now given room to move. If it projects beyond the articular edge, the tautening of the ligaments joining the bones exerts beneficial centripetal force. So does the suction created by the distraction. Moreover, if the joint is held at mid-range during the traction, i.e. in a position that ensures that every ligament is lax, the bones are pulled apart and pressure on the displacement ceases. Pain is thus relieved and the muscles cease to guard the joint. Traction is particularly valuable at the cervical and thoracic joints, where it not only has the effects set out above, but also protects the spinal cord and the anterior spinal artery. Traction is essential for one type of displaced loose body at the knee, which cannot be shifted, even during anaesthesia, by ordinary forced movements. The same applies to a carpal subluxation. Gentle forcing at almost any joint is tolerated better if the movement is carried out during traction.

Traction Alone

This is used at the spinal joints and at the shoulder. At the *neck* intermittent traction can be given by suspension. It serves to settle a protrusion already reduced more accurately in place. A Zimmer machine can be employed to ease pain in an ambulant patient and to maintain reduction in cases of great instability. Sustained traction in bed is the only effective treatment for the rare small nuclear disc protrusion at a cervical level. At the *thorax*, the indication is the uncommon nuclear type of disc protrusion, a disc lesion at a very kyphotic joint or one adjacent to a wedge fracture of a vertebral body. At the *lumbar spine*, the position is different. These large joints are so strong that manual traction is no longer effective as an adjuvant. Moreover, nuclear protrusions are quite common at the lumbar joints, in contradistinction to cervical and thoracic levels. It is now a question of manipulation *or* traction—manipulation for a displaced fragment of cartilaginous annulus, traction for a soft nuclear protrusion. Traction applies continuous suction to a pulpy herniation and, unless it is too large, draws it back into place a little more each day. Hence at least thirty minutes' treatment is required daily, with between 40 and 80 kg distraction force.

At the *shoulder*, many cases of arthritis are unsuited to forcing. They require intra-articular hydrocortisone. If this is unobtainable, the physiotherapist's best alternative is distraction of the humeral head from the glenoid. This lasts some seconds, then is released, and repeated again many times. During the first few attempts, muscle spasm keeps the bones in contact but, after a few minutes, they are felt to come apart. Relief ensues which continues after each session ceases.

CONTRA-INDICATIONS TO FORCED MOVEMENT

It is most unwise to manipulate a joint merely because it hurts and the radiograph reveals no abnormality. On the contrary, movement at a joint should be forced only when clinical examination has revealed that a disorder suited to such treatment is present. This positive attitude of manipulating for good reason bears no relation to forcing movement because no contra-indication has been discovered, no one can think what else to try, and a friend was recently relieved by this means.

1. Symptoms of Activity

Peripheral Joints

Pain in the absence of movement, especially at night, wide reference of pain and inability to lie in bed bearing weight upon the affected joint, all indicate that the lesion is in the active stage. In such cases, the end-feel is hard, muscle spasm springing suddenly into play to protect the joint. These phenomena show that forced movement, particularly under anaesthesia will merely serve to increase the trouble.

Spinal Joints and Knee

At these joints the situation is reversed. Internal derangement at a spinal joint may well set up constant pain and inability to bear weight on the affected joint. These symptoms are no longer any reason for avoiding manipulation; on the contrary, the more severe the symptoms, the more urgent manipulative reduction becomes, as long as the attempt can be made tolerable to the patient. It must be remembered that, in my view, the only reason for manipulating any spinal joint between the third cervical and the sacrum is to reduce an intra-articular displacement. Patients with diseases like rheumatoid arthritis, osteitis deformans, myeloma, chordoma, metastasis are, of course, unsuited.

2. Signs of Activity

Peripheral Joints

Local warmth, effusion and muscle spasm all demonstrate that the lesion is in the active stage. Though the joint may or may not be suited to gentle stretching, it is certainly unsuited to forced movement. Synovial swelling occurs in rheumatoid arthritis and in the analogous conditions that complicate disorders like spondylitis, gout, non-specific urethritis, lupus erythematosus or psoriasis and provides a permanent contra-indication to even gentle stretching.

Spinal Joints

In internal derangement at a spinal joint, the muscles may guard the joint, holding it in a deviated position. This does not contra-indicate an attempt at reduction, but suggests that the manoeuvres to be employed first are those which do not force the joint in the restricted direction. Only when reduction is almost complete can manipulation towards the restricted range be cautiously attempted.

Knee

In arthritis or a sprain, the situation is identical with that at the other peripheral joints. If a part of the meniscus or a loose body is displaced, the situation is the same as at the spinal joints, and reduction should be attempted, even in the presence of fluid in the joint, warmth and muscle spasm.

3. Lapse of Time

Ligamentous adhesions do not consolidate themselves in under six weeks. Hence gentle stretching rather than strong forcing is required during this period. If traumatic arthritis at the shoulder has not been abated by early stretching, it often becomes too active for forced movement at the end of three or four weeks. Unless intra-articular hydrocortisone is employed, it may well be six months before stretching becomes worth while once more. It is in these cases that distraction of the humerus from the glenoid provides the physiotherapist's alternative to steroid therapy.

4. Special Joints

Forced movements of any sort should never be used for post-traumatic stiffness at the elbow-joint. Passive attempts at stretching out the joint are apt to diminish rather than increase the range of movement; moreover, there is the ever-present danger of setting up myositis ossificans in the brachialis muscle. In fact, the only common objects of manipulating the elbow are the relief of tennis elbow—an extra-articular condition—and the reduction of a loose body. Traumatic arthritis at the hip is best treated by rest in bed; osteoarthrosis is somewhat benefited by stretching out and internal derangement is, of course, fully relieved if the loose body can be shifted to a neutral part of the joint. The digital joints of the hand and foot respond badly. Trouble at the lower radio-ulnar joint is aggravated by forced movement or even active exercises.

Mobilization is contra-indicated in the treatment of those joints and ligaments the tension on which is not under voluntary control. These are the acromio-clavicular, sterno-clavicular, sacro-iliac and sacro-coccygeal joints, the symphysis pubis, the cruciate ligaments at the knee and the superior and inferior tibio-fibular joints.

5. Special Ligaments

Naturally, the ligaments that span the joints (see above) at which no muscles exist to control mobility cannot develop adhesions requiring rupture. On the contrary, any traumatic overstretching leads to ligamentous laxity which forced movements can only increase.

Ligamentous sprain at the shoulder- and elbow-joints does not remain localized but rapidly leads to months of traumatic arthritis. Stretching the shoulder-joint helps if it is carried out soon enough, but is harmful at the elbow at all times. A strained ulnar collateral ligament at the wrist gets well of itself in a year and is aggravated by mobilization, but is lastingly abolished by one local infiltration with hydrocortisone. Adhesions about the capitate bone at the wrist cause chronic pain that can continue indefinitely. Manipulation is harmful, yet a few sessions of deep massage afford permanent cure.

The coronary ligaments at the knee provide the outstanding example of ligaments whose mobility can be maintained or restored by deep friction. Manipulation moves the femoro-tibial joint, not the menisco-tibial joint, and is therefore useless, whereas the physiotherapist's finger-tip can apply therapeutic movement to the exact spot with great success, even after many years' disability. The cruciate ligaments can become overstretched; painful laxity can be converted into painless laxity by topical hydrocortisone but only operative intervention can achieve shortening. All manipulative endeavours are harmful.

In contradistinction to the talo-fibular ligament at the ankle, which often develops adhesions that require manipulative rupture, sprain of the tibio-navicular (deltoid) ligament is aggravated by such mobilization. The same applies to the anterior tibio-talar ligament. Adhesions may form at a hypermobile mid-tarsal joint, but in spite of the long-standing ligamentous laxity, manipulation is effective.

6. Unsuitable Intra-articular Spinal Displacements

It is true that in the treatment of internal derangement, the first thought is always the feasibility of reduction. However, at the spinal joints, the protrusion of disc substance may become larger than the aperture whence it emerged; if so, reduction is impossible. Alternatively, the displacement may consist of soft nuclear material incapable of being shifted by manipulation, whereas traction may succeed. However, neither manipulation nor traction is effective if the protrusion becomes really large, and is dangerous when the fourth sacral root is menaced.

7. Radiographic Appearances

Considerable change visible on the radiographic indicates the presence of structural alterations that cannot be overcome, but it is important to define their relevance to the symptoms present. Manipulation cannot help a patient's osteoarthrotic knee, but is the treatment of choice for a small cartilaginous loose body, formed secondarily to the degenerative process and displaced within the osteoarthrotic joint. The presence of osteophytosis can be ignored if internal derangement is present; for if a fragment of cartilage has shifted in an osteoarthrotic joint, reduction should be attempted, just as it would at the same joint devoid of osteophytes. This is so particularly at the spinal joints where evidence of osteoarthrosis provides no bar whatever to an attempt at manipulative reduction.

A useful proviso to manipulation is, of course, an X-ray photograph demonstrating the absence of serious disease of bone, e.g. malignant deposits, tuberculosis, etc. Normal radiographic appearances must not, however, be thought to indicate that manipulation is safe. Early invasion of bone due to secondary neoplasm, sacro-iliac laxity and fragmentation of an invertebral disc, for example, may all be made worse by manipulation; yet the radiograph may well reveal no abnormality.

8. Rheumatoid Arthritis and its Analogues

In the acute or subacute stages, every manipulative procedure is strongly contra-indicated. In the chronic stage, when fibrous fixation of a peripheral joint has taken place in a bad position, the deformity may be slowly corrected by forcing under anaesthesia followed by immobilization in plaster in the improved position. This may be repeated several times at intervals. This treatment should not be attempted if the radiograph shows such juxta-articular rarefaction of bone that the bone is more likely to fracture than the joint to move.

9. Bony Block

When forcing movement at a joint ends with the sensation of bone against bone, it is impossible to increase the range beyond this point.

10. Children

Congenital deformity often calls for manipulation in infants and children. On the other hand, adhesion formation after sprain of a joint does not occur; hence, forced movement after an articular sprain should be avoided.

7
Rehabilitation After Injury

SUMMARY OF TREATMENTS

1. Injury to Bone

Alternatives:

    (a) Ignore the fracture and treat only the soft parts by passive movement, then by exercises.

    (b) Reduce and splint the fracture and treat the soft parts by exercises.

Local anaesthesia may need to be induced between the bone ends for:

    (a) Manipulative reduction.

    (b) Pain at the site of fracture.

    (c) Encouraging mobility of the soft parts.

2. Injury to Muscle

    (1) Partial rupture.

        (a) Aspirate the haematoma.

        (b) Induce local anaesthesia during the first week only, and follow by active off-weight exercises.

        (c) Deep massage to the torn fibres while the muscle is held in full relaxation, followed by active exercises without resistance.

        (d) Avoid resisted exercises until recovery is well established.

        (e) Stretch out if necessary.

    (2) Complete rupture
Operative suture.

3. Injury to Tendon

    (1) Complete rupture.

        (a) Suture.

        (b) Transplantation.

    (2) Partial rupture or strain.

        (a) Massage to the site of injury and avoid painful movement.

        (b) Local infiltration with hydrocortisone.

    (3) Teno-vaginitis and teno-synovitis.

        (a) Injection of steroid suspension.

        (b) Massage and avoid painful movement.

        (c) Operation, i.e. slit up the sheath.

(4) Snapping.
    (a) Leave.
    (b) Operation.
(5) Trigger.
    (a) Acupuncture with injection of steroid suspension.
    (b) Plastic operation on the tendon sheath.
(6) Teno-periosteal tear.
    (a) Stretch out by manipulation.
    (b) Splint in relaxation.
    (c) Deep massage or injection of steroid suspension.

N.B.—Local anaesthesia is useless in every type of tendinous lesion except calcification.

4. Injury to Ligament
(1) Partial rupture.
    (a) Local anaesthesia: first day only.
    (b) Deep massage or steroid suspension where accessible.
    (c) Passive movements to the joint and then the same movements repeated actively.
    (d) Resisted exercises for the muscles; first off-weight, then weight-bearing.
    (e) Mobilization, perhaps under anaesthesia, and after-treatment.
(2) Complete rupture.
    (a) Suture.
    (b) Treatment as above, but with slower progress to exercises and weight-bearing.
(3) Permanent laxity.
    (a) Leave; prescribe exercises to compensate.
    (b) Operation.
(4) Ossification.
    (a) Wait; e.g. Stieda–Pellegrini's syndrome.

5. Injury to Joints
(1) Dislocation.
    Reduce and follow by exercises.
(2) Recurrent dislocation.
    (a) Resisted exercises to one muscle; stretch out the antagonist.
    (b) Operation.
(3) Haemarthrosis.
    Aspirate.
(4) Joints and ligaments unsupported by muscles. These are:
    Acromio-clavicular joint.

Sterno-clavicular joint.
Sacro-iliac joint.
Sacro-coccygeal joint.
Symphysis pubis.
Cruciate ligaments of the knee.
Superior and inferior tibio-fibular ligament.

(*a*) Rest.
(*b*) Support.
(*c*) Injection of steroid suspension.
(*d*) *No* exercises or forced movement.

(5) Joints with muscles about them.

N.B.—Each joint is different.

(*a*) *Shoulder :*
  (1) Recent injury: gentle forcing and exercises. If fails, intra-articular hydrocortisone.
  (2) Capsular contracture: forcing (perhaps under anaesthesia) and exercises.
  (3) Subdeltoid bursitis:
    (i) Recent: rest and steroid infiltration.
    (ii) Chronic: local anaesthesia.
    (iii) No exercises.

(*b*) *Elbow :* splintage in flexion; intra-articular hydrocortisone.

(*c*) *Wrist :* massage to sprained structure.

(*d*) *Trapezio-first-metacarpal joint :* massage to capsule; intra-articular silicone; arthroplasty; arthrodesis.

(*e*) *Finger-joints :* wait, often for a year.

(*f*) *Hip :* rest in bed until the full range of movement returns.

(*g*) *Knee :*
  (1) Massage to the site of ligamentous sprain; then movements, passive and active. Instruction in gait.
  (2) Rupture of adherent scars.

(*h*) *Tarsus :*
  (1) Massage; then passive and active movement; then instruction in gait.
  (2) Injection of steroid suspension.
  (3) Manipulative rupture of adhesions.

(*i*) *Toes :* protect; intra-articular hydrocortisone.

6. Internal Derangement of Joints

This occurs at:
Jaw (meniscus).
Elbow (loose body).

Wrist (carpal subluxation).

Spinal joints (disc lesion).

Knee (meniscus or loose body).

Tarsus (loose body).

(*a*) Reduce the displacement by manipulation, often during traction, and maintain reduction by posture and/or appliance.

(*b*) Reduce by sustained traction (nuclear protrusion).

(*c*) Ligamentous sclerosis (lumbar and thoracic joints).

(*d*) Excise loose fragment.

(*e*) Arthroplasty (hip-joint).

(*f*) Arthrodesis (spinal joints).

(*g*) Epidural local anaesthesia (lumbar joints).

(*h*) Sinu-vertebral block (lumbar and thoracic joints).

(*i*) Posterior ramus sclerosis or neurotomy (lumbar joints).

(*j*) Chemonucleolysis (lumbar joints).

8
Schools of Thought in Manipulation

There are five different attitudes towards spinal disorders, and consequently five different intentions in manipulation. The different types of manipulation consist of osteopathy, chiropractice, bonesetting, oscillatory techniques, and the methods evolved by myself and now forming part of the every-day practice of orthopaedic medicine. All five have their successes; hence, in a simple case it does not seem to matter much what theories the manipulator has on the nature of the disorder or what technique he employs. Sometimes any manoeuvre will do and even those laymen who have never had any tuition at all possess satisfied clients. Though treatment based on an erroneous idea sometimes affords relief, the situation is hit-or-miss. Clearly, an open mind on the nature of spinal lesions and full clinical examination leading to conclusions consistent with anatomical fact are required for uniformly good results. Unbiased diagnosis leading to selection of the most effective technique makes all the difference between success and failure.

In theory, the five different schools of thought each possess different ideas on the nature of spinal lesions. In practice, however, it is well to realize that anyone can call himself an osteopath, a chiropractor or a bonesetter. Hence many people using these labels are wholly untrained and may have given no thought at all to the theoretical side of their work. They really subscribe to no particular hypothesis, merely using any terms that appeal to them or are found best to satisfy their clients.

Intention
The different intentions behind spinal manipulation, as I see it, are as follows:

Osteopathy: To restore a full range of movement to the spinal joint.
Chiropractice: To shift the vertebra back into place.
Bonesetting: To click the bone back.
Oscillation: To abolish signs and symptoms without involvement in theoretical arguments on the nature of the lesion.
Orthopaedic medicine: To get the loose fragment of disc back into place.

Tuition of Lay Manipulators

The concepts put forward by lay manipulators today are based on the views of two British doctors (Harrison, 1820; Riadore, 1843). There are two schools of osteopathy in Britain. The British School takes on lay students for a four-year course. The London College offers a nine-month course of postgraduate training to doctors.

However, most laymen calling themselves osteopaths have not been to the British School. Of the seventy-seven non-medical osteopaths listed in the London telephone directory, only twenty-four are accepted by their fellows and included in the osteopaths' register (M.R.O.). These letters are protected by law and indicate recognition by a limited company (The General Council and Register of Osteopaths Ltd). Young (1969) has pointed out that these letters constitute a trademark, but that they have no legal bearing on professional competence. A rival register was started, but a High Court injunction forbade the use of the same letters and the new organization now uses M.G.O.N. (Member of the Guild of Osteopathy and Naturopathy). Even so, if a patient insists on visiting an osteopath rather than a physiotherapist or a doctor skilled in spinal manipulation, the designation M.R.O. is at least a guarantee that the layman has followed a course of tuition. In 1976 a bill was put forward in the House of Commons whereby those who had attended these two institutions were to be afforded state registration, but it was pointed out that it is difficult officially to accept people who regard diseases as caused by spinal derangement, since the Health Service is based on contrary medical concepts.

Osteopaths and chiropractors are in the happy position of making a diagnosis by palpation, and then deciding, again by palpation, if spinal alignment and mobility are now restored. Hence they manipulate at any level where they can perceive limited movement or muscle spasm, no matter how anatomically impossible it is for a lesion there to cause the patient's symptoms. This explains how (it puzzled me for years) a layman can unashamedly manipulate the neck in a patient whose only complaint is sciatica. Once the layman is satisfied that the previously affected joint moves normally, no more treatment is required. This explains how a patient can be told he is 'cured' when his symptoms continue unabated.

OSTEOPATHY

This is a system of healing originally based on the idea that all disease results from vertebral displacements. This was Still's original postulate, announced a hundred years ago. He argued that the displaced bone pinched a spinal artery, depriving the relevant organ of blood and thus provoking disease in it. When it was pointed out to him that this was anatomically impossible, he altered his hypothesis to pressure on a nerve. This, so he averred, stopped transmitting life-force, with the result that function at the organ to which the nerve ran became impaired. Hence, the essential difference between osteopathy and medical manipulation (merely a method of treatment) lies in the fact that its adherents follow an alternative single-minded system of medicine, running counter both to the tenets accepted by doctors throughout the world and to the evidence provided by the many medical discoveries of this century. No positive evidence is offered by them in support of their theories, nor any disproof of the facts doctors are agreed on. It is not manipulation as such that the scientific mind rejects but its expansion to include the treatment of non-spinal disease.

Still had, in fact, hit on a partial truth, which he misinterpreted. Spinal displacements do occur, though it is a fragment of disc that moves, not the vertebra itself. They can result in local symptoms or, if the nerve-root is compressed, pain felt anywhere within the relevant dermatome. No visceral disturbances result, however, and Still's main hypothesis—that all disease stems from spinal displacements—is a wholly false extension from the fact that some pains in the trunk have a spinal origin.

The 'Osteopathic Lesion'

Doctors are often accused of unwillingness to change their ideas, but, in the end, when a theory has been shown to conflict with fact, they do give way. Osteopaths' conservatism is far more rigid. They still cling to the 'osteopathic lesion' as the main cause of bodily disease, upholding a notion put forward a century ago as if it were an unalterable edict. Yet the entire body of medical research over the whole of this century has shown the causes of disease to have no connection with spinal derangements. Conversely, those who do suffer alterations in their spine do not develop disease elsewhere.

Osteopaths palpate the spinal joints in search of limited spinal movement and muscle spasm. The lesion that they detect is fixation of a spinal joint in a faulty position within its normal range of movement, occurring without irreversible change.

There is no doubt that such fixation occurs, as inspection of the back in many cases of acute lumbago will show, but the cause does involve irreversible change. When the disc cracks and a mobile fragment forms, the lesion cannot be reversed. Cartilage is an avascular tissue and therefore cannot unite or regenerate.

The joint may be fixed in flexion or side-flexion by the shift of a loose fragment of disc blocking one aspect. This can be confirmed radio-graphically (see Plates XVIII and XX in the sixth edition of *Textbook of Orthopaedic Medicine*, Volume I). The only way a joint can become suddenly fixed within its normal range (i.e. without actual dislocation of the bones) is by internal derangement. But the osteopaths will have none of so obvious an explanation. A broken fragment of disc displaced and jamming the joint is too simple a concept for their purposes; anyone can grasp such a mechanism. Moreover, it rests on a discovery made, not by themselves, but by doctors.

In my view, osteopaths have for years been treating disc lesions, often successfully, without realizing it. They have obscured a simple disorder by giving it a meaningless name—the 'osteopathic lesion'.

Facet-Locking

Osteopaths lock the facet joints before manipulating the spinal joint they hold to be at fault. Naturally, when the bones engage at the extreme of range at any joint, no further movement is possible and they regard it as locked, but this has nothing to do with locking in the medical sense (e.g. at the knee). In fact, crowding the vertebrae together is the worst manoeuvre possible. If something is to be moved, distraction of the joint surfaces facilitates any manoeuvre. As the facets are wedge-shaped, the further they are pulled apart the greater the range of movement at the joint. Manipulation during traction has the virtue not only of separating the facet joint surfaces but of abolishing pain (so that the patient relaxes spontaneously), giving room for the loose fragment to move, and applying suction (so that any shift that does occur is towards the centre of the joint).

The reason why chiropractors, even in suitable cases, need so many sessions of manipulation is not far to seek. In consequence of this refusal to recognize the displaced fragment of disc as the cause of most neck troubles, they are led to jamming the vertebrae together (locking the facets) instead of pulling them apart. Here lies the cause of their slow effect and physiotherapists' opportunity to secure startling successes (Coldham, 1975).

Specificity

Laymen criticize my manoeuvres for lack of specificity. In fact, of course, what matters is effectiveness not elegance. They take pains to palpate each spinal joint to find out at which one the restriction of movement is the greatest. This laudable endeavour leads to two errors. Statistics have shown that in two cases out of three the lesion lies not at the joint where the movement is limited or osteophytes are visible radiologically, but at a joint that appears normal. In any case it is not possible to restrict a manipulative thrust to one joint only. This is fortunate for laymen, since they often relieve a patient even though their intention has been directed at the wrong level.

My methods are unavoidably specific for quite a different reason. They consist of taking all the relevant joints as far as they will go, until resistance is felt and the overpressure is applied. In other words, the normal joints move as far as they will, whereupon the manipulative thrust inevitably falls on the blocked joint.

'*Hypermobile segment*'. That the stress must finally fall on the blocked joint is equally so whether the joint is hypo- or hyper-mobile. Hypermobility is a bogy invented by lay manipulators to scare physiotherapists, and it has proved quite successful. They quite forget the hundred years of osteopathy, and eighty years of chiropractice, during which this entity was not put forward. It was only when physiotherapists began to threaten the earnings of laymen that this cautionary tale was adumbrated. A hypermobile joint, e.g. genu recurvatum, may well move further than another individual's but when the extreme range is reached it stops in exactly the same way as an ordinary joint.

What is often hypermobile is a small fragment of intra-articular disc. Such instability is not uncommon and implies that reduction is particularly simple, but that redisplacement will prove equally so. This situation by no means calls for the avoidance of manipulation, but indicates the immediate need, as soon as it has been effected, for measures to stabilize the joint containing the unstable fragment.

Cure by Manipulation

Cure by manipulation does not prove that the theory held by the manipulator is well-founded. It proves merely that manipulation was the correct treatment, though the patient is naturally prone to believe in the ideas of the man who put him right. In fact, cases of pain referred from spinal structures may cause considerable difficulty in diagnosis. Pain felt in the anterior thorax or abdominal wall may be attributed to a visceria lesion, since the resemblance to angina, pleurisy, chronic cholecylstits, appendicitis or renal colic may be considerable. Clearly, the lesions actually present could be relieved by manipulation of a spinal joint. The layman, hearing that a medical practitioner has made a diagnosis of some visceral lesion and finding that his manipulations have cured the patient, so far from suspecting the accuracy of the doctor's diagnosis, may quite honestly believe that he has cured visceral disease. This is just ignorance; but the step from the supposed cure of a visceral lesion by manipulation to the postulate that all lesions have a spinal origin is a small one.

CHIROPRACTICE

Whereas osteopaths palpate for lack of spinal mobility, chiropractors palpate for vertebral displacement. Oddly enough, this puts them into the position of more direct followers of Still's original idea than osteopaths. Chiropraxy was modestly described in 1935 during the enquiry in the House of Lords as 'the science of palpating and adjusting the articulation of the human spinal column by hand only'. This is a perfectly acceptable statement, but more recent chiropractic assertions have not stopped at that. They too claim to influence visceral disease and in the U.S.A. the following list was issued by the Parker Chiropractic Research Foundation, based on analysis of a quarter of a million cases. Suitable disorders included acne, angina, appendicitis, diabetes, epilepsy, haemorrhoids, hyperpiesis, jaundice, obesity, paralysis agitans, pneumonia, renal disease, rheumatic fever, ulcer. I regard such claims as a real menace and a number of cases of permanent damage, even death, have been reported.

In general, osteopaths force a joint by distant leverage, whereas chiropractors apply their pressure directly to the bone itself. They employ a strong thrust at one particular joint. Sometimes they fix the joints above and below by locking the facets before applying a direct manual thrust on the vertebra they hold to be at fault, again as a result of palpation. They make a speciality of manipulating the occiput, atlas and axis, and there exists an extreme sect among them which regards manipulation of the upper two joints of the neck as enough for all purposes.

BONESETTING

This craft started centuries ago and continues now. The manipulators who call themselves bonesetters are largely untutored countrymen who have an inborn flair for manipulation, or come from a family that has practised manipulation for generations. The bonesetter does not set bones in the meaning of today, i.e. reduce dislocations or fractures, but manipulates, alleging that he adjusts minor bony subluxations only. In general, bonesetters manipulate the joints near the place where symptoms are felt. They occasionally reduce a displaced fragment of disc and also, as Hood pointed out in 1871, rupture adhesions. They regard the click as the cartilaginous fragment shifts, or the snap as an adhesion ruptures, as audible evidence that the 'bone has been put back'.

OSCILLATORY TECHNIQUES

Percussion cadencée (rhythmic percussion) was employed by Seguin in France in 1838 for acute torticollis. Manual vibrations were used by

Kellgren, a Swedish physiotherapist, and by my father, Edgar Cyriax, M.D., who used them in a wide variety of disorders, but it seemed to me that they were too fine and too gentle to have much effect on tough tissues. More recently, Maitland, a physiotherapist in Australia, has been employing repetitive thrusts of lesser frequency but with more strength behind them. They are not identical with the mobilizing techniques that osteopaths misname 'articulation', nor are they as jerky as chiropractors' pressures.

The great virtue of Maitland's work is its moderation. He has *not* expanded his manipulative techniques into a cult; he claims neither autonomic effects nor that they are a panacea. Indeed, he goes out of his way to avoid theoretical arguments and insists on the practical aspect of manipulation. He says: if such and such a movement is painful and/or limited, let manipulation be employed by the physiotherapist to restore painless range. He leaves it to doctors to decide what the pathological entity was and how it benefited from manipulation.

This welcome attitude enables physiotherapists to put patients right without awaiting a consensus on academic matters among medical men. It avoids physiotherapists appearing to join one faction or another, and thus prevents any hostility arising from either side. This tactful policy benefits patients enormously and is speeding doctors' acceptance of effective measures.

The Techniques

These are described in Maitland's book (1964). The method consists of antero-posterior pressures and releases given to the affected joint as the patient lies prone. In the neck and lumbar spine, lateral oscillations can also be employed. First, each spinal joint is tested in turn in order to ascertain where pain is provoked or resistance encountered; treatment is correctly concentrated at this level. The manipulator places both thumbs on the tip of the appropriate spinous process and applies his oscillations at the rate of about two a second. Movement is generated by alternately flexing and extending both elbows synchronously, so that a series of little thrusts is delivered to the bone. As a result, the joint is extended slightly at the same time as the bone is pressed anteriorly. An antero-posterior glide is imparted during slight extention. The elasticity of the tissues brings the joints back to the neutral position again, ready for the next little thrust.

A number of variations exist. The thrusts can be applied with different degrees of amplitude and force, and the pressure extending the joint can be fully or only partly relieved between thrusts. They can be applied centrally, on both sides, on one side, and from the lateral or postero-lateral aspect as well as in the case of neck and lumbar region, the thrust then applied to the transverse process. The joint may be supported in side-flexion or rotation (or both) before the mobilizations are begun. These oscillations are used without traction and many hundreds are given at one session. The patient is examined at short intervals during the session, to enable the manipulator to assess the result of his treatment so far. He continues or alters his technique in accordance with the change, or absence of change, detected.

These mobilizations clearly provide the physiotherapist with a useful addition to those of orthopaedic medicine and, better still, with an introduction to them. She gains confidence from using gentle manoeuvres and, if the case responds well—albeit in longer time—need seek no further. They cannot be expected to be as quickly effective in considerable displacement; but having gained confidence in carrying out the oscillatory techniques, she does not hesitate to pass on to stronger measures if they are seen to be required. Ending with more forcible manoeuvres is very different from having to plunge straight into effective manipulation in a case where the physiotherapist is uncertain of her skill, or of the exact lesion present or of the doctor's backing.

SPINAL MANIPULATIVE METHODS OF ORTHOPAEDIC MEDICINE

These measures are perfectly straightforward and possess an explicable intention directed to a factual lesion. They are based on the discovery of disc lesions as the primary cause of degenerative change and pain of spinal origin. This novel concept obliged us to think out new methods adapted to it. Osteopaths' techniques originated as a way of shifting a vertebra that they now no longer regard as displaced. Our methods, as far as the spine is concerned, have been devised with a different intention—the reduction of a small intra-articular displacement consisting of cartilage.

Our manoeuvres possess no autonomic effects and can, therefore, be employed on healthy people suffering merely from a spinal subluxation. (Not that I believe that osteopathic or chiropractic techniques really alter autonomic tone.) They are not directed to altering the position of a vertebra; the radiograph shows that it is not displaced. They are not intended to restore a full range of movement, for osteophytosis often makes this impossible, but merely to render painless such movement as can be performed. They do not directly affect muscle spasm, but of course spasm secondary to articular trouble subsides as soon as the causative joint lesion is relieved. The patient is examined by clinical assessment of function at the deranged joint, of the muscles that control it and of the nerves that lie close to it; moreover, the lesion found present is correlated with the patient's symptoms. Once reduction has been achieved, all discomfort ceases, both local and referred. The criterion of success is cessation of symptoms and the restoration of painfree movement. The patient, not the manipulator, is the arbiter.

Our methods rely on the fact that, when a series of spinal joints is moved each to its extreme of range, the normal joints move freely, the blocked joint not. The unaffected joints are thus moved as far as they can go; now the final over-pressure falls inevitably on the deranged joint. Moving the normal joints is carried out gradually over a wide range and continued until the resistance of the blocked joint makes itself felt. Then a final thrust of tiny amplitude is given acting on the displacement itself.

Many of our spinal manipulations for internal derangement are carried out during traction. This makes them much more likely to succeed quickly than oscillatory techniques or lay methods. Traction (a) increases the distance apart of the vertebrae, giving the loose fragment room to move; (b) relieves pain, thus enabling the patient to relax; (c) tautens the posterior longitudinal ligament, exerting centripetal force; and (d) applies suction, again with centripetal effect.

The main advantages of these methods are first, that they are more successful and secondly, that they do not take long to learn. In my view it is not the elegance or the elaborate nature of a manipulation that matters, but its effectiveness. Though the methods are so much simpler, they are at least as effective as laymen's, which are hampered by lack of adequate traction and, often, by mistaken localization of the lesion. If our manoeuvres during traction get patients well more quickly, the need for the more subtle techniques of osteopaths and chiropractors will dwindle. The other advantage is that our methods, which can be learned in a few months, fit well into the physiotherapist's curriculum. By contrast, osteopaths' and chiropractors' manoeuvres take, so they aver, years of undergraduate practice to master.

It is worth noting that in countries where physiotherapists are not taught manipulation, laymen are ousting them from this field at an alarming rate. The latest convert is Medicare, in the U.S.A., where scarcely any manipulation is taught to physiotherapy students. In Australia and Denmark, where state recognition has lately been accorded to chiropractors, the tuition of physiotherapy students has concentrated on 'mobilization'. This policy unhappily leaves them with methods which cannot be compared in rapid success with laymen's manoeuvres.

I have in my day taught a thousand students—three times the number on the osteopaths' register in Britain—methods that have proved both safe and more quickly effective than laymen's treatments. Yet the principal of the

School of Osteopathy in London has stated that my efforts to transfer public recourse from manipulation from osteopaths to physiotherapists has failed. He may prove right, but I still hope that the strong trend towards laymen can be reversed. If the methods of examination and manipulation that were standard tuition at St Thomas's Hospital for thirty years were now taught at every school, we might win yet, but time is short.

9
Should Physiotherapists Manipulate?

Divergent opinions exist on whether or not physiotherapists should manipulate. The controversy can be simply resolved by pointing out that the past policy of withholding such tuition from physiotherapists has in no way diminished the public demand for manipulation; it has merely forced potential patients to go to the bonesetter. Even those doctors who resent the idea of physiotherapists manipulating must surely prefer manipulation by trained personnel working under doctors' guidance to the indiscriminate recourse by patients to all sorts of largely untrained laymen without doctors' prior approval. Come what may, the patients are going to be manipulated; at least let manipulation be sought from trained physiotherapists who give treatment ethically to patients sent to them by doctors.

In 1938, when I started teaching physiotherapists manual techniques, I found them most suited to performing manipulation. The know their anatomy well; they study movement in all its branches; they learn the function and the feel of joints and muscles; they develop strong, sensitive and skilful hands; they have a practical bent; they possess time and patience and are accustomed to working with doctors. Moreover, unlike laymen and bonesetters, they also practise many of the other methods that are called for in soft-tissue lesions not amenable to manipulation. In fact, they are the very people to whom patients needing manipulation have been sent for years, but alas, not with this request.

Manipulation by physiotherapists is by no means novel. It was introduced in 1916 by Mennell, my predecessor at St Thomas's Hospital, who was for many years the chairman of the Chartered Society of Physiotherapy. All his students were taught his techniques, but other schools did not follow suit. His teaching could not extend to the rationale of spinal manipulation since, in those days, disc lesions had not been recognized. When sciatica (Mixter and Barr, 1934) and pain in the back (Cyriax, 1945) were respectively ascribed to disc lesions, the way in which manipulation relieved pain became obvious. Though Mennell taught empirical manipulation, and we teach its theoretical basis too, the benefit to the patient is the same. There is, however, an important difference. Current appreciation of the pathological entity present has enabled a soundly based system of clinical examination to be formulated which can be relied upon to determine the nature and position of any lesion of the moving parts. Such a diagnosis indicates clearly whether manipulation is called for or not, and, if not, what alternative approach should be chosen.

In the past, spinal manipulation has suffered from the extreme positions taken up by its advocates and detractors. The former have been apt to manipulate all-comers with cheerful dogmatism. The latter have refused in any circumstances to countenance an attempt at manipulative reduction when a fragment of cartilage is displaced within a spinal joint, while remaining quite happy about its performance for, say, a torn cartilage at the knee. Such irrational attitudes have naturally thrown a cloud about manipulation which, like any other medical treatment, should be adopted or avoided on rational grounds only. This is exactly the informed selectivity that evolves naturally from collaboration within the doctor–physiotherapist team. Neither purveys a single method of treatment; between them they can practice every approach that medicine offers.

Physiotherapists offer another advantage. It is clearly undesirable that there should exist five variations on the theme of spinal manipulation— osteopathy, chiropraxy, bonesetting, oscillatory techniques and the methods that were taught at St Thomas's. Only when these different methods are all practised by one person will it become possible to determine if one is more quickly successful than another and which type of disorder responds best to one particular set of techniques. The only group of people undoctrinaire enough to allow themselves to be grounded in the most effective fraction of each of these methods is the physiotherapy profession, and I for one would welcome such expanded tuition. The only physiotherapy teacher who has achieved this eclectic status is Kaltenborn in Oslo. His approach offers an example that deserves to be followed in physiotherapy schools throughout the world.

OBJECTIONS

It must be realized that the objections are theoretical and rest largely on inexperience of manipulation by trained physiotherapists. In practice, wherever our graduates have travelled they have been warmly received and their special skills have been commended by doctors and patients. Moreover, their successes have happily served to transfer the gratitude that some members of the public accord to laymen to the manipulating physiotherapist and the doctor instructing her. However, emphasis must be laid on the fact that our students have always been taught, not just manipulation as a manual craft, but how to identify the lesion present, how to determine whether manipulation is called for or not, how to vary technique according to the type of lesion, and what safeguards to employ.

Doctors' Disagreement

Not all doctors agree with manipulation, it is true, but if the Chartered Society of Physiotherapists is to wait until all doctors are agreed on any subject, it will wait till doomsday. I am by no means alone in regarding radiant heat as a futile treatment, but this does not stop our students from being taught how to use a lamp. When a rational manual treatment, now in use for a century, is shown tó have a wide application, to be successful and to possess a logical justification, it must be made available within the medical sphere. The alternative is to let the public go on being treated by all sorts of laymen—a solution abhorrent to doctors and, one must suppose, to teachers of physiotherapy too, since it redounds to the detriment of both professions. In 1962, Wilson distributed a questionnaire to all family doctors in his county. Seventy-five out of ninety-two answered 'Yes' to the question: 'Is there a place for manipulative treatment in orthodox practice?' This is four doctors out of five and surely provides a proportion high enough for the Chartered Society of Physiotherapists to act upon. He found that thirty-eight doctors themselves manipulated, largely for lack of a suitable medical auxiliary to whom to depute the work. Indeed, some doctors find themselves in such straits that they may give a patient an unofficial tip to try a bonesetter. It should be a point of honour with the physiotherapy profession to close this gap with the minimum of delay, if only to save our patients from laymen's hits and misses.

Danger

All effective treatments are dangerous. They possess indications and contra-indications; only wholly inert measures are as incapable of harm as they are of good. Since the physiotherapist manipulates only at the doctor's request, the bonesetters' bugbear—the unsuitable case—is avoided. Moreover, all my cervical and thoracic manipulation, i.e. along the extent of the spinal cord, is carried out during traction, which exerts a strong centripetal force on the contents of the joint being treated; in addition, no movements towards flexion are ever included. As a further safeguard, the articular signs (determined before manipulation starts) are assessed afresh after each manoeuvre, thus affording a clear pointer to what is happening inside the joint. It is on these consecutive findings that a decision was based on what to do next and whether to go on or stop. Manipulation by laymen, in spite of their lack of precautions, is remarkably lacking in danger. Poor technique means many avoidable failures, and lack of medical knowledge leads to much expenditure of time, effort and money on futile treatment for unsuitable disorders, but lasting harm is rare; otherwise, these men would be for ever in serious medico-legal trouble.

In spite of this very unsatisfactory state of affairs, there are many people who swear by 'a wonderful bonesetter'. I want this esteem to pass to physiotherapists, as has already happened to many of our graduates. Safe and effective manoeuvres, which so often secure dramatic relief, cannot fail to commend physiotherapists to patients and doctors alike. It is those who never saw the work at St Thomas's who most readily decried it. Visitors gained full reassurance when they noted the great trouble taken both by the medical staff and by the physiotherapists to make sure of proper selection of cases and of correct treatment, correctly given.

TUITION

To learn when to manipulate and when not, and what sort of manoeuvres to use, is a diagnostic problem involving years of study. By contrast, manipulation itself is not hard to learn, as is evidenced by the many entirely untutored individuals who earn a successful living this way. Nevertheless, before it is taught to students, it must be learned and practised by the teachers. Here lies a very real bottleneck. There are forty schools of physiotherapy in Britain, all short of teachers, whom it is difficult to second elsewhere for lengthy periods of tuition and practical work. Courses in localization and manipulative technique were started by me in 1942 and still continue now. Six years ago, when I retired from St Thomas's, I offered to give a series of weekend lectures to provide an introduction to assessment and manipulation for all final-year physiotherapy students who cared to come. The Education Committee of the Chartered Society of Physiotherapy forbade the publication of this announcement in their journal and the embargo continued until 1976, when it was modified. The statement in *Physiotherapy* reads that students are 'at liberty to take up Dr Cyriax's offer themselves and ask him to lecture to them out of school hours'. In fact in 1973 manipulation was withdrawn from the syllabus and replaced by 'mobilization'. Students are now faced with the situation—difficult to sustain with logic—that in their undergraduate days they are not to be grounded in manipulation, though it is a suitable postgraduate activity on which courses are given to selected individuals. Presumably the trouble is that nothing can be taught until the practical assessment of the candidate's skill is made possible by the creation of a panel of competent examiners.

EXPERIENCE IN OTHER COUNTRIES

The first country to show interest was New Zealand. In 1952, my senior physiotherapist, Miss J. Hickling, lectured and demonstrated at every main hospital there in the course of a year. Manipulation by physiotherapists has been taken for granted there ever since. Next came a report from Dublin (1956). Pringle, working in industry, found that the time off work with lumbago was halved after he had sent two physiotherapists to St Thomas's for a fortnight's tuition. Two other doctors, both of whom started by employing one of our graduates, have described similar experiences in Paris (Troisier, 1962) and in Bremen (Hirschfeld, 1962). Miss J. M. Ganne, one of our graduates, now Vice-Principal of the Physiotherapy School in Adelaide, teaches the preliminary examination and manipulation to her students as standard practice.

The Norwegian Achievement

The next country to encourage manipulation by physiotherapists was Norway. After some months at St Thomas's in 1952, a physiotherapist from Oslo named Kaltenborn devoted his considerable energies to getting their Physiotherapists' Charter enlarged to include manipulation. He won over the medical profession and his application was approved by their National Health authorities in 1957. Meanwhile, he had taught two groups of physiotherapists who were examined by me in consecutive years. The successful candidates were placed on an official register of manipulating physiotherapists to which doctors referred when seeking such treatment. Within two years, the Health Service statistics showed the recovery from a number of common disorders to be so much more rapid that it was decided to pay a double fee for a session of manipulation. The same happened in Bremen, where the Health Service actuary found the period of disablement to be so much shorter when the patient was treated by Dr Hirschfeld and Miss Longton that, within four years, a new hospital department had been built for them, large enough to accommodate all suitable cases from the whole city and district.

In Norway, an association of manipulative physiotherapists was founded in 1957, and in 1962 a similar association of doctors. Under the medical leadership of first Schiotz and now Koefoed, the advantages of manipulation were kept under constant review and presented to their colleagues. In due course, understanding increased and the doctors of Norway, Denmark, Sweden and Finland looked at the matter scientifically and in large measure approved. In 1962, Hult lectured in Stockholm on the results of employing a St Thomas's graduate, Miss A. Nixon as she was then, at his hospital.

With doctors' participation, Kaltenborn started courses on the localization of lesions and on manual treatment for doctors and physiotherapists in 1962. As from 1964, all physiotherapy students in Norway were examined in these techniques at their qualifying examinations. In 1966, a book by, and for, doctors and physiotherapists was published—*Manipula-*

tion av Ryggraden by Brodin, Bang, Bechgaard, Kaltenborn and Schiotz—
and in 1967 Kaltenborn's next illustrated book for physiotherapists
appeared, *Frigjoring av Ryggraden* (freeing of the spine).

To give some idea of Kaltenborn's indefatigable determination to get
manipulation accepted on a sound basis, it suffices to say that, in the twelve
months ending May, 1967, he gave eleven courses in Norway, twelve in
Sweden, three in Denmark and one in Iceland. They were attended by
180 doctors from all over Europe (of whom I was one) and 769 physiotherapists (counting a participant at more than one course as a fresh
individual). It is evident that one dedicated physiotherapist with en-
lightened medical support has, in the course of only fifteen years, reversed
the medical climate in the whole of Scandinavia as regards manipulation
and has secured widespread medical approval for his work with physiotherapists. (In consequence, there is only one bonesetter practising in the
whole of Norway.) At his courses, Kaltenborn teaches what he has found
best in osteopathy, chiropraxy and orthopaedic medicine without a trace
of fringe indoctrination. He uses the orthopaedic medical approach to
clinical examination, but prefers manipulative methods with unisegmental
effect. This is perfectly satisfactory, for the clinical examination is what
matters. Manipulation done one way or the other is less important than
how to identify lesions suited to manipulation. The physiotherapists who
have learnt from him are now teaching in most of the schools in Scandinavia. Miss Hickling and Mr Preastner, my two senior physiotherapists,
have also devoted much of their leisure to further courses, but spare-time
teaching has obvious limits and has the important defect that it never
reaches undergraduates at all.

The position today is that a method of treatment, first advocated by
Hippocrates more than two thousand years ago, practised by laymen for
over a hundred years, and at St Thomas's since 1916, was shown to have
a logical justification in 1945. In my view, the time has come for these
methods to be included in normal medical and physiotherapeutic practice,
so that they become available at all hospitals. Though my techniques are
novel, it must not be thought that there are any fresh principles involved.
What has changed is the selection of cases—the insistence on exact
measures for precise reasons restricted to suitable cases. Physiotherapists
doing the sort of work I expect of them are nothing new either. A surgeon
in Oxford, J. Grosvenor, who died in 1823, advocated friction, passive
movements, then active exercises. He employed a staff of female assistants,
one of whom in 1826 was taken on at the Radcliffe Infirmary as a 'rubber-
nurse'. He was also the father of rehabilitation, saying to his patients, as he
took their sticks and crutches away: 'Your own constant exertions are
necessary as well as mine.'

Physiotherapists who manipulate are abiding by principles of treatment by movement established more than two millennia ago and are following a sequence in manual medicine dating back since before Christ. This progress was reversed during the first half of this century and they must now make up for lost time. Only then will laymen's virtual monopoly be broken.

Taped Lectures

Interested readers can obtain a tape-recording by myself entitled 'Should Physiotherapists Manipulate?' from the Medical Recording Service Foundation (an educational branch of the Royal College of General Practitioners) at Kitts Croft, Writtle, Chelmsford, Essex. There is another very informative taped lecture by Dr G. Symonds entitled 'Backache and Lumbar Disc Lesions', recorded by Medikasset (volume 7, no. 1) and available from Winthrop Laboratories, Winthrop House, Surbiton-on-Thames, Surrey KT6 4PH.

10
Steroid Therapy

Until 1952, no alternative had existed to deep massage in the treatment of musculotendinous lesions. When a painful scar had formed in a muscle, it had to be broken up by accurately directed deep friction. This remains so now, but in tendinous lesions this monopoly has ceased. For scarring in a short tendon or for roughening of the gliding surfaces in teno-synovitis there has existed for the last twenty years an alternative approach (Cyriax and Trosier, 1953): topical steroids, which provide the medical profession with a potent agent for abating a localized area of unwanted inflammation. Since the reaction to overuse or an aseptic injury is always excessive, a way to reduce traumatic inflammation has been sought for years. It has now been found. However, steroids are a suspension of insoluble particles. Hence their action is confined to the cells with which they lie in contact; there is no effect elsewhere nor any spread to adjacent structures. The lack of solubility carries the advantage that an intense anti-inflammatory effect is exerted at the point of application. It also implies that great precision in diagnosis and injection technique must be maintained. The following factors must be considered before an injection of a steroid suspension is given:

1. In what tissue does the lesion lie?
2. What part of that tissue, in a horizontal plane?
3. What part of that tissue, in a vertical plane?
4. What posture should the patient adopt to facilitate palpation of the tissue at fault?
5. How should the doctor place his finger on the relevant structure?
6. Where shall the needle be inserted, in what direction and how deeply?
7. How long a needle is required, and what sort of syringe?
8. How much of the suspension is needed to cover the whole affected area?

Between arriving at a decision on which is the tissue at fault, then which part of it, and then actually infiltrating at the point the doctor intends to reach, there is obviously room for a number of minor errors. Unhappily, merely one minor error vitiates the result. For example, when words like 'frozen shoulder', 'rotator cuff syndrome', 'painful arc syndrome' are considered viable diagnoses, it is clearly impossible to use this method; for no indication has arisen of exactly where the lesion lies. Steroids, like deep friction, need a diagnosis accurate within a millimetre or two. Hence the positions illustrated in this book that were devised forty years ago for rendering various structures accessible to massage are also the ones required for facilitating injection into the right spot. They bring the affected tissue within finger's reach, show how the digit is best applied, thus aiding delineation of boundaries and palpation of extent.

When triamcinolone is used for short tendons, the strength containing 10 mg/ml is to be preferred, since rupture has been reported after using the 40 mg strength. With the weaker solution this has not occurred in any of my cases, and the effect is just as good.

SUITABLE DISORDERS

The disorders that respond particularly well to local steroid therapy are: localized subdeltoid bursitis, supraspinatus tendinitis, infraspinatus tendinitis, subscapular tendinitis, arthritis at the shoulder, tennis elbow (teno-periosteal only), golfer's elbow (teno-periosteal only), traumatic arthritis at the elbow, arthritis of the lower radio-ulnar joint, traumatic arthritis of the acromio-clavicular joint, osteoarthrosis of the sterno-clavicular joint, recent sprain of either collateral ligament at the knee, cruciate ligament strain (no other treatment exists), supra-patellar and infra-patellar tendinitis, recent sprain at ankle or tarsus, achilles tendinitis, plantar fasciitis, traumatic arthritis of a metatarso-phalangeal joint (no other treatment exists), and overuse arthritis of sesamo-first-metatarsal joint (no other treatment exists).

In order to give the anti-inflammatory effect of the hormone the most favourable environment in which to act, the patient is asked not to exert the limb for the week after the injection, however well he may appear to himself to be. Too early violent exertion may lead to relapse.

Many hospitals exist where steroids are not used in the manner indicated above. Moreover, many family doctors regard injections of any steroid suspension as outside their scope. Hence, physiotherapists need have no fear that their precise massage techniques will be overtaken to an appreciable extent during the foreseeable future.

Rheumatoid Arthritis

The insoluble steroids have also brought within the scope of orthopaedic medicine the rheumatoid type of arthritis. Intractable for centuries, rheumatoid arthritis has now been shown to respond very favourably to intra-articular injection. In cases without irretrievable damage to the joint and in a reasonably chronic phase, steroids can be relied upon to bring immediate relief lasting many months. This relief can be maintained by further injections at whatever intervals prove necessary; they can often be semi-lastingly discontinued. Naturally, the fewer the number of joints requiring treatment, the more practicable this becomes. In acute cases, flaring at many joints at the same time, local treatment is useless. Rheumatoid teno-synovitis responds particularly well. The peripheral joints in ankylosing spondylitis, psoriasis and lupus erythematosus respond well, but in Reiter's disease steroids are without effect. These injections have no systemic effect and are thus free from the serious objections to prolonged courses of cortisone. However, there is a limit to the number of intra-articular injections that can be given to a weight-bearing joint, for fear of setting up a steroid arthropathy. At the joints of the upper limb this does not apply.

Intra-articular injection is simpler than infiltration of some part of a deeply placed tendon. As soon as the needle can be felt to pass between the joint surfaces, the injection is given. Traction applied by an assistant is helpful at the small joints of the fingers or toes.

STEROID PHONOPHORESIS

An important discovery has been made which will entirely change the situation of physiotherapists as regards steroid therapy. It was shown twenty years ago that hydrocortisone could be driven through the skin and deposited unaltered in the deep tissues. In 1963, Griffin and Touchstone showed that phonophoretic penetration reached 6 cm through the intact skin of pigs. Kleinkert and Wood (1975) applied 1% and 10% hydrocortisone ointment spread 0·5 mm thick and employed ultrasonic waves with a frequency of 1 MHz. The maximum intensity was 2 W/cm² from a quartz radiating crystal of 10 cm² area. Excellent results were secured.

Now for the first time it has become possible for a physiotherapist herself to apply a steroid suspension to the site of a lesion. She no longer needs to ask the doctor to inject it for her. Obviously the best results will be achieved by aiming the steroid at the affected part of the tissue at fault and using the localizing method of selective tension described in Volume I. She also puts the patient into the position that brings the tissue closest to the surface in the same way as for massage.

Here we have a great advance in therapeutics, putting within the physiotherapist's scope many lesions which previously lay outside it, e.g. rheumatoid arthritis. This is an opportunity that every physiotherapist must hasten to grasp, but with discretion. It will prove of no help to call an internal derangement at the spinal joint a ligamentous sprain in order to treat that alleged sprain with ultrasonic waves. Such wishful thinking will, as always, redound to the benefit of the manipulative layman.

Part II
The Illustrations

General Remarks on the Illustrations

All except a few photographs (cervical manipulations) are taken with the patient on a couch about 40 cm high. This is the height most generally useful for giving deep friction, since the physiotherapist can sit comfortably at her work, keeping her forearm horizontal and not bending her back. A low couch is also essential for those manipulations in which the final thrust is imparted by the momentum of her thorax, poised above the patient, transmitted via the arms held vertically. However, some manipulations, especially those at the neck, require a high couch and the physiotherapist must be provided with both sorts of couch if she is to do her work properly.

DESCRIPTION OF PHYSICAL SIGNS

A list of the physical signs identifying each lesion has been included for each condition. This information tells the physiotherapist what to look for before starting treatment and enables her to confirm the suitability of the lesion present. Having ascertained the relevant signs she can watch for significant alterations as the session progresses or from day to day at each pre-treatment examination. The other important advantage is negative. If the signs present show that the disorder is not suited to the types of treatment that physiotherapists give, this becomes evident to her at once. It may always happen that the patient's state, and hence the signs, change between the doctor's examination and his first attendance, perhaps some days later, to the physiotherapist. For example, a patient with sciatica may be ordered manipulation or traction but, in the interval between seeing doctor and physiotherapist, may develop a root palsy. Since this event contra-indicates both measures, it is the duty of the physiotherapist to be aware of this possibility and to test for impaired conduction each time the patient comes. Or it may happen that a patient referred for massage to the supraspinatus tendon is found at his first attendance no longer to have pain on resisted abduction of the arm. Clearly, this patient too requires reference back to the doctor for renewed examination. The physiotherapist who knows the physical signs that ought and, equally importantly, ought not to be present can greatly help doctor and patient. I for one have derived much benefit from the informed clinical care always exercised by both my staff and student physiotherapists.

MANIPULATIVE TECHNIQUE

Readers will note that the manipulations described include all suitable lesions at the peripheral as well as the spinal joints. This is not a book devoted to spinal manipulation alone and the methods used are not those of osteopathy or chiropractice. Osteopathy is based on methods elaborated a hundred years ago for shifting a vertebra. Our techniques were thought out, as far as the spinal joints are concerned, on the basis of reduction of a small fragment of disc. The methods are therefore different, especially at cervical and thoracic levels, where each manoeuvre is carried out during strong traction. Separation of the joint surfaces gives the loose piece room to move, while centripetal force is acting on it.

Manipulation for internal derangement is not 'set', i.e. the operator does not know in advance exactly what manoeuvre will prove effective, but merely how to set about the attempt. This involves ascertaining the physical signs first, performing one manoeuvre and then examining the affected part again to assess the result. The session continues until the patient's symptoms and signs have been modified to the greatest extent possible. This approach is again quite different from laymen's, who continue until they —not the patient—decide that all is well.

Throughout, the operator's assistant is a physiotherapist. Obviously, those who work single-handed can devise simple mechanical devices for keeping a patient still during traction. Patients do not much like being strapped into position and the assistant, by altering the angle of her pull at the precise moment of overpressure, can help the operator. Human assistance is therefore much to be preferred.

The sequences described are not inviolable. If one manipulation helps, it is repeated. Then another is tried, and so on. But experience, the result of each particular manoeuvre, end-feel and the estimate of a patient's tolerance all affect the number and type of manoeuvres contemplated.

No two people manipulate in exactly the same way. (My patients tell me that even mechanical traction is given differently by different physiotherapists.) Allowance must be made, therefore, for minor individual variations, for one individual prefers to use one grip rather than another, depending on which finger is the stronger, what is the span of the hand and what is the range of movement at the wrist and digital joints.

MASSAGE TECHNIQUE

There are, with few exceptions, several ways of giving manual treatment to any one structure. The method chosen for illustration has been the one that best suits most physiotherapists' hands, and is the simplest, the least open to misconstruction and the most suitable for photographic representation. No claim is made that the best method has been illustrated throughout, since for many structures there is no one way that markedly surpasses others. In many instances the physiotherapist can, by reversing her position, approach the same tissue in the same way from the opposite direction. Often the same structure can be given massage alternately with the finger or thumb of either hand. Sometimes, too, several different grips can be employed to apply pressure to the same tissue. Depending on the shape and size of the hand and on the respective strengths of the fingers and thumb, different physiotherapists prefer to accomplish the same movement in different ways. It is my hope that physiotherapists will try the methods set out in this book and, once fully familiar with the movement to be imparted, modify them to suit their own preference. In the case of deep massage this latitude does not apply to the position in which the patient is placed or the exact siting of the tip of the operative digit or digits. There are structures that are out of reach of the physiotherapist's finger unless the patient is first put into a special position. This position is then unalterable. Moreover, the position of the physiotherapist's finger-tip is equally invariable. But whether she prefers to sit facing the patient or to stand behind him when giving friction to a tissue is a matter which each physiotherapist decides for herself. Indeed, one of the ways of making deep friction less tiring is to apply it first from one position with one hand, then from another with the other. Hence, within the rigid framework of the position of the patient and the placing of the physiotherapist's operative finger or thumb, there is often much scope for individual choice on exactly how the identical frictional movement is to be imparted to the structure at fault. Since the posture that the patient must adopt for receiving adequate friction is the very one that brings the tissue at fault best within reach of the physiotherapist's finger, it follows that the same position is often the one ensuring the greatest accuracy in an injection of hydrocortisone. When the medical man can feel clearly the structure he is aiming at, maximum precision can be attained. Hence the postures for massage that we devised thirty years ago are as relevant as ever. Physiotherapists will do doctors a valuable service by explaining the situation and putting the patient into the best position before the infiltration starts.

INJECTION TECHNIQUE

The best way to find an exact anatomical spot, often without reference to local tenderness, may well involve the patient's adopting the same posture, and the doctor using the same palpatory technique, as the physiotherapist employs. Hence, included in this volume now is a series of descriptions of how a structure is found and infiltrated. Variations in technique make all the difference to the result, for hydrocortisone, an insoluble powder, does not spread within the tissues. It works only where it is placed, and must therefore be made to lie in contact with all the affected fibres. The tissue at fault is infiltrated all over, not merely injected at one point along the affected extent. No other publication offers this information. For the first time a standard technique is set out for most of the lesions that respond well to topical steriod infiltration or phonophoresis.

Note

Clarity is maintained in the textual description by regarding the manipulator always as male and the patient as female. The same applies to the physician giving an injection. When deep massage is described the operator is always 'she' and the patient 'he', whatever the photograph may show.

PLATE 1

TEMPORO-MANDIBULAR JOINT

Injection Technique

Lesion—Monarticular rheumatoid arthritis.

Physical Sign—Limitation of movement of slow onset.

Differential Diagnosis—Sudden displacement of the meniscus. Sympathetic arthritis secondary to lesions in adjacent bone, e.g. following dental extraction. Tetanus. Hysteria.

Patient's Posture—She lies on the side with the affected jaw uppermost. A felt pad in the mouth keeps the mouth open as far as possible.

Injection Technique—The lower edge of the zygoma is identified and just below, level with the tragus, the physician can feel the condyle of the mandible moving as the mouth is opened and closed. A thin needle attached to a syringe containing 1 ml of hydrocortisone suspension is inserted at the base of the tragus and pointed slightly forwards, aiming at the space left behind when the condyle has shifted anteriorly as far as possible by the patient opening his mouth as wide as he can. The needle becomes intra-articular at about 1·5 cm.

Result—One or two intra-articular injections of 25 mg hydrocortisone usually restore full painless range in cases not too chronic.

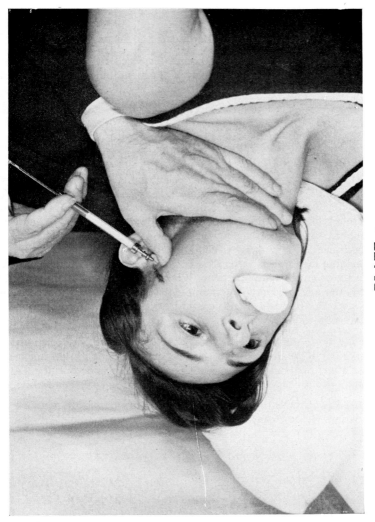

PLATE 1

TEMPORO-MANDIBULAR JOINT

Reduction of Displaced Meniscus

Site of Lesion—The meniscus becomes displaced forwards within the joint, blocking the movement anteriorly of the mandibular condyle. Hence the patient can separate her teeth by about 2 cm only.

Physical Signs—Limitation of movement of sudden onset. Opening and deviation to the painless side are blocked.

Patient's Posture—The patient lies supine on a high couch and opens her mouth as wide as possible. Her head is well supported on a firm cushion.

Technique—The manipulator winds a substantial length of ordinary bandage round his thumb for protection and stands level with the patient's thorax facing her. If the right temporo-mandibular joint has suffered derangement, he stands on the patient's left side; he puts his right hand on her forehead for counter-traction and his left thumb against her right lower back teeth. The fingers of his left hand grip her chin.

By pressing downwards as hard as he can on her molars, the mandible is distracted from the temporal bone. When adequate separation has been achieved after a few seconds' traction, the mandible is rapidly moved from side to side. Full rightward and leftward deviation are forced alternately as quickly as possible by the fingers round the chin.

Duration of Treatment—This manoeuvre is repeated as often as is necessary. If full painless range towards opening the mouth has not been achieved after, say, six repetitions, it is wise to stop and continue a few days later.

Result—Reduction is nearly always possible in one or two sessions of manipulation. Relapse can, of course, occur but is uncommon.

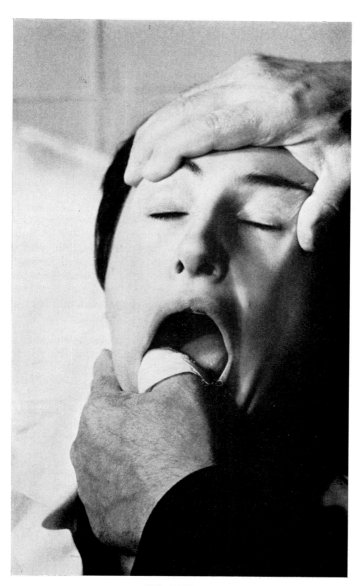

PLATE 2

SPLENIUS CAPITIS MUSCLE: OCCIPITAL FIBRES

Massage Technique

Site of Lesion—Bilateral and unilateral post-traumatic fibrosis occurs at the occipital insertion of the splenius capitis muscle with about equal frequency. Lesions here follow immobilization after concussion and set up pain, often felt radiating to the temple.

Physical Signs—The passive movements of the neck are painless, but resisted extension and side-flexion towards the affected side both hurt at the occiput.

Patient's Posture—The patient lies prone on the couch, his forehead supported on a low pillow so that he can breathe easily.

Technique—The physiotherapist sits level with the patient's neck facing his head and on the side distant from the lesion. She steadies his head with one hand. She places the index finger of the other hand, reinforced by the middle, on the affected spot, which is usually placed well forwards and under the occiput. She presses upwards as well as forwards, thus catching the muscle against the bone. Her forearm follows a line at 45° to the vertical, and the friction is imparted by her drawing her forearm and hand to and fro in this alignment.

Duration of Treatment—Twenty minutes' treatment two or three times a week is adequate. Two to six weeks' treatment may be required in chronic cases.

Results—Uniformly good.

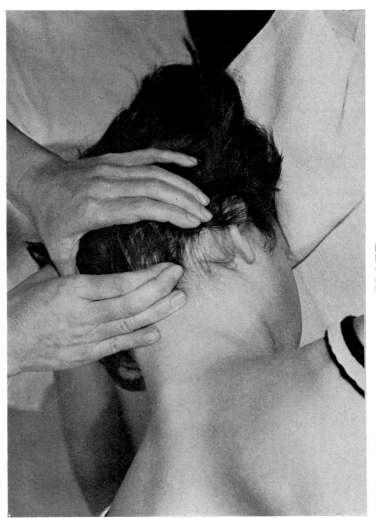

PLATE 3

SPLENIUS AND SEMISPINALIS CAPITIS MUSCLES: MID-CERVICAL EXTENT

Massage Technique

Indication for Massage—To inhibit voluntary contraction of the muscles about the affected cervical joint. This should be done just before manipulative reduction is attempted.

Patient's Posture—The patient lies face downwards on the couch, his forehead supported on a pillow so that he can breathe comfortably.

Technique—The physiotherapist sits facing his head. She places her thumb on the affected area while the fingers supply counter-pressure on the far side of the neck. This grip avoids pressure on the trapezius muscle, which is not involved in the restriction of movement. The physiotherapist imparts her friction by alternately flexing and extending her wrist. By keeping her fingers still and using them as a fulcrum, the thumb is made to move over the muscles.

Duration of Treatment—This should last about fifteen minutes. The attempt to effect reduction by manipulation should follow at once.

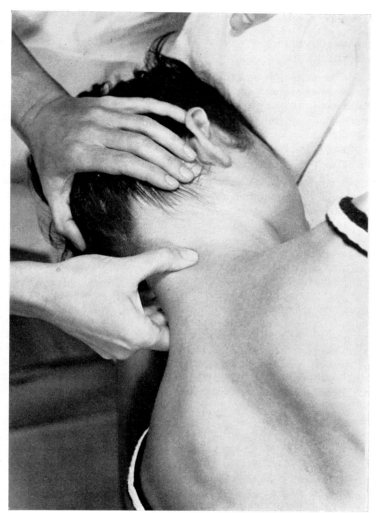

PLATE 4

CERVICAL SPINE: FORCED ROTATION

Indications—Limitation of, or pain on, the extremes of movement at the cervical joints due to:

(*a*) Early osteoarthrosis or diffuse capsular adhesions following trauma. In this case the movement is a quick one, intended to break adhesions.
(*b*) Advanced osteoarthrosis or ankylosing spondylitis. In this case the movement is a slow stretching, intended to lengthen the contracted ligaments.
(*c*) The matutinal headache of elderly men.
(*d*) Osteoarthrosis with ligamentous contracture at a facet joint.

Contra-indications—Displacement of part of a cervical intervertebral disc. In this case the manipulation must be carried out during traction. Basilar ischaemia.

Patient's Posture—The patient lies supine on the couch.

Technique—The physiotherapist stands or half-kneels (depending on the height of the couch) at the patient's head. If his neck is to be rotated to the right she hooks the fingers of her right hand round the right side of the mandible. By exerting traction here the neck is extended, thereby bringing the occiput into prominence. Her left hand now obtains a better purchase. Rotation is forced—during slight traction—by the right thenar eminence, which is pressed (suddenly or gradually, according to the lesion present) against the patient's left maxilla.

Some soreness may result lasting a few days. Patients should therefore be treated once a week until reasonable relief has been secured (two to four sessions). Headache should be entirely relieved (one or two sessions).

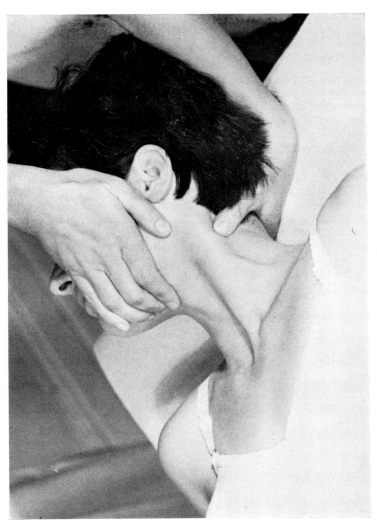

PLATE 5

CERVICAL SPINE: FORCED SIDE-FLEXION

Indications and Contra-indications—As for forced rotation of cervical spine (see Plate 5).

Technique—The physiotherapist must take the weight of the patient's head with the least possible amount of her fingers under his occiput, since she must lay her thenar eminence on the side of his head above the ear. Her other hand is used purely as a fulcrum, so as to ensure that it is movement at the cervical spine which is forced. Unless such a fulcrum is provided, a general side-flexion movement is imparted to the whole cervicothoracic spine.

Assuming that his neck is to be bent to the right, the physiotherapist supports the patient's head by the finger-tips of the left hand passed under the patient's occiput; she lays her thenar eminence on his temporal bone. This is feasible only if the hand is held vertically. She places her right hand, fingers pointed vertically downwards, against his right clavicle in such a way that the base of her index finger lies against the transverse process of the sixth cervical vertebra. So as to avoid the patient's trachea, her thumb is either tucked away in her palm or kept well extended.

Movement is now forced—suddenly or gradually depending on the nature of the lesion present—by the physiotherapist strongly pushing her two hands towards each other simultaneously, scissors fashion. By this means the patient's head is forced to the right and her neck towards the left. A side-flexion movement confined to the neck therefore results.

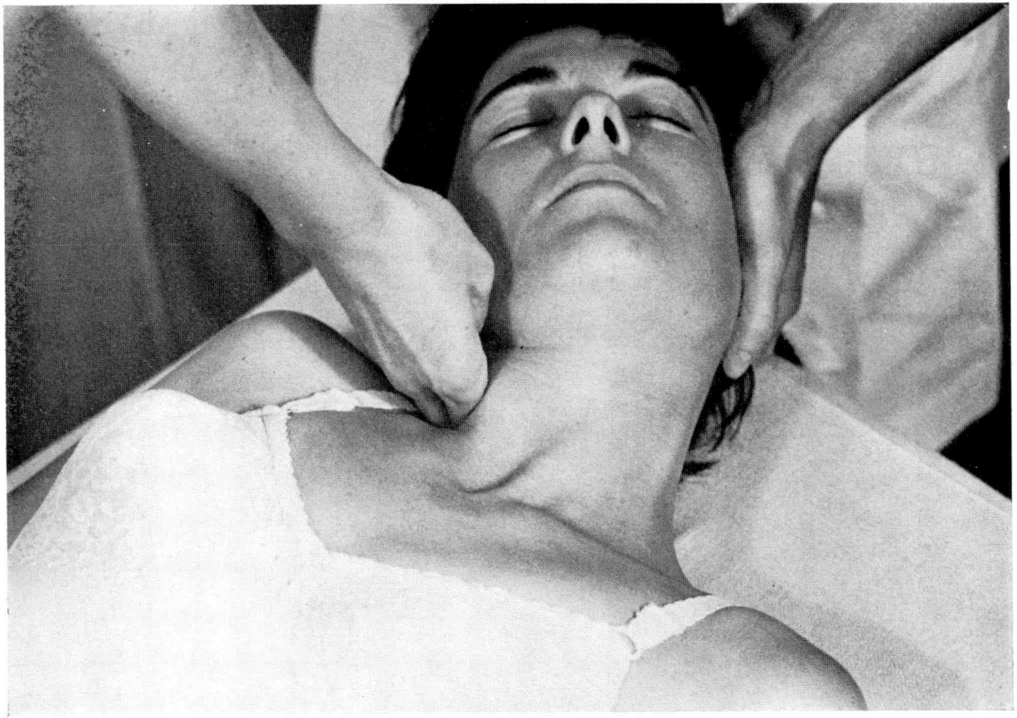

PLATE 6

MANIPULATOR'S POSTURE FOR APPLYING TRACTION

General Remarks—Before any attempt is made to reduce an intra-articular displacement at a cervical intervertebral joint strong traction must be applied. By this means the joint surfaces are separated as widely as possible and a suction effect produced; in addition, the stretched ligaments exert centripetal force. Moreover, during such traction, the patient's pain is largely or wholly relieved; as a result she relaxes, now permitting movements which would otherwise have provoked severe pain and such resistance as to render manipulation impossible. Manipulation without traction may lead to an increase of the displacement within the joint, but this disaster cannot in my experience occur if strong traction is exerted and maintained during the whole time that movement at the affected joint is being forced. It must be remembered that not only may root pressure be set up or increased by injudicious manipulation, but even pressure on the spinal cord itself may result. If manipulation were to enlarge or bring about such a central protrusion, damage to the cord might result, from which the patient might never fully recover. Thus, the likelihood of success and the avoidance of undue pain are much enhanced by traction, which also provides the only safeguard against making the patient worse (see Volume I).

The Couch—This should stand 80 to 90 cm high. The manipulator should be able, while pulling, to get his centre of gravity on a horizontal level with the patient. It must be strongly built, for the legs have to withstand repeated use as supports for the manipulator's feet. Square legs are preferable to round, for on occasion the manipulator may wish to press his knee against one leg of the couch so as to pull harder. The floor must be carpeted lest his foot slip.

Assistants—One or two are required, depending on the manipulator's strength and the degree of traction found necessary in any particular case. At times they stand at the foot of the couch, each grasping one of the patient's ankles. At other times they stand level with the patient's thorax, combining counter-traction with steadying him against lateral strains.

Manipulator's Posture—The position of his feet controls that of his body. The most comfortable stance is with one thigh medially and the other laterally rotated so that purchase is taken with the outer midtarsal area of one foot and the inner midtarsal area of the other, held against the legs of the couch. Stout shoes prevent the feet being hurt. The feet point in the same direction as the rotation movement to be performed, but in the opposite direction during side-flexion.

Adjuvant Traction—The reasons for traction are:

1. The pressure on the displacement eases; it recedes somewhat. Hence the pain abates and the patient is happy to relax his neck muscles, thus greatly aiding the manipulator.

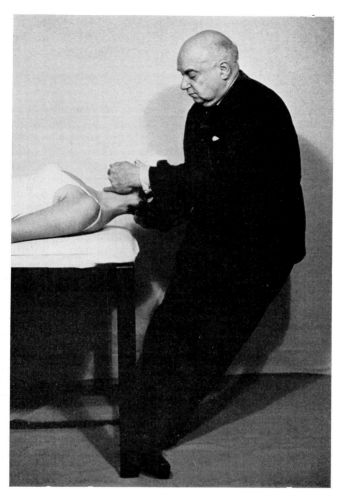

PLATE 7

2. The vertebrae come apart (see Plate 7 in Volume 1).

3. The facets are disengaged and thus allow more movement at the intervertebral joint.

4. Suction results with centripetal effect.

5. The posterior longitudinal ligament becomes taut again with centripetal effect.

Technique—The manipulator's hands grasp the mandible and occiput as shown, and the patient is asked to let him take the weight of the head. The manipulator's body weight is now used for traction, which can be increased by his leaning farther backwards until his elbows are straight and at the same time extending both knees, or even more by flexing one knee and pressing it against the leg of the couch, i.e. abducting his thigh. The straighter the manipulator's arms are held, the farther backwards he can lean, and the stronger the traction. Hence, he must keep his abdomen as far away from the patient's head as possible. When the manipulator feels the patient's neck muscles relax and that good traction has been secured (this may take two to four seconds) the manoeuvre is carried out.

Many variations are imposed by what happens at each manoeuvre, and greater and lesser degrees of extension can be used during the preliminary traction. Obviously, if one technique is found to help, it is repeated, perhaps many times at slightly different angles. If a manoeuvre does harm, or shoots pain down the patient's arm, it is avoided. If two or three manoeuvres are without effect, or increase symptoms, manipulation is abandoned. Manipulation is never carried out during flexion.

Result—Traction of the order of 140 kg is obtained by me in this way. Several experienced staff physiotherapists have reached 100 kg when tested against a spring balance. X-ray photography before and during manual traction of the order of 100 kg has shown that the distance between the upper borders of the first and fourth thoracic vertebrae increases from 7 to 8 cm during traction. This amounts to 2·5 mm distraction at each joint. This clearly provides an effective increase of the space within which the loose fragment is made to move.

The Click

All normal necks click when manipulated; when students practise on each other, clicks devoid of any significance are felt. If a patient with a displaced fragment of disc is manipulated, his neck is bound to click. Some of these clicks are meaningless, others indicate a beneficial movement of the loose fragment. This is ascertained when the patient sits up and is examined afresh. Cervical disc displacements seldom shift with one resounding click, as so often happens at a lumbar joint. First one, then another of the painful movements become painless, each with a click. Hence, some clicks mean nothing, others are significant; this is discovered only when the patients sits up for re-examination. But if there is no click, there will be no improvement; hence, the click is clearly relevant.

PLATE 7 (continued)   99

Caution

Manipulation should be avoided, or carried out with due caution in the following types of case. It must be remembered that the medical literature on both sides of the Atlantic is littered with warnings against manipulation of the cervical spine, but most doctors have observed only the results of manipulation either under anaesthesia or carried out by laymen. Hence, though plenty of true contra-indications exist, the idea that the mere existence of osteophytosis ('cervical spondylosis') makes manipulation dangerous is entirely erroneous. The criteria are quite different.

1. *Marked Articular Deformity*—Patients with gross cervical deformity must not be treated by the standard manipulation at first, for fear of injuring the spinal cord. This is a very real danger if general anaesthesia is used. Cases of marked flexion or side-flexion deformity must be treated by repeated traction in the line of deformity until this has been overcome. To this end, the patient lies on the couch and the manipulator moves the head towards the corrected position until pain is just starting. He then pulls his hardest in that line, and repeats this manoeuvre again and again until the head can be held painlessly in the neutral position. Only then can reduction by the ordinary methods be safely begun.

2. *Increased Brachial Pain*—If the patient feels the slightest increase in the brachial pain, or even twinges in her arm as the movement reaches its extreme, manipulation must stop at once. The same applies if she begins to feel discomfort in the upper limb not previously present. An increase in the cervical pain when the patient sits up and is examined is not uncommon after the first or second manoeuvres, and must not dismay the manipulator; if he carries on the new pain will cease as the original ache abates. If the manipulation causes the pain to change sides, over-reduction has been effected; the loose fragment has been shifted too far. This calls for further manipulation with considerably less traction.

3. *Acute Torticollis*—During the first few days of acute torticollis in young persons, examination is apt to disclose no range at all of one side-flexion movement of the neck and of rotation in the same direction. It is quite useless to try to force the cervical joint in either of these directions; it increases pain and does not alter range. The neck must be manipulated in the direction in which range is full, during very strong traction. This leads to more movement and less pain when the limited directions are tested. The technique of gradual increase in range described on page 122 should follow. The patient should leave an hour or two later with full movement. She is apt to relapse slightly and should therefore be seen the next day, when manipulation in the ordinary way is usually possible and quickly effective.

4. *Nuclear Protrusions*—These do not respond to manipulation. They recede slowly during measures for gradual reduction (see Plates 16 to 18); they cannot be clicked back into place like fragments of cartilage. If

manipulative reduction of a pulpy protrusion is attempted, an elastic rebound is experienced when rotation is forced during traction. Though the manipulation proceeds to full range, when the patient sits up for re-examination, the same degree of limitation of rotation is found as before. Once this recoil has been felt and the difference in range of passive and active rotation noted, it is useless to go on.

5. *Early Cervical Myelopathy*—Cases occur of compression of the spinal cord from a cervical protrusion. When this is exerted by a central posterior disc protrusion, manipulative reduction may still prove possible. In such cases, pins and needles in the hands and/or feet provide the only symptom, and examination reveals merely limitation of neck movements without interference with conduction along spinal cord or nerve roots. A maximum of traction must be exerted with a minimum of joint movement. Rotation is especially undesirable and often aggravates the condition. Osteopathic or chiropratic types of manipulation must not be employed since they too are useless and occasionally dangerous.

If the impact on the spinal cord and, later on, the anterior spinal artery is caused by an osteophyte, manipulation is futile and may well prove most harmful.

6. *Basilar Ischaemia*—Arteriosclerosis of the vertebral or basilar arteries leads to cerebellar ischaemia. The main symptom is vertigo on changing posture, e.g. sitting up from lying down, and pins and needles, often in the face, precipitated by moving the neck. Since the vertebral arteries can be compressed against the atlas, particularly on rotation, manipulation can cause thrombosis; paralysis, even death, has been reported (see Volume I). Manipulation is best avoided unless the operator is very experienced, and I would never ask a physiotherapist to carry it out in such a case. If it must be attempted, the technique for cervical myelopathy (see above) is adopted.

Contra-indications
Manipulation must not be attempted in the following conditions:

1. *Evidence of Impaired Pyramidal Function*—A spastic gait, inco-ordination or an extensor plantar response shows that manipulation is dangerous and, at best, sure to fail. This does not apply, of course, if the nervous disease is unconnected with the lesion in the neck.

2. *Basilar Insufficiency*—Unless the manipulator is very sure of his ground and eschews lay techniques, it is better to desist (see above).

3. *Drop Attack*—In patients with a congenital deformity leading to marked instability, the bone may suddenly shift far enough to obliterate both vertebral arteries. In consequence of the sudden ischaemia the patient from time to time falls to the ground inexplicably without losing consciousness. A history of drop attacks is an absolute bar to manipulation.

PLATE 7 (continued) 101

4. *Rheumatoid Arthritis of the Spinal Joints*—Especially at a cervical level, this must never be treated by manipulation. The ligaments become stretched, hypermobility leading to subluxation takes place. The spinal cord is endangered, even without the added risk of manipulation, which is, in any case, always useless.

5. *Anticoagulant Therapy*—Intraspinal bleeding can compress the spinal cord and require urgent evacuation.

Failure is Probable

In the following conditions, manipulation is not dangerous, merely very seldom of any use.

1. *Root Palsy*—Minor pins and needles do not count. A weak muscle, an absent reflex, or cutaneous analgesia—often all three together—indicate that the protrusion has become larger than the space through which it emerged; hence, it cannot be put back.

2. *Primary Postero-lateral Onset*—When the symptoms appear in the reverse to usual order, reduction is very seldom feasible in cases of unilateral pain. Paraesthetic digits followed by pain in one forearm, then arm, then scapula, are seldom benefited by manipulation.

This unfavourable prognosis does not apply to slight *bilateral* root pain preceded by pins and needles in both hands.

3. *Cervical Movement provokes Brachial Pain*—If any cervical movement, instead of setting up merely scapular pain, causes or increases pain in the limb itself, manipulation seldom succeeds.

4. *Brachial Pain of over Two Months' Standing*—When unilateral brachial pain has lasted longer than two months, manipulation seldom increase the rate of spontaneous recovery over the next two months. However when, contrary to normal expectation, root pain has failed to get well after six months, manipulation may well restart the mechanism of spontaneous recovery, as from a few days later.

Novice's Routine

The order in which a manipulative sequence is carried out may make a large difference to the result. On the first occasion, a routine must be followed until it becomes clear which manoeuvres help and which do not, and what is the end-feel in each direction.

A reasonable start would be as follows:

1. Rotation to less than full range in the direction that does not hurt, using the method of Plate 8.
2. Full rotation in the same direction, using the method of Plate 8.
3. Rotation to full range in the direction that does hurt, using the method of Plate 8.

4. Full rotation in the direction that does not hurt, using the method of Plate 9.
5. Full rotation in the direction that does hurt, using the method of Plate 9.
6. Side-flexion towards the painless side (Plate 10).
7. Lateral glide (Plate 12).

RESULTS OF THESE MANIPULATIONS

Nine out of ten of all cervical disc protrusions found suitable on clinical examination prove quickly reducible by means of these methods. One session lasting perhaps twenty minutes often suffices; at the most three to four such treatments given on alternate days. This provides a happy contrast to laymen's endless sessions. Fifty to a hundred are not uncommon in chiropractice. Pain felt in the upper limb naturally implies a greater degree of displacement; in such a case success is less certain and several sessions may well be required.

If a patient has not begun to improve after two sessions of adequate manipulation, it is not worth while going on. As long as each session affords some lasting improvement, continuation is justified, but it is very rare for more than six to eight sessions to be required. Physiotherapists must not lapse into the ways of lay manipulators, blithely manipulating once or twice a week for as long as the patient cares to keep up her visits.

First Manipulation for a Cervical Disc Lesion

Lesion—Postero-lateral protrusion of the intervertebral disc causes at first unilateral cervico-scapular pain. A fragment of the cartilaginous disc becomes displaced, most often at the sixth cervical joint, occasionally at the fourth, fifth or seventh joint; rarely at the second or third. Protrusion of the pulpy nucleus is very uncommon; if so, manipulation is useless and continuous traction is the only effective measure.

Physical Signs—When the active and passive neck movements are tested, the partial articular pattern of the internal derangement emerges. Since the displacement passes towards one side of the joint, the pain is unilateral and some movements are blocked (and therefore painful), others not. Hence the expectation is that two, three or four of the active neck movements will evoke the ache, whereas four, three or two will not cause any discomfort. The same passive movements hurt rather more; the resisted movements not at all. In cases suitable for manipulation, signs of root pressure or of impaired conduction along the spinal cord are both absent.

Before the manipulative attempt starts, the neck movements are memorized so that the operator knows which movements hurt and which not, where the pain thus provoked was felt and what degree of limitation of movement (if any) was present.

Anaesthesia—General anaesthesia is contra-indicated. It is easy to do harm unless the patient is conscious and able to help the manipulator by informing him, step by step, of the result of each manipulative attempt. Nor can he find out which manoeuvres prove beneficial and which not, nor can he decide what to do next and whether to go on or stop. Local anaesthesia has no place in treatment. By contrast, deep massage to that part of the semispinalis capitis muscle overlying the affected joint (see Plate 4) often greatly assists manipulative reduction carried out immediately afterwards. Hence, in resistant cases, this preliminary is well worth a trial.

Patient's Posture—The patient lies face upwards on the couch; her feet are held by one or two assistants, depending on the amount of distraction likely to be required. If she wears dentures, she must not remove them but bite on a thick pad of folded lint, otherwise the jaw may be overclosed disagreeably. Her shoulders should lie level with the end of the couch, thus enabling the neck to extend a little. This is essential, for the manipulations are all carried out with the neck held either in the neutral position or in very slight extension. If any degree of flexion is permitted, further protrusion is encouraged. Muscular relaxation and the patient's confidence are maintained throughout by the manipulator, who never ceases to support the patient's occiput.

Technique—It is vital to keep up the greatest possible traction throughout each manipulation; neglect of this injunction may well lead to aggravation. It is by observing the results of manipulation carried out (as most laymen do) without adequate traction that many doctors have come to the mistaken conclusion that manipulation of the neck is dangerous. It is; but not if the right case is chosen and strong traction applied to ensure that, if the fragment shifts at all, it does so towards the centre of the joint.

The manipulator stands at the patient's head, with both his feet firmly planted against the couch. One of his hands is hooked under her mandible and traction here keeps her neck extended. Pressure on the trachea with the little finger must be avoided. His other hand grasps the lower occiput, supporting and pulling at the same time. Slow rotary movements, not approaching the full range, are now carried out during traction. This enables the manipulator to get the feel of the patient's neck and to judge how she is going to stand the slight discomfort. This gradual beginning also allays the patient's fears of sudden twists and agonizing pains.

The circumduction during traction should be maintained for some seconds, whereupon the tension is gradually released. Cracks will be felt when a neck is manipulated in this way whether there is any lesion present or not.

Assessment of Progress

The patient then sits up, moves her head in each direction and reports the result (or lack of result) of this first manoeuvre. At the same time, the manipulator judges the effect on the range of movement. If any benefit accrues, the same manoeuvre should be repeated, the patient sitting up for re-assessment of the result at the end of each attempt. If symptoms persist he should pass on to the second manipulation (see Plate 8).

As the manipulations proceed, the scapular pain tends to move upwards and medially and to become smaller in extent. Thus a pain felt all over the scapular area moves to the base of the neck; the tender area of muscle (what used to be called 'fibrositis') moves too. When a full and painless range of movement has been restored to the cervical joint, the tender spot disappears, thus proving that it is a secondary phenomenon. While the pain and the tender spot are moving in this manner, the neck movements one by one become painless. The manipulator judges which manoeuvre to adopt next by noting end-feel and the result of each manipulation on the extent and severity of the pain, as well as on the range and painfulness or not of the neck movements.

CERVICAL SPINE: ROTATION DURING TRACTION I

Second Manipulation for a Cervical Disc Lesion

See general remarks at p. 96

Patient's Posture—The patient lies on a high couch, her shoulders level with the edge. An assistant holds her feet.

Technique—The operator supports the occiput with one hand, maintaining the neck in the neutral position. He hooks his other hand under the jaw, his fingers spanning the mandible and the tips curled over on the far side. His little finger must avoid pressing on the trachea. The neck is now ready to be turned in the direction that has been found not to hurt. If the rotation is towards the right, the right hand lies under the chin, the left spans the occiput and his body and feet face towards the right. He leans backwards until his arms are straight, stays pulling for a second or two and feels the slack being taken out of the intervertebral ligaments. He then goes on turning the head smoothly until a click is felt. When this manoeuvre is attempted the first time, the click is likely to be felt at about two-thirds range, certainly before full range is reached. As soon as this intra-articular sensation is felt, the traction is relaxed and the head turned back simultaneously. The patient now sits up for reassessment of the articular signs.

The rotation during traction is now repeated in the same direction as before. When the resistance is felt that indicates that full range is approached, a quick thrust of small amplitude is made, forcing another degree or two of rotation. A second click is usually felt; the patient again sits up for re-examination.

The point has now been reached when it is improbable that a third rotation will help further; the end-feel helps here. The harder it is, the less likely it is that repetition will prove beneficial. The operator therefore reverses his hands and posture, and this time turns the head to the left (the direction known to hurt). It is probably only with over-pressure at full range that a third click will be elicited.

Advantage—This grip makes strong traction easy to maintain. Since the pull of the hand under the mandible has the greater leverage, flexion is simple to avoid. Moreover, not much power is available to the operator at the extreme of rotation; this ensures a gentle beginning.

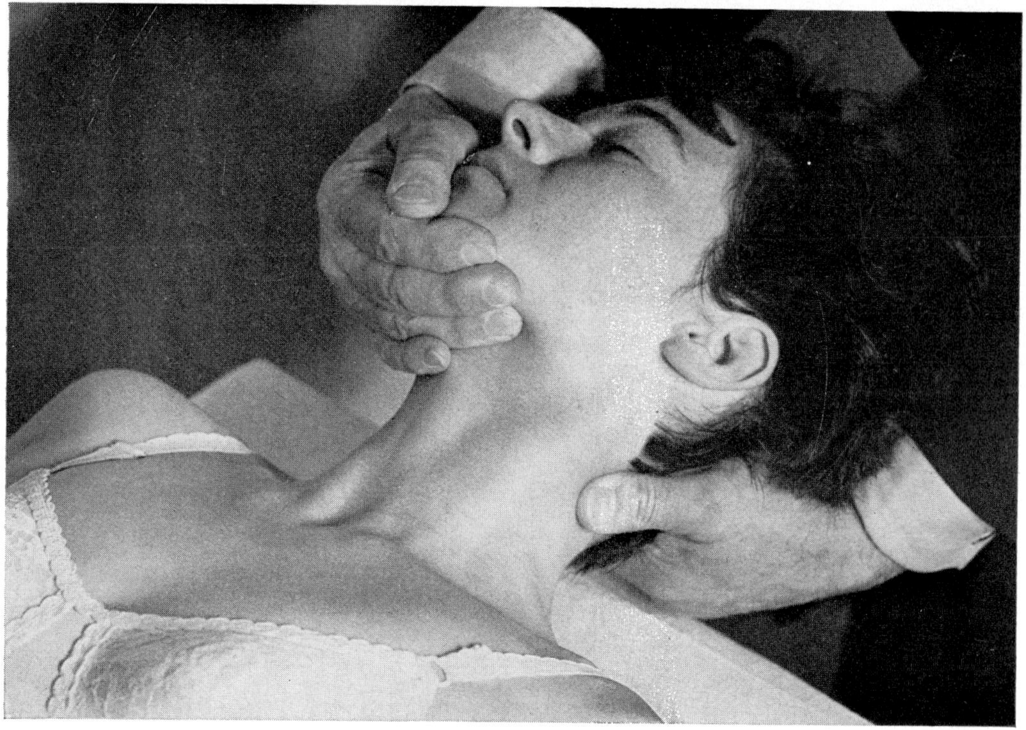

PLATE 8

PLATE 9

CERVICAL SPINE: ROTATION DURING TRACTION II

Third Manipulation for a Cervical Disc Lesion

See general remarks at p. 96

Indication—When repetition of the second manipulation ceases to afford benefit, this technique follows. This method gives the operator much greater power at the extreme of the rotary range.

Direction—First in the direction that has been found not to hurt, then, if necessary, in the painful direction.

Patient's Posture—The patient lies on a high couch, her shoulders level with the edge. An assistant holds her feet.

Manipulative Technique—If the head is to be turned to the right, the manipulator applies his right hand to the patient's left cheek, so that he can press on her maxilla with his thenar eminence. His fingers are hooked under the mandible; the traction there forces the patient's occiput into his other hand and a solid grip of the head is secured. He now leans backwards and stays so until he feels that the slack has been taken up.

During considerable traction, the rotation is continued until a click is felt, or mounting tension indicates that the extreme of range is approaching. A further thrust is now given—quite a hard jerk but of very small amplitude. The head is now turned back and the traction simultaneously slackened. The patient sits up for re-examination. If benefit accrues and the operator felt that the full over-pressure range was not reached, this movement is repeated. If he felt that the neck would move no farther that way, the same manoeuvre is repeated, now in the direction that causes pain in the scapular area, but not if it is known to set up brachial pain.

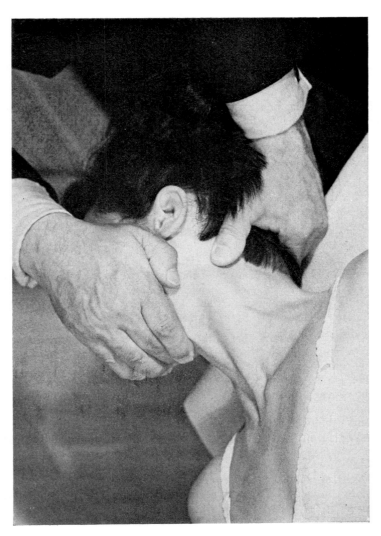

PLATE 9

CERVICAL SPINE: SIDE-FLEXION DURING TRACTION

Fourth Manipulation for a Cervical Disc Lesion

See general remarks at p. 96

Indication—The first two manipulations will probably have improved the position of the loose fragment, but if they have not succeeded in securing full reduction, this method follows. It is difficult to carry out, since the body has to be correctly balanced to maintain traction at the extreme of range.

Direction—It is now no longer a question (as in rotation) of which movement hurts and which not; the criterion is the position of the patient's pain. Side-flexion is always performed *towards the painless side,* since it is unwise to pinch a protruded fragment of disc lest it displace itself further.

Patient's Posture—The patient lies face upwards, her shoulders level with the edge of the couch. If lateral flexion is to be forced towards the right, counter-traction is applied at her left shoulder. There are two ways of doing this: with one or two assistants. One suffices if only moderate traction is required (Plate 10); really strong traction calls for two (Plate 10a).

Technique—Assuming that side-flexion is to be forced towards the right, the operator stands at the patient's right shoulder, his body and feet facing towards the left. He has to perform three tasks with two hands; for this reason he must use his forearm applied to the postero-inferior aspect of the patient's parietal region to force full side-flexion at the last moment. Traction is maintained by the manipulator's left hand hooked under the patient's mandible. The base of his right index finger applies counter-pressure against the mid-cervical transverse processes, and by curving over the fingers of this hand under her occiput he is able to support the patient's head and pull at the same time. His left forearm, pressing against the skull just above the ear, forces side-flexion while both hands continue to apply firm traction for a second or two, until the play in the joints is taken up. His right foot is pressed against the leg of the couch and he now kicks his left leg out backwards and to the right so that the momentum of the limb carries his whole body round to the right with it. The left leg bears no weight; it is merely used to swivel the operator's body. He goes on turning until he feels tissue tension heralding the extreme of range, letting his elbow be drawn a short distance away from his side. He now draws his left elbow towards his side sharply. This adduction movement applies a sudden strong side-flexion, by means of his forearm pressing against the side of her skull just above the ear. Inexperienced manipulators tend to stand upright at the final moment, their body weight supported by their feet rather than supplying traction.

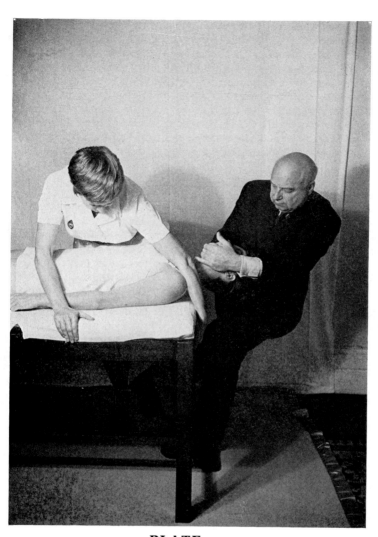

PLATE 10

Assistants' Position—If two are available, they stand facing each other level with the patient's thorax. If the neck is to be flexed to the right, the assistant to the patient's right grasps her shoulder with her left hand and draws the thorax towards herself until the arm engages against her abdomen. She now leans forwards and keeps her trunk applied to the edge of the couch by pulling with her right hand grasping the far side of the couch. The assistant to the patient's left turns to face the head and puts her right foot against the leg of the couch. She clasps her hands round the shoulder. This assistant keeps the shoulder from shifting up the couch; the former prevents the trunk from moving to the right at the moment of forcing.

If only one assistant is available, she stands at the side of the couch towards which lateral flexion is to be forced, level with, and facing, the patient's thorax. She leans well forwards and grasps the upper end of the couch about midway. This forearm is now held vertically, just beyond the base of the patient's neck. She now leans well forward, her abdomen against the patient's arm, and holds the far side of the couch. Her one forearm now stops the patient slipping up the couch and her abdomen prevents the thorax moving sideways as traction, then side-flexion, are carried out.

Repetition—If improvement is noted, the manoeuvre is repeated. If the articular signs have almost ceased, only side-flexion towards the painful side remaining uncomfortable, side-flexion in this direction may be carefully carried out, with a maximum of traction and the movement carried to less than full range at the first attempt. If all the previous manoeuvres have afforded no benefit, forcing side-flexion towards the painful side is contra-indicated.

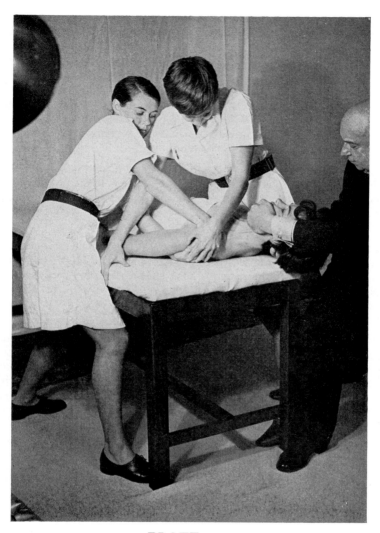

PLATE 10a

PLATE 11

CERVICAL SPINE: ANTERO-POSTERIOR GLIDE

Fifth Manipulation for a Cervical Disc Lesion

See general remarks at p. 96

Indications—This manipulation should be adopted if (1) considerable limitation of the range of extension at the neck remains after the other neck movements have been rendered painless by the previous manoeuvres or (2) the displacement lies postero-centrally.

Patient's Posture—The patient lies face upwards, her shoulders level with the end of the couch. One assistant suffices to hold the feet, for really strong traction cannot be exerted. The neck is in the neutral position and must not be allowed to extend when the operator applies pressure downwards.

Manipulator's Posture—The outer side of the nearer of the operator's knees presses against the leg of the couch. The hand at the occiput is used both to support the patient's head and, as he leans backwards, to apply traction to her neck. His other hand rests on her chin; his elbow is flexed to a right-angle. The forearm is vertical, ready to thrust hard downwards.

Technique—The patient's chin bears the brunt of this manipulation. Since this is a tender area in everyone, a layer of sponge rubber is interposed between the patient's mandible and the palm of the manipulator's hand. While his one hand at the occiput maintains traction and the position of the patient's head, strong downward pressure is exerted momentarily by means of his other hand on the chin. In this way, during traction, a backward gliding is induced of each cervical vertebra on the adjacent one.

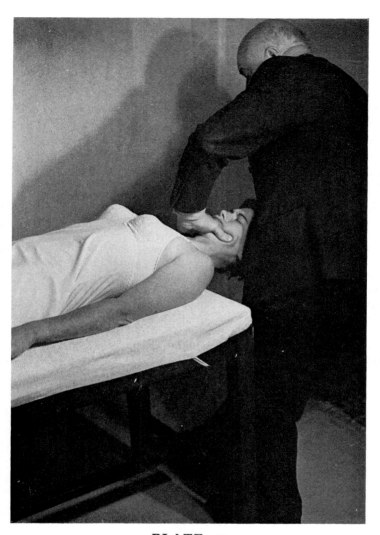

PLATE 11

CERVICAL SPINE: LATERAL GLIDING

Sixth Manipulation for a Cervical Disc Lesion

See general remarks at p. 96

Indication—When reduction is almost complete, but a fine adjustment remains to be made, this manipulation is very useful. It also serves to remove the generalized ache that often follows the previous five manoeuvres.

Patient's Posture—The patient lies face upwards on the couch, her shoulders level with the edge. An assistant holds the patient's trunk still by grasping her far arm and pulling until her near arm is pressed against the assistant's abdomen.

Technique—The movement to be carried out is a pure lateral gliding of one vertebra on the other, while the head retains its vertical relationship to the trunk. The operator stands at the patient's head supporting it in both hands. His thenar eminences apply alternating pressure at the left and right temples. His thumbs, aligned on her mandibles and pressing near each angle of the jaw, keep her head in line with her body. Side-flexion of the neck is thus prevented. Note that each thumb-nail is kept horizontal, since abduction of the thumb is much stronger than extension when the alternating pressure is exerted. The patient must relax well, but she should not find this difficult for the manipulation is virtually painless. It is a smooth movement, carried out without traction. The motive force is produced by the operator swaying his body from side to side at the hips.

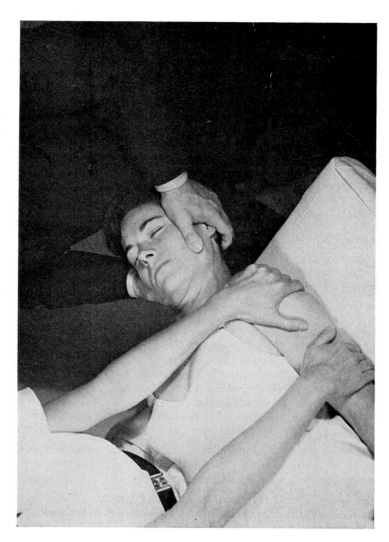

PLATE 12

CERVICAL SPINE: TRACTION WITH LEVERAGE

Indications—Central cervical disc protrusions. These are potentially dangerous for, however slight to start with, they menace the spinal cord, either of themselves or by drawing out osteophytes that compress the cord and eventually the anterior spinal artery. Left in place for long enough, they can cause severe crippledom. They may set up bilateral scapular aching, often referred to both upper limbs, with pins and needles in hands (acroparaesthesia) and/or feet.

Tinnitus not caused by ear disease may prove relievable by the technique described below, as may postural vertigo.

Contra-indication—Signs of pressure on the spinal cord. If the lower limbs are paraesthetic without objective evidence of pressure on the spinal cord, the manipulation can still be carried out. If there is any spasticity, inco-ordination, or the plantar response is extensor, manipulation is strongly contra-indicated.

Patient's Posture—The patient lies on the couch with her occiput exactly level with the edge of the couch. Two assistants hold her feet.

Technique—The operator places his hand under the patient's occiput and a layer of sponge rubber half an inch thick between the back of his hand and the edge of the couch—otherwise he hurts the back of his hand later. He grasps the patient's jaw with his other hand, holding the neck in slight flexion. With both feet against the legs of the couch, he swings backwards until the whole of his body weight is sustained by the hand under the mandible. He now bends his knees, thus extending the patient's neck to the neutral position with a jerk. He uses the chin-occiput lever to apply traction at the foramen magnum. In this way he can double his pulling force. No traction is applied via the hand under the head, which only steadies and is squeezed between occiput and couch, providing the fulcrum.

Caution—Rotation during traction, especially under anaesthesia, is dangerous in postero-central disc protrusion. The techniques of osteopathy and chiropractice are also contra-indicated.

Results—Most sufferers from this type of protrusion are thick-set elderly men, and the condition has often been allowed to get slowly worse for a year or two, owing to neurologists' widespread misconception that no effective treatment exists. Hence, many patients have passed beyond the scope of manipulation. In some of these it is no longer the disc protrusion but the resulting osteophytes that cause the pressure; in these cases manipulation is, of course, useless. But many can be largely or wholly relieved. Some, once symptom-free, require maintenance manipulation each few months. By contrast, we have had patients with paraesthetic hands and feet who, ten years after reduction, have suffered no recurrence. If manipulation fails, or has only a temporary effect, and pressure on the spinal cord mounts, myelography and laminectomy must be considered.

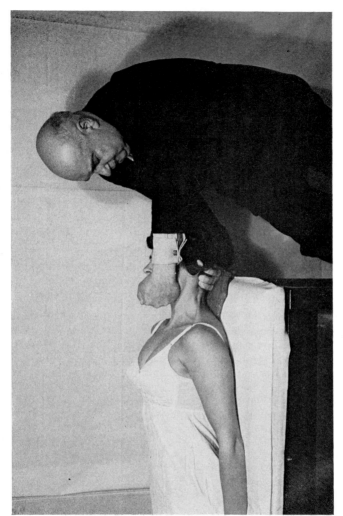

PLATE 13

CERVICAL FACET JOINT: INTRA-ARTICULAR INJECTION

Lesion—All elderly people have osteophytes visible radiologically at the zygo-apophyseal joints of the mid-cervical spine, but they do not usually set up discomfort. When symptoms do appear, they originate from the axis-third and third-fourth joints.

In ankylosing spondylitis all the facet joints become involved. It is only when one joint is hurting alone, or much more than the others, that the injection is worth their while.

Physical Signs—Osteoarthrosis of a facet joint is difficult to identify as a cause of symptoms, for pain at one side of the mid-neck so much more often results from a minor disc lesion within an already osteophytic intervertebral joint. The articular signs are similar and in fact it is really only after the first session aimed at manipulative reduction has failed that this diagnosis comes to the fore.

Patient's Posture—The patient lies prone on a low couch. Her head is supported slightly flexed and held by an assistant in full side-flexion away from the painful side. In this position the two articular processes lie as far apart as possible, presenting a 0·5 cm extent of articulating surface.

Injection Technique—The operator sits facing the patient's neck and identifies the bony posterior aspect of the tender facet joint with his left thumb. The joint lies 2 to 2·5 cm from the midline. A 1 ml tuberculin syringe is half-filled with the steroid suspension and fitted with a thin needle 3 cm long. At the level of his thumb the needle is thrust vertically downwards. If it hits bone, the point is on the lamina; if it traverses a tough ligament and then abuts against cartilage, the point lies intra-articularly and the injection is given.

Result—though the condition is non-inflammatory, i.e. merely degenerative osteoarthrosis, most patients lose their symptoms for at least some years after one or two injections.

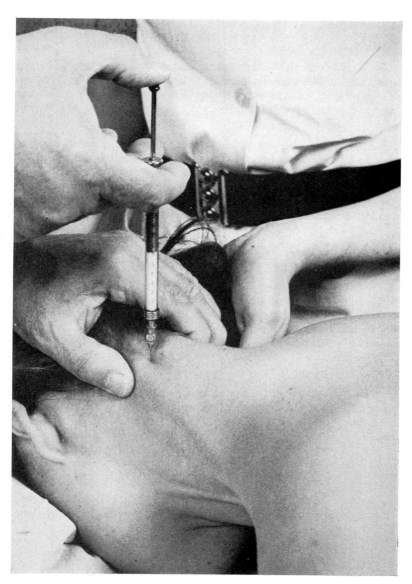

PLATE 14

CERVICAL SPINE: SUSTAINED ROTATION AND SIDE-FLEXION

Lesion—Acute torticollis in patients under thirty years old. This may result from sudden displacement of a large fragment of intervertebral disc, or may appear gradually during a night's rest, the patient going to bed comfortable but being transfixed by pain as soon as he wakes and moves.

Physical Signs—The patient has lain with her head tilted all night and wakes with 'a crick in her neck', which is held with visible deformity. The pain is unilateral in the upper scapular area and lower neck. Flexion, extension, one side-flexion and one rotation movement may increase the symptom, but are of full range. By contrast, one side-flexion movement and the rotation in the same direction are entirely blocked; no movement these two ways exists.

Contra-indications—Lay manipulative techniques and all forms of traction tend to make the patient worse if performed in the acute stage.

Technique—A beginning is made by carrying out full rotation, then full side-flexion, several times with very strong traction, only in the painless direction. These two manoeuvres are repeated until the patient can sit up with the head held in the neutral position and has lost constant pain. The temptation would now be to manipulate in the painful directions, but this hurts the patient and may make her worse; it certainly confers no benefit in patients under thirty.

Further Technique: The patient lies on the couch, the head supported on it. The head is now rotated passively until pain just starts. A sandbag is placed fixing the head in this position. After five minutes the head is turned a little more, and so on (Plate 15). It may take half to one hour before full painless rotation is achieved. The same is now performed in side-flexion (Plate 15a).

Result—The patient should leave after two hours, able while standing to move her neck painlessly and fully in any direction. There is a tendency to minor recurrence. She should therefore attend the next day, when manipulation in the ordinary way is usually all that is necessary.

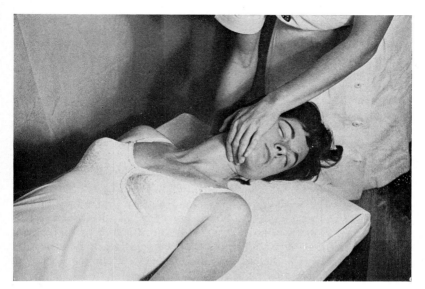

PLATE 15

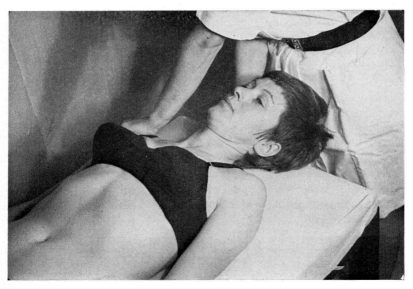

PLATE 15a

HEAD-SUSPENSION

Head-suspension is used far too often. It is nothing like as successful as manipulation during traction. Hence, my advice to a physiotherapist asked to give suspension for the ordinary case (with unilateral scapular pain and the partial articular pattern) is to request permission to add passive movement. However, 'passive movement during suspension' deprives the operator of all finesse since she cannot adjust her pressure according to the sensation imparted to her hand and she is deprived of end-feel. But it is better than mere traction, and the physiotherapist must do her best that way. Better still would of course be 'passive movement after suspension', i.e. manipulation after the neck had been stretched.

Indications

Early nuclear protrusion: Long-standing nuclear protrusions respond only to sustained traction in bed, but the early case may do well on suspension. Nuclear protrusions are recognized by a soft end-feel with rebound, and by the fact that, in spite of a full range being secured at the moment of forcing during traction, the range of movement is shown on re-examination to have been unaltered by the manipulation.

Minor central protrusion: Small *postero-central* protrusions do better on suspension than *postero-lateral* displacements. In the former case, this treatment is well worth a trial. Four to eight daily sessons should suffice. Alternatively, a minor displacement in a patient too nervous to accept manipulation may prove reducible in the end by suspension. Again, postero-central displacements do better than postero-lateral.

Stability: When a patient returns with complete relapse after full reduction the previous day, the fragment of disc is clearly very unstable. Reduction by manipulation is repeated, followed by suspension in the hope that a further shift to a more stable position can be secured.

Maintenance of reduction: Another way of dealing with the unstable fragment that shifts every few days is daily suspension at home. This is particularly successful when the chief pain is upper cervical. Suspension is carried out for, say, ten minutes every morning and reduces the incipient displacement before it has given rise to appreciable symptoms. This policy enables a patient to keep himself comfortable indefinitely.

Diagnostic suspension: Suspension can also be used in diagnosis. Difficulty may arise in distinguishing between pain and pins and needles arising from a cervical disc lesion, from the thoracic outlet syndrome or from the carpal tunnel syndrome. If suspension stops the pain and paraesthesia for the time being, a cervical lesion is clearly responsible.

Contra-indications—The neck may not be able to withstand the body weight in elderly or fat patients. If suspension brings on paraesthesia in hands or feet, the dura mater has probably become adherent to the cervical

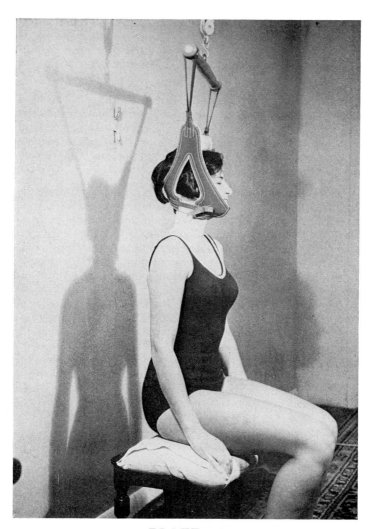

PLATE 16

vertebrae and it is dangerous to go on. If suspension causes or increases pain in the arm, it must be stopped.

The real contra-indication, however, is trying in vain to reduce an ordinary small disc displacement by suspension alone when all that is needed is manipulation during traction.

Patient's Posture—The patient sits on a stool with a small cushion under his thighs. His feet remain on the ground throughout. If these two precautions are observed no harm can well come of head-suspension; for, if the cord breaks, the patient merely falls an inch or so back on to the cushion and, if the pain becomes unexpectedly severe, he can at any moment rise to his feet instantly.

Technique—By adjustment of the length of the occipital strap, the collar is so arranged that the anterior portion clears the trachea while supporting the mandible. When the strain is taken on the cord, the patient's head must be found held in the neutral position; if not, the straps have been sewn on to the collar in the wrong place or at the wrong angle. The spreader must be wide enough to stop the straps squeezing the ears.

The physiotherapist stands by the patient, observing his expression. She pulls gradually on the cord until the patient's buttocks are just clear of the stool and holds him there for as long as is tolerable, i.e. one to five minutes as a rule, but the longer the better. When the patient indicates that he has had enough, she lets him down again equally slowly. Letting a patient down too quickly may set up severe pain. After a minute or two's rest he is suspended once again for as long as he can bear. Daily treatment for up to a fortnight is reasonable. If he is to be manipulated afterwards, ten or fifteen minutes should be spent thus; if suspension forms the whole treatment, at intervals for up to half an hour.

CONTINUOUS TRACTION IN RECUMBENCY

It must be realized that once a root palsy has developed all endeavours to effect reduction are doomed to failure, since the size of the protrusion has now come to exceed the aperture whence it emerged.

Indications

Postero-lateral protrusion : These may cause severe pain in the upper limb without a root palsy ensuing. If manipulative reduction fails, and the symptoms are too pronounced for the patient to wait several months pending spontaneous recovery, traction in recumbency affords the only hope of swift relief.

Nuclear protrusion : Usually a young adult. The patient has suffered months of inability to turn the neck one way because of scapular pain. Examination shows all the cervical movements to be of full range and painless except rotation, which can be carried out through 90° one way but only 45° the other way. When manipulative reduction is attempted an elastic recoil is felt at the extreme of range. Though full passive movement is attained, the restriction is found unaltered when the patient sits up afterwards and moves the neck actively.

Central disc protrusion : In early cases the patient may merely experience paraesthesia in his limbs on neck flexion, signs of pressure on the spinal cord not yet having appeared. Reduction is an urgent necessity, but manipulation is dangerous except by the method shown in Plates 11 and 13. Should these fail sustained traction is indicated at once.

Contra-indication

Small cartilaginous displacements : Naturally, if the protruded fragment is small and cartilaginous, manipulative reduction is as quick and easy as traction in recumbency is slow and troublesome. Not only that, but continuous traction may not succeed in bringing about reduction. Thus, I have more than once reduced a displaced fragment of cartilage by one manipulation after weeks' continuous traction (carried out elsewhere) had failed.

Technique—The head of the bed is raised on 30-cm blocks and a pulley is screwed to the bedrail. A leather collar (the same as that used for head-suspension—see Plate 16) is strapped loosely under the patient's chin and occiput. Strips of sponge rubber 1 cm thick are inserted between the mandible and the leather. The straps on the collar are attached to a special spreader 50 cm wide. The extra width ensures that the straps clear the patient's ears, which soon become painfully squeezed if an ordinary spreader is used. The weight hangs by a cord passing over the pulley to the centre of the spreader. For the first twenty-four hours 4 or 5 kg are required. If the chin gets sore or the temporo-mandibular joint begins to ache, a metal bit engaging against the patient's upper teeth can be sub-

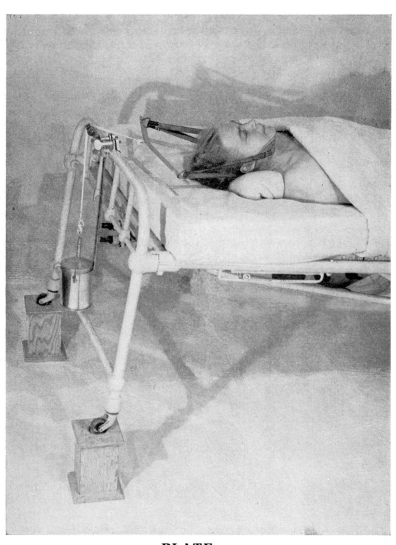

PLATE 17

stituted for some hours. The patient is kept under heavy sedation for the first day or two, i.e. until the severe brachial pain has abated. Vomiting must be avoided, if necessary by cyclizine.

Patient's Posture—The patient's neck must not be allowed to flex; hence the back of the head lies directly on the mattress, a small folded towel supporting the nape of the neck. The straps and cord run roughly parallel with the mattress, and care must be taken, day and night, that the patient does not slip up the bed far enough for the spreader to catch against the bedrail. The patient may rotate her head whenever she likes. She requires full nursing: feeding, washing, bed-pan, etc.

Progress—Once the pain in the scapular area and upper limb has wholly ceased the weight is diminished; finally it is removed for, say, half an hour at a time. If nothing untoward happens the weight is left off for longer periods by day, a small weight (e.g. 2 kg) being retained for a further few nights, since it is during sleep that the neck muscles relax best. In due course the patient tries sitting up for a few minutes at a time; these periods are then lengthened, provided that the pain remains absent.

Result—The patient may expect to leave hospital, pain-free, in seven to twelve days.

COLLARS

These are best made of plastic and are scarcely visible if they are made of transparent material and a scarf is worn.

Immobilizing Collar

Indications

1. Unstable fragment. When reduction proves very unstable, relapse ensuing within a day or two, retentive apparatus is called for. As soon as the collar is ready, manipulative reduction is repeated and the collar put on at once. It has usually to be worn for six months, while stability slowly returns to the loose fragment. If the displacement recurs during the period that the collar is worn, reduction is repeated.

2. Adherent dura mater. When adhesions bind the dura mater to the vertebral bodies, every time the neck is flexed, the spinal cord is stretched and further damage is caused. A collar maintaining the neck erect must be worn permanently.

Contra-indication—It is obviously useless to apply a collar while the displaced part of the disc remains protruded. This is often done, but merely adds further discomfort to that already caused by the displacement. Wearing a collar neither hastens nor retards the rate of spontaneous recovery in cases of cervical disc lesions setting up brachial pain.

Construction—The plastic is strong, rigid and light. Two anterior bolts secure the back piece to the breast plate. A plastic strap, detachable in front, joins the occipital support to that for the mandible. The collar maintains the head in very slight extension.

Weight-relieving Collar

Indications

1. Pressure on the spinal cord or on the anterior spinal artery caused by central cervical disc protrusion or by osteophytes in cases unsuited to laminectomy.

2. Scapular or brachial pain, with or without paraesthesiae in the hands, caused by the mushroom phenomenon at a cervical level. Relief from compression strain on the joint is now essential.

3. Intractable pain or paraesthesia felt in the neck, ceasing when the examiner lifts the seated patient's head, so that its weight is no longer borne by the cervical spine.

Construction—The illustration shows a collar devised for me. The chest piece and the collar supporting the chin and occiput are separate and held apart by four adjustable screws. As these are lengthened, the weight is taken off the neck enough to make the symptoms cease. The screws are then held in that position by fixing bolts.

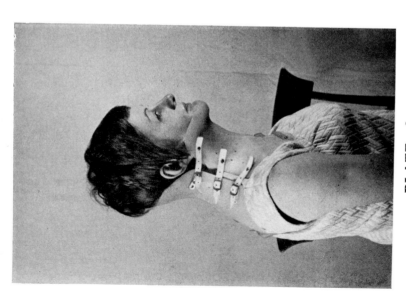

PLATE 18a

PLATE 18

SERRATUS ANTERIOR MUSCLE: SCAPULAR INSERTION

Massage Technique

Strain appears to occur only at the fibres of insertion at the deep aspect of the inner border of the scapula. Rarely one or other of the digitations on the lateral aspect of the thoracic wall is injured by direct violence.

Physical Signs—Unilateral scapular pain unaltered by movement at the cervical or thoracic joints. Full active but not passive elevation of the arm hurts, as does resisted abduction with the patient's arms held out horizontally in front of him. Examination of the shoulder and the rest of the upper limb reveals no abnormality.

Patient's Posture—The patient lies prone. The physiotherapist brings his forearm behind his back so as to rotate the arm medially; this lifts the vertebral edge of the scapula away from the chest wall.

Technique—The physiotherapist stands at the patient's head, facing his thorax. She grasps the edge of the scapula, her thumb applied to the anterior aspect of the vertebral border of the bone at the site of the lesion. Her fingers supply counter-pressure at the dorsum of the scapula. The friction is imparted by an adduction–abduction movement of her thumb along the insertion of the serratus muscle. As with all pure thumb movements, massage carried out in this way is very tiring, but other techniques are apt to prove ineffective.

Thoraco-scapular Crepitus—The photograph illustrates the best way to lift the scapula off the chest wall. This position also seems to give access to the affected area when massage is given for painful thoraco-scapular crepitus.

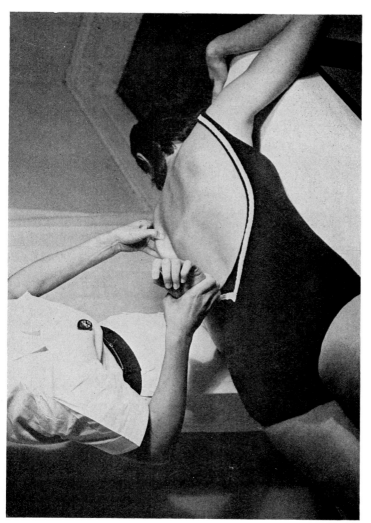

PLATE 19

PECTORALIS MAJOR MUSCLE: OUTER EDGE

Massage Technique

Lesion—This is traumatic, as a rule the result of an overstrain during heavy lifting, sometimes directly from a blow. Repeated stresses, e.g. in carrying a baby, may be responsible. The common site is that shown in the illustration. The other fibres that may be affected are those lying just below the outer half of the clavicle (not illustrated).

Physical Signs—Unilateral pectoral pain brought on by full passive elevation of the arm and by resisted adduction, medial rotation and forward movement of the arm at the shoulder.

Patient's Posture—The patient adopts the half-lying position on the couch. He abducts his arm somewhat so as to bring the muscle into prominence; his hand may suitably rest on his hip.

Technique—The physiotherapist sits by his side, facing him. She grasps the edge of the muscle, which would otherwise be apt to move as a whole with the physiotherapist's hand. By maintaining her grip and pulling her hand bodily towards herself, she imparts the required friction.

Results—Good. Since the pectoralis major muscle is one of those responding well to the induction of therapeutic local anaesthesia the patient should be referred back to his doctor if he does not recover quickly.

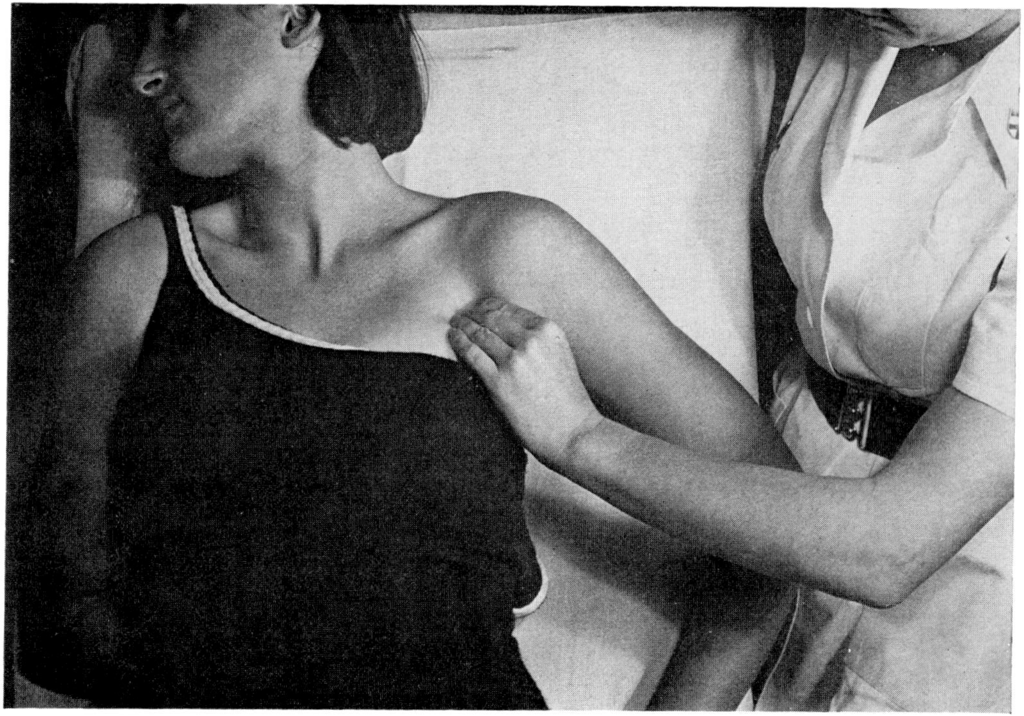

PLATE 20

ACROMIO-CLAVICULAR JOINT

Massage Technique

Lesion—This is nearly always traumatic. Osteoarthrosis in elderly patients is a common radiological finding, but is often symptomless. If an injury results in ligamentous laxity and a tendency to subluxation, these persist, but do not necessarily cause pain.

Physical Signs—Pain felt *only* at the point of the shoulder at the extreme of scapular range and on gentle forcing of passive movement at the shoulder-joint. Often the most painful movement is full passive adduction of the arm across the front of the chest. No resisted movement hurts.

Indication for Massage—Trauma to the joint followed by persistent symptoms. Osteoarthrosis causing pain.

Patient's Posture—The patient adopts the half-lying or sitting position.

Technique—The physiotherapist stands behind him at his shoulder. She presses one finger on the joint and gives her friction by a horizontal to-and-fro movement of the whole hand in the sagittal plane. Exercises afterwards are to be avoided.

Results—Full relief is usually attained, even in cases in which the tendency to subluxation of the joint persists.

N.B.—When the deep aspect of the joint is affected, the physiotherapist's finger cannot reach the right spot. Phonophoresis or an injection of steroid suspension is then called for (see Plate 22) and is very effective.

Sterno-clavicular Joint
This responds so well to intra-articular injection of steroid suspension that other methods of treatment are scarcely worth considering.

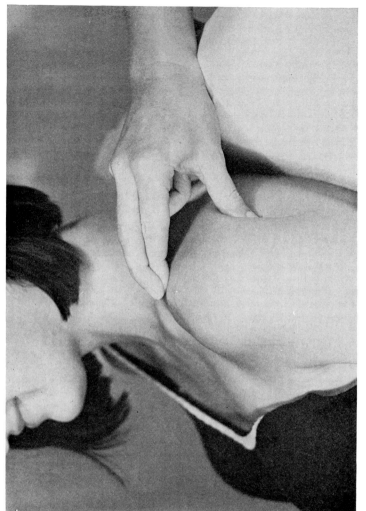

PLATE 21

ACROMIO-CLAVICULAR JOINT

Injection Technique

Lesion—In young people trauma strains the acromio-clavicular ligaments. In older people with osteoarthrosis overuse may set up a clinical arthritis in an otherwise symptomless joint. If an injury results in ligamentous laxity a tendency to subluxation results, but this is not necessarily painful.

Physical Signs—Since the acromio-clavicular ligaments are derived from the fourth cervical segment, the pain is localized to the point of the shoulder and cannot radiate to the arm.

Active scapular elevation often hurts, but pain is set up at each extreme of passive range at the shoulder, especially full adduction across the front of the chest. A painful arc is uncommon; if present it indicates that the inferior ligament is tender. No resisted movement hurts.

If the joint is found to be tender, the superior ligament is at fault, but the inferior may well be affected also. If there is no tenderness, the inferior ligament is affected alone.

Patient's Posture—The patient lies with his arm by his side and the lateral edge of the acromion is identified; 2 cm medial to this line the gap between acromion and clavicle is palpated.

Injection Technique—If only the inferior ligament needs infiltration, a 1 ml syringe suffices; if the superior ligament has to be dealt with as well, a 2 ml syringe is required. It is filled with steroid suspension and a thin needle 2 cm long is fitted.

The needle is thrust vertically downwards. If it hits bone at less than 1 cm depth, the tip does not lie intra-articularly and slightly different spots are tried until the needle slips in to its full length. If only the deep ligament requires infiltration, five or ten drops are injected about it fanwise when the resistance of the ligament is felt. If the superior ligament is also affected, the second ml of suspension is injected along each side of the joint line.

After-treatment—The shoulder is sore for the rest of the day. The arm is used as little as possible for two or three days, whereupon the patient returns to ordinary activities and to games at the end of a week.

Result—One injection is nearly always curative after recent or long-standing trauma. Patients who overstrain an osteoarthrotic joint afresh require a further injection.

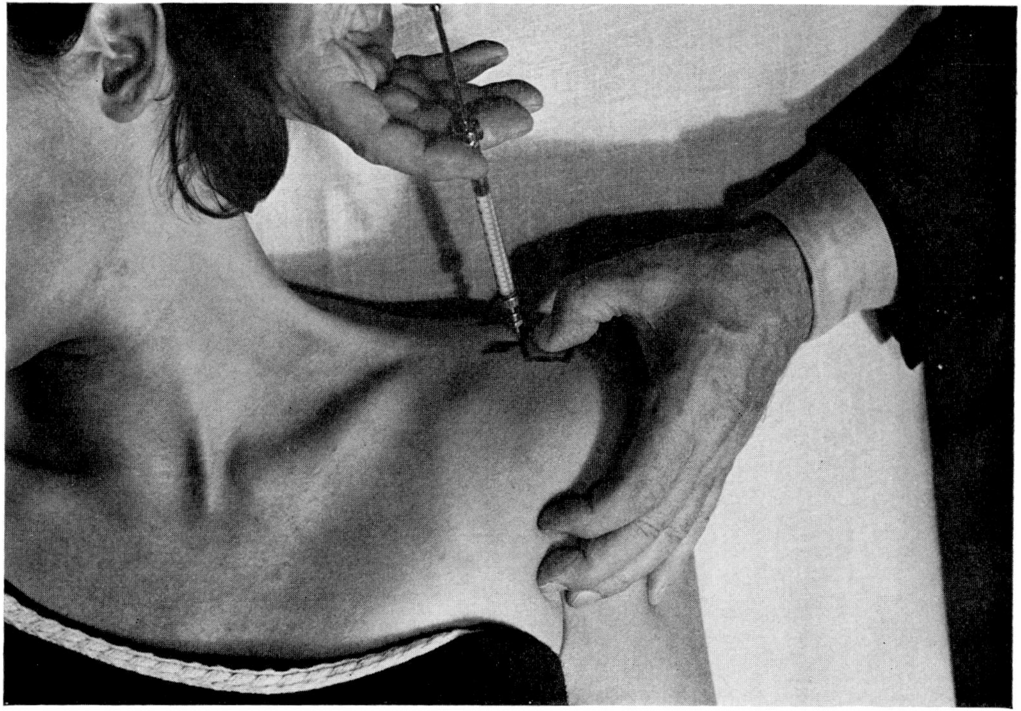

PLATE 22

SUPRASPINATUS TENDON

Massage Technique

Lesion—Painful scarring within the substance of the supraspinatus tendon. This is a very common condition, caused by heavy lifting. One memorable sprain is less frequent than prolonged repeated overstrain.

Indication—Supraspinatus tendinitis without calcification.

Physical Signs—A full passive range of movement is present at the shoulder-joint. Resisted abduction is painful and the other resisted movements are not.

Accessory signs are:

1. If full passive elevation hurts, the lesion lies where it can be pinched between the humeral tuberosity and the upper edge of the glenoid. This indicates that the scar lies at the distal end of the tendon and deeply.

2. If a painful arc is present (i.e. pain appearing as the arm passes the horizontal and ceasing *at each side* of this point), the lesion lies where it can be pinched between acromion and greater tuberosity. This implies that the scar lies superficially at the distal end of the tendon. Naturally, such cases improve more quickly, since the physiotherapist's friction can be applied directly to the lesion.

3. If full passive elevation does not hurt and a painful arc is not detected either, the musculo-tendinous junction of the supraspinatus is probably at fault (see Plate 25).

Patient's Posture—The patient bends his elbow to a right-angle and puts his forearm behind his back, his elbow well into his side. He then leans back in the half-lying position, thus fixing his arm in adduction and medial rotation. In this position of the arm the supraspinatus tendon is bent through a right-angle and lies in the sagittal plane, passing from the base of the coracoid process directly forwards over the head of the humerus to the greater tuberosity, emerging under the anterior edge of the acromion.

Technique—If the patient's right shoulder is to be treated, the physiotherapist must use her right hand; if his left shoulder, her left hand. She sits facing his shoulder and makes sure that the patient's arm has not moved from the adducted position. She places the tip of her index finger on the patient's tendon, flexing it at the distal joint but keeping it extended at the proximal interphalangeal joint. She reinforces with the middle finger. Her thumb is used for counter-pressure; in order that it shall be well placed for this purpose, it must be applied as far down the patient's arm as the physiotherapist's span will allow, i.e. as nearly opposite her index as is possible.

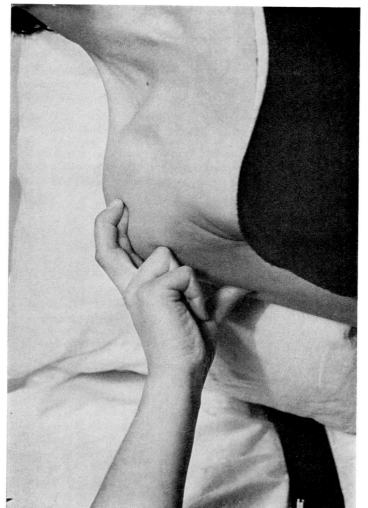

PLATE 23

While this posture is held, the anterior edge of the tendon is easily palpable. The physiotherapist finds the right spot, not on the bone of the greater tuberosity, but directly posterior to this point. Her finger is made to traverse the tendon from side to side by her alternately flexing and extending her wrist, using the thumb both as a fulcrum and to maintain pressure. The sweep is 2 cm from one edge of the tendon to the other. A physiotherapist's greatest strength just suffices to break up the scar in the tendon.

Duration of Treatment—About a quarter of an hour's friction twice weekly suffices. Two to six weeks' treatment is required as a rule.

Results—No matter how long-standing the tendinitis, few patients fail to get well in two months; the average period has been one month. An occasional case of relapse after resumption of heavy work is encountered.

Caution—*The tissues overlying the bony tuberosity are more tender than the adjacent supraspinatus tendon itself, even when tendinitis is present.* If, therefore, the physiotherapist enlists the patient's help and applies her friction to the most tender area instead of to the site of the tendon, her treatment will be directed to the wrong spot. The criterion is, as always, palpation of the tissue containing the lesion, not the discovery of tenderness.

SUPRASPINATUS TENDON

Injection Technique

Steroid suspension is particularly successful in abolishing supraspinatus tendinitis. Friction breaks the scar up, whereas steroid suspension renders the scar incapable of maintaining the inflammation in it, to which the pain is due. Since scar tissue and the fibrous tissue of which a tendon is composed are so similar, the former causes no trouble once its persistently inflamed state has been abolished.

Indication—Supraspinatus tendinitis with or without calcification. There is a considerable tendency to recurrence if calcification is present.

Intention—To infiltrate the entire extent of the scar, which must be thought of as a cubic lesion and dealt with on a three-dimensional basis.

Physical Signs—These are studied to ascertain first that supraspinatus tendinitis is present, then which part of the tendon, then which aspect of that part (see p. 142).

Patient's Posture—He is put into the same posture as for friction and for the same reason—to bring the tendon into the most easily palpable position.

Injection Technique—There is not much room to feel the anterior edge of the tendon passing forwards from under the acromion to the tuberosity. It is best therefore to use the little finger for palpation. The edge is identified. A 1 ml tuberculin syringe with a needle 2 cm long and as thin as possible is thrust vertically downwards into the tendon. No resistance is felt for the first 1 cm or so, then the point of the needle reaches the tendon and the operator recognizes the tough tissue. Considerable resistance is encountered to intratendinous injection; hence a long thin syringe is essential to provide enough purchase to force the suspension into the dense tissue. If no resistance is encountered at the correct depth, a partial rupture is present and the intact part of the tendon must now be sought with the point of the needle. The operator injects about twenty droplets along the teno-periosteal junction, deeply or superficially according to the accessory signs. This involves half-withdrawing the needle and reinserting it at a slightly different angle, until the whole width of the tendon (1·5 cm) has been infiltrated.

After-treatment—The patient avoids exerting his arm for seven days. He is free to do everything after two weeks.

Results—One-half of all cases are cured by one injection. Most of the rest get well with two or three. If relief lasts six to twelve months and then recurrence becomes manifest several times running, a sclerosing injection is substituted. If the tendon is calcified, the injection may relieve for a

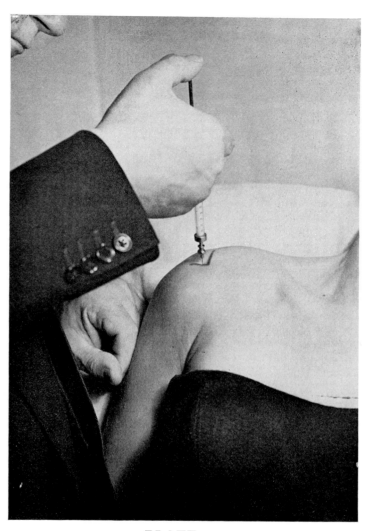

PLATE 24

month or two only; if so, 2% procaine is substituted, to dissolve the deposit. If necessary the calcified material can be curetted out.

If the injection fails completely, the question of a mistaken diagnosis arises. If local anaesthesia proves the ascription to be correct, the deduction must be made that the tendon cannot be disinflamed. If so, the scar must be broken down by deep friction—our standard treatment before hydrocortisone became available in 1952.

Theoretical Difficulties—Many doctors believe in an entity called 'the rotator cuff syndrome'. This term includes the supraspinatus, infraspinatus and subscapular tendons under one blunderbuss label. Clearly, no treatment can be given until the affected one of these three tendons has been singled out. This is not difficult, since each tendon possesses a different function (see Volume I).

Other doctors believe in primary contracture of the rotator cuff, causing limitation of movement at the shoulder. This idea is easily disproved. By contracting, opposing action of the subscapularis and infraspinatus muscles would cancel each other out. But no tendon exists passing beneath the head of the humerus to offset the effect of contraction of the supraspinatus muscle. The shoulder would therefore fix in full abduction. It never does.

Others regard 'painful arc syndrome' as possessing localizing significance. It does, of course, imply that the lesion lies in a pinchable position between the acromion and one or other of the humeral tuberosities, i.e. the supraspinatus, infraspinatus or subscapular tendon, or the subdeltoid bursa. The first three hurt when the tendon is tested by the appropriate resisted movement; if the bursa is affected, no resisted movement hurts. Hence differentiation presents no difficulty.

Finally, the word 'periarthritis' may be used. If this has any meaning at all, it would be to indicate that some tissue adjacent to the joint, but not forming part of it, is at fault. All the periarticular tissues have names, and which one must be stated.

SUPRASPINATUS MUSCLE: MUSCULO-TENDINOUS JUNCTION

Massage Technique

Lesion—This is either traumatic or due to prolonged overuse. Lesions of belly itself are very rare.

Physical Signs—A full and painless range of passive movement is present at the shoulder-joint. Resisted abduction hurts; the other resisted movements do not. Pain on full passive elevation is absent; there is no painful arc. This combination draws attention to the proximal end of the tendon.

Patient's Posture—The patient sits with his arm held in passive abduction by support at the elbow. This relaxes the belly of the supraspinatus muscle and brings the affected part within reach.

Technique—The physiotherapist stands by the patient's unaffected shoulder with her forearm passing behind his neck. She presses the front of her middle finger-tip, reinforced by the index, deeply into the angle formed by the spine of the scapula and the back of the outer part of the clavicle. She imparts the transverse friction by keeping her finger at this spot and rotating the forearm to and fro by alternate supination and pronation movements.

Duration of Treatment—A quarter of an hour's friction thrice weekly.

Results—Cure has so far proved invariable after four to eight treatments. If a patient does not improve and the physiotherapist shows her technique and it is found correct, the probability is that the diagnosis is mistaken. Local anaesthesia should be employed to confirm or disprove this ascription. Steroid suspension has no value in treatment at this site.

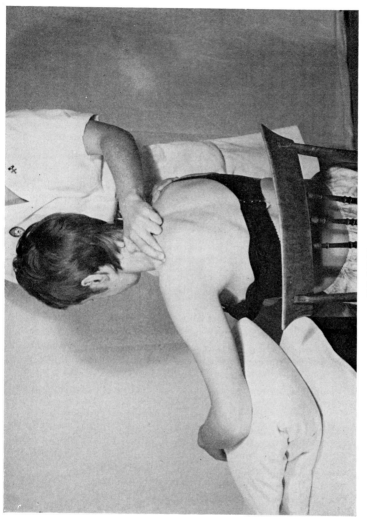

PLATE 25

INFRASPINATUS TENDON

Massage Technique

Lesion—The painful scar lies close to or at the insertion of the infraspinatus tendon into the greater tuberosity of the humerus.

Physical Signs—A full range of passive movement is present at the shoulder. Resisted lateral rotation hurts and the other resisted movements do not. Accessory movements are:

1. Full passive elevation hurts. This indicates that the lesion can be pinched between the humeral tuberosity and the edge of the glenoid, i.e. that the deep aspect of the distal end of the tendon is affected.

2. A painful arc. This shows the painful scar to be pinchable between acromion and tuberosity, i.e. that the superficial aspect of the distal end of the tendon is affected.

3. If neither of these signs appears the lesion lies in the body of the tendon (not at the musculo-tendinous junction).

Patient's Posture—The patient lies face downwards, propping himself up on his elbows. The weight of his thorax acting downwards ensures that his scapula lies at right-angles to the humerus; in this position the acromion is drawn away from the greater tuberosity, uncovering it. Slight lateral rotation of the arm is maintained by the patient's holding on to the edge of the couch. This combination of flexion and slight lateral rotation brings the tuberosity backwards. The arm is now pushed into slight adduction, which brings the humeral tuberosity out from under the acromion. Running along, just below the most lateral extent of the spine of the scapula, the infraspinatus tendon is easy to feel on its course towards the head of the humerus.

Technique—The physiotherapist sits facing the patient's head and places her fingers on the front of his shoulder. She feels for the tendon with her thumb which she flexes until good pressure is obtained. Alternate abduction and adduction of the thumb now draw it to and fro across the tendon. At the extreme of the adduction movement, she feels the tip of her thumb engage against the posterior acromial edge.

Duration of Treatment—Twenty minutes two or three times a week.

Results—The main difficulty is to ensure that the massage is given exactly to the spot in the tendon where the strained fibres lie. When this is found, some six or eight sessions of massage suffice to bring about recovery. Since, however, there is about 2 cm of latitude in the placing of the operative finger, the physiotherapist cannot avoid occasionally making a false start slightly to one or other side of the lesion. The physician cannot help her direct her finger within this limit, hence allowance must be made for some trial and error during the first few sessions.

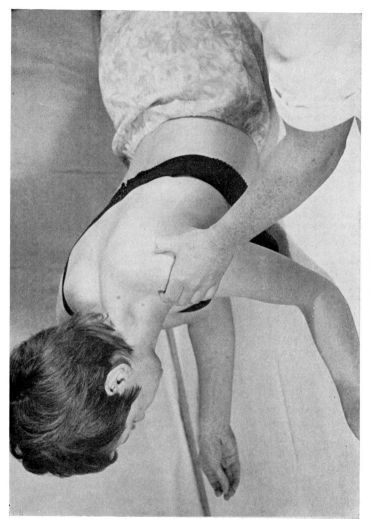

PLATE 26

INFRASPINATUS TENDON

Injection Technique

Steroid suspension is particularly successful in abolishing infraspinatus tendinitis. The scar remains, but is no longer inflamed. Hence tension on it no longer hurts.

Intention—To infiltrate the entire extent of the scar, right across the tendon, superficially or deeply, according to the accessory signs found present (see Plate 26).

Physical Signs—These are studied, first to ascertain that infraspinatus tendinitis is present, then for the accessory movements that single out one part of the tendon. Unfortunately, they are less often as clear as is to be expected in supraspinatus tendinitis. When in doubt, the physician should induce local anaesthesia (2 ml) at the part of the tendon that appears affected, and make a localized diagnosis that way.

Patient's Posture—This is the same as when friction is required, because in either case the tendon needs to lie in the best position for palpation.

Injection Technique—The entire length of the infraspinatus tendon is easily felt and, in cases of doubt, the tendon can be palpated not only to define its position but also to discover if one point along it is more tender than elsewhere. The operator uses his flexed thumb for palpation, identifies the upper and lower edges of the tendon, and its point of insertion into the tuberosity. It lies farther from the skin, especially in thick-set people, than the supraspinatus tendon, and the thinnest possible needle is used, but now 3 to 4 cm long. It is fitted to a tuberculin syringe containing 1 ml of steroid suspension and he thrusts it vertically downwards until the resistance of the tendon is felt. He injects twenty or so droplets along the affected area, close to the surface and deeply, by half-withdrawing the needle and then reinserting it at slightly different angles and to slightly different depths.

After-treatment—The patient should use the arm sparingly for the first seven days, and resume full activities after two weeks.

Result—Most patients get well after one or two injections. If a failure is encountered and the diagnosis is correct, friction must be substituted.

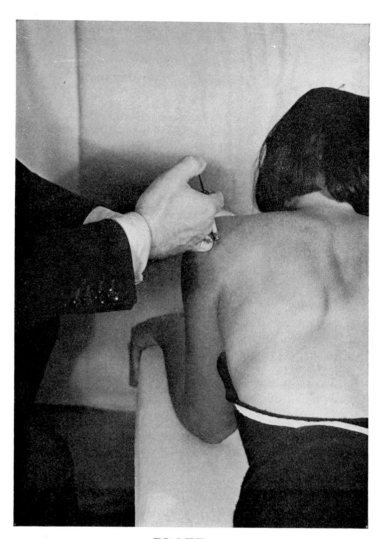

PLATE 27

SUBSCAPULARIS TENDON

Massage Technique

Lesion—Scarring at the teno-periosteal junction with the lesser tuberosity. It may follow a single overstrain or repeated overuse.

Physical Signs—A full range of passive movement is present at the shoulder. Resisted medial rotation hurts. The other three medial rotator muscles—pectoralis major, latissimus dorsi and teres major—are chiefly adductors. Hence, when resisted adduction is found not to hurt, that leaves the subscapularis. The accessory movements are:

1. A painful arc exists. The tendon is affected at the uppermost part of the lesser tuberosity.

2. Full passive adduction of the arm across the front of the chest hurts. The lower part of the tendon is pinched against the coracoid process.

Since the tendon is always affected (in my experience) at the insertion into bone, these two signs differentiate between a lesion lying at the upper end of the tuberosity from one along the shaft of the humerus.

Patient's Posture—The patient adopts the half-lying position on the couch. He holds his arm close to his side and bends his elbow, putting his hand on his thigh.

Technique—The physiotherapist sits at the patient's side facing him. She puts her thumb on the head of his humerus and identifies the bicipital groove, rotating his arm to and fro using the forearm as a lever, to identify the two edges. Immediately medial to the inner edge of the groove lies the subscapular tendon, but it cannot be palpated: it feels as hard as bone. She notes the spot. She then bends her thumb to a right-angle and hooks it round the medial edge of the upper part of the deltoid muscle, and draws the belly laterally, letting the short head of biceps slip under her finger. She can now apply her thumb to the subscapular tendon without the intervening mass of deltoid belly. She now moves her thumb vertically up and down applying counter-pressure with her fingers at the back of the shoulder. In this way transverse friction can be given to the upper or lower part of the tendon. Massage here is extremely disagreeable.

Duration of Treatment—Twenty minutes twice a week is as much as the patient or the physiotherapist can stand. Treatment usually has to be continued for one month.

Results—Not more than two-thirds of the patients are fully relieved by massage. Hence, if the patient is not much better at the end of one month it is not worth while going on. However, it is best to avoid massage altogether in these cases, since it is my experience that a single injection of steroid suspension is regularly curative.

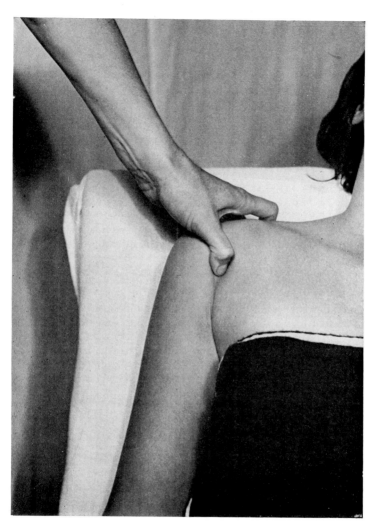

PLATE 28

SUBSCAPULARIS TENDON

Injection Technique

Hydrocortisone is extremely successful in abolishing subscapular tendinitis. The scar continues intact but, being deprived of inflammation, no longer hurts when tension falls on it during muscular contraction.

Intention—To infiltrate the length of scar tissue at the upper or lower teno-periosteal junction, depending on the accessory signs found present (see Plate 28).

Patient's Posture—He lies supine on the couch, his hand on his thigh. In this position the bicipital groove faces directly anteriorly and is identified by palpation with the thumb, the finger behind the shoulder applying counter-pressure. If difficulty is experienced the humerus should be rotated, using the forearm as a lever, to enable the two sharp edges of the groove to be identified. Immediately medial to the groove lies the sub-scapular tendon. The insertion is some 3 cm long.

Injection Technique—A tuberculin syringe is filled with 1 ml of steroid suspension and fitted with a fine needle 2 cm long. The medial edge of the bicipital groove is palpated and the tendon infiltrated at points $\frac{1}{2}$ to 1 cm medial to that line, at the upper or lower extent. The injection, unlike the friction, can be given directly through the deltoid muscle, and the substance of the tendon is recognized by considerable resistance it offers to the progress of the needle and to the infiltration itself. Some twenty droplets are injected at the affected area of tendon, superficially and deeply.

After-treatment—The patient should avoid all exertion for a week; after a fortnight he can do anything he likes.

Result—Full relief after one adequate infiltration is the rule; few patients require a second.

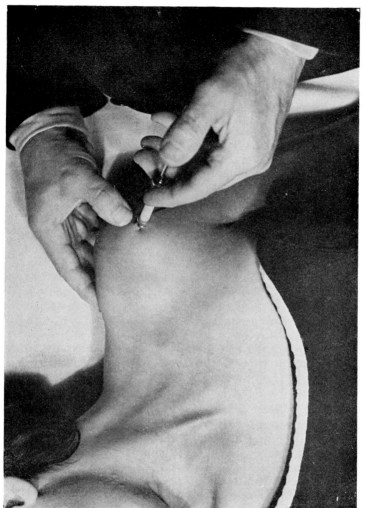

PLATE 29

SHOULDER-JOINT: FORCED ELEVATION

Lesion—This is of three types:

1. After an injury, direct or indirect, adhesions form about the capsule of the shoulder-joint just as at other sites. They differ, however, from post-traumatic adhesions at other joints for they result in limitation of movement in *every* direction. When ruptured by manipulation, these adhesions are felt and heard to tear as if they were thick bands, whereas at other joints adhesions give way in a manner suggesting more numerous and much slighter strands of tissue.

2. Osteoarthrotic capsular contracture. This is the same as occurs in osteoarthrosis elsewhere. The existence of osteoarthrosis makes the joint very sensitive to mere overuse or slight injury, traumatic arthritis supervening for minor cause; in such cases adhesions form about the already contracted capsule of the joint and the two types of disorder are present together.

3. Non-specific arthritis.

Indications for Manipulation—Limitation of movement in the capsular pattern, when the criteria set out below are satisfied.

Capsular adhesions causing movement limited in one direction only. This is rare, but may follow a reduced dislocation provoking anterior contracture.

Stretching the shoulder-joint in the manner described here is called for in all cases of recent capsular trauma in patients over forty-five years of age. Many such injuries eventually result in a severe traumatic arthritis; this is preventable by immediate stretching of the capsule, repeated until a full and painless range of movement has been restored. Under the age of forty-five, traumatic arthritis does not supervene.

In established arthritis, stretching the joint out is called for when:

(a) The pain does not reach beyond the elbow.
(b) There is no pain except on movement.
(c) The patient can lie on that side at night.
(d) The end-feel is elastic.
(e) When the joint is forced, the resistance to movement is perceived before appreciable pain is evoked.

If these criteria are observed, cases unsuitable for stretching (and they are many) will be singled out.

The next precaution observed by the physiotherapist is to stretch the shoulder out fairly gently on the first occasion. At his next attendance she asks how long the shoulder felt sore for after treatment. If the patient denies any added discomfort this is an encouraging sign, indicating that stronger stretching is required. If he answers that the arm hurt more for one to two hours, the correct amount of force was employed and must be repeated. If the soreness lasted longer, perhaps for a day or two, the case is unsuitable (see Plate 32).

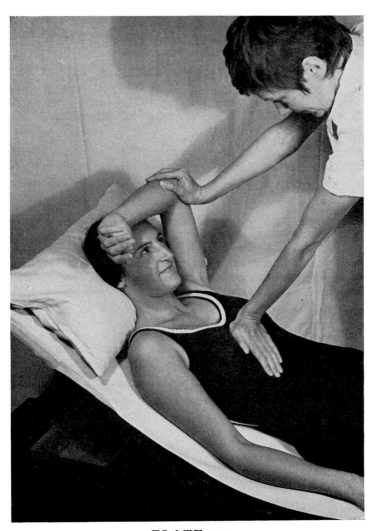

PLATE 30

Alternative Treatment—If the capsular pattern is present but the criteria contra-indicate forcing, one alternative is to inject hydrocortisone intra-articularly. Two injections at a week's interval usually bring the joint into the stretchable stage. The other alternative is the technique described overleaf (Plates 32 and 33).

Patient's Posture—The patient lies face upwards on the couch, the end of which is slightly raised. He brings his arm up as far as he can, keeping his hand in front of his forehead.

Technique—The physiotherapist must be ready to devote at least fifteen minutes daily to forcing elevation. Short-wave diathermy given *just* before the manipulation affords heat analgesia and diminishes the patient's discomfort. Throughout the physiotherapist watches the patient's face and tries him as hard as is reasonable.

Her one hand on his lower sternum keeps the patient's thorax on the couch; otherwise he will eventually arch his back, thus appearing to achieve an increase in the degree of elevation of his arm. Her other hand presses hard against the patient's elbow, slowly forcing elevation at the shoulder, now slackening her effort enough to afford some respite, now increasing her pressure again. No jerk is given. To start with, only elevation is forced. When progress has been made, adduction and rotation can be cautiously added. In long-standing cases, after perhaps a week's forcing, a large adhesion is felt and heard to part; from this moment the pain eases and the range of movement increases. Two or three such bands may require rupture before a full range of movement is restored to the joint.

After-treatment—Exercises in every direction follow, in order that the patient may retain actively the added range of movement afforded him passively.

SHOULDER-JOINT
Injection Technique

Lesion—Arthritis at the shoulder (sometimes misnamed 'periarthritis' on account of the absence of X-ray changes).

Physical Signs—Limitation of passive movement at the shoulder-joint in the capsular proportions, i.e. a certain amount ot limitation of abduction range, more limitation of lateral rotation, less limitation of medial rotation. These findings indicate arthritis. A common pattern would be: 45° limitation of abduction range, 70° limitation of lateral rotation, 10° limitation of medial rotation.

Indications—The common causes of restricted movement on the capsular proportions are traumatic arthritis and monarticular rheumatoid arthritis. Both respond very well to intra-articular hydrocortisone. However, osteoarthrosis is not helped by intra-articular steroid therapy. All three are apt to be lumped together under the label 'frozen shoulder' which is therefore an unhelpful term.

Patient's Posture—She lies prone, her forearm under her upper abdomen. The arm is now fixed in some degree of medial rotation, which turns the articular surface of the humerus to face posteriorly, thus affording a larger target. Moreover, she cannot readily move her arm nor watch the puncture.

Technique—There is more than one way of reaching the cavity of the shoulder-joint, but this is the simplest. The physician places his index finger on the point of the coracoid process and his thumb on the point where the acromion and the spine of the scapula meet at right angles. The line joining his fingers crosses the glenoid cavity. A 2 ml syringe is filled with steroid suspension and a 5 cm thin needle is fitted. (The thinner the needle, the more readily the physician can feel its point traversing the capsule of the joint.) It punctures the skin at the physician's thumb, aimed just lateral to the tip of his index. At first the needle passes freely but the capsule offers a characteristic resistance. Now impingement against cartilage is felt and the injection given.

The shoulder-joint bears no weight and no case of steroid arthropathy has been observed whatever the number of injections.

Progress—After the first injection the spontaneous pain ceases thirty-six hours later and the patient gets his first good night's rest for months, finding that he can lie on that side at night. At the extreme of possible movement pain is still evoked and the range has not altered. The intention is now to give further injections at increasing intervals, keeping the joint continuously under the disinflaming action of the steroid. To this end, the next injection must be given just before the effect of the previous one wears off. Hence in a fortunate case the interval might be one week, ten

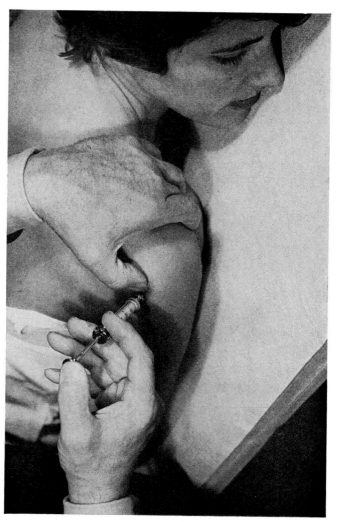

PLATE 31

days, two weeks, three weeks, four weeks; a total of six injections. Four is the least, and ten the greatest number of injections required.

The range of movement begins to increase after the third or fourth injection. Once the patient can move the arm freely, the end-feel is soft and no relapse is noted a month after the previous injection, no more need be done; final complete recovery now proceeds spontaneously.

Comment—Twenty-three years ago Troisier and I pointed out that what was then called 'frozen shoulder' was no longer incurable; intra-articular steroid injection was regularly successful. The pain was abolished as from the first injection. Yet today this disorder is still regarded as intractable, and all sorts of useless treatments are given prolonged trial, for lack of the simple procedure set out above.

SHOULDER-JOINT

Distraction Techniques

This method was devised by Miss J. Hickling, MCSP, in a search for suitable treatment at the shoulder when the joint was too irritable to respond to ordinary stretching. She appears in the photographs.

Lesion—Limitation of movement at the shoulder-joint in the capsular pattern, i.e. arthritis.

Indication for Distraction—Unsuitability for the ordinary type of stretching, i.e. the pain is constant and spreads below the elbow; the patient cannot sleep on that side at night. The end-feel is sudden spasm.

Accessory movements* in the neutral position carry the important advantage of increasing range and sedating pain without the exacerbation of symptoms and spasm that is provoked when an irritable joint is stretched out in the ordinary way.

Patient's Posture—The patient lies on a high couch in the position of maximum comfort, so that each aspect of the joint capsule is equally relaxed. This involves holding the arm in slight flexion and medial rotation. The pillows are arranged with this in view.

Physiotherapist's Posture—She sits facing the patient, as close as possible to him. One corner of the pillow is curled round the patient's elbow and the physiotherapist leans against it, curbing any tendency towards abduction. She slides one hand up the inner aspect of the arm as far as the axilla and accommodates the shaft of the humerus in her rounded palm.

Distraction Technique—Distraction of the humeral head from the glenoid surface in a lateral direction is now attempted by pulling both with the hand in the axilla and with the lower forearm as it lies along the inner aspect of the humerus. No abduction occurs. The other hand cups the head of the bone and helps to judge the degree of distraction.

The physiotherapist should not attempt distraction by flexing her wrist and applying pressure lower down the arm to prevent abduction. This results in a degree of angulation at the joint which may be sufficient to upset the quality of the passive movement which is being sought.

Progress—In severe arthritis no distraction proves possible at the first attempt, muscle spasm keeping the joint surfaces in apposition. Any attempt to overcome this spasm is vain; it merely hurts the patient and increases spasm. The physiotherapist simply coaxes distraction of minimal amplitude, intermittently and with slight irregularity in depth and timing, for up to half an hour.

---

* The term 'accessory movement' denotes those movements which form an integral part of any normal joint movement, but are not under voluntary control.

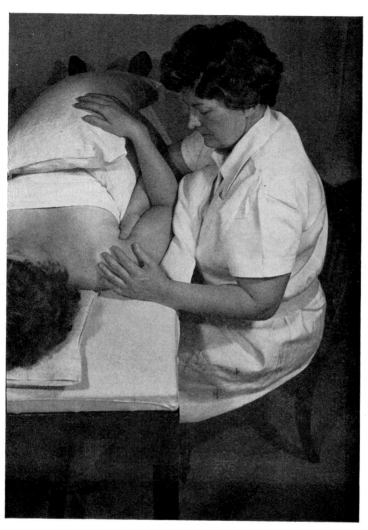

PLATE 32

Typical Response—In a severe lesion, the response to be expected is set out below.

First day: No effect, but no flare afterwards. No attempt is made to carry out movements that are under voluntary control, e.g. elevation, and as much rest as possible is enjoined. Exercises are contra-indicated.

Second day: About half-way through the session the joint suddenly relaxes and normal distraction is felt. From this moment the constant ache in the arm may be expected to ease, and night pain to become steadily less.

Third day: The muscles relax as from the beginning of the session. Dosage is increased by following up the easy distraction that is now obtained, both by increasing this movement and by adding a slight forward or circumduction movement to it. If any movement increases the pain or leads to a return of muscular spasm decreasing range, these extra measures are diminished.

Fourth and fifth day: Treatment on these lines is continued, each distraction being maintained for a longer time and with greater amplitude. By now the continuous ache in the arm should largely have abated.

Further Measures—Once the pain–spasm cycle begins to be broken, movements of the humeral head on the glenoid surface can be increased, especially posteriorly and inferiorly. Examination will soon begin to show that the movements under voluntary control (e.g. elevation and rotation) increase spontaneously in range, without any direct forcing. Once elevation is beginning to yield, the humeral head can be moved with mounting vigour (see Plate 33). In addition the basic position may be changed; for example, the arm may be held in 90° of flexion while accessory movements are used, suitable grips being devised for each individual. In due course the joint loses its irritability. At this stage, little spasm is provoked whenever the movements under voluntary control are gently forced, and the end-feel becomes elastic. Now for the first time forcing the extremes of range becomes indicated and speeds recovery (see Plate 30). Even so, the accessory movements should be continued.

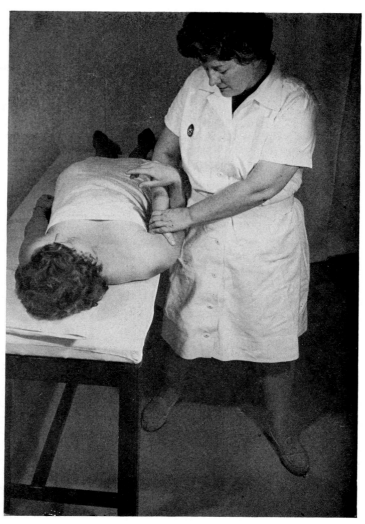

PLATE 33

PLATE 34

SUBDELTOID BURSA

Injection Technique

No physiotherapy avails in subdeltoid bursitis; it can be treated only by injection or phonophoresis, whether calcification is present or not.

Lesions—The subdeltoid bursa is liable to acute and chronic inflammation. They are separate disorders, not merging from one to the other.

The exposed part of the bursa lying under the deltoid muscle may be affected, or the sub-acromial part beyond finger's reach, or both.

Physical Signs—Acute bursitis leads to increasing pain in the arm reaching to the wrist in about three days. Passive scapulo-humeral abduction is grossly restricted by severe pain, but the range of lateral rotation is little diminished: the non-capsular pattern. The whole extent of the bursa accessible to palpation is extremely tender and often thickened. Spontaneous recovery takes six weeks; the severe pain lasts seven to ten days.

There is no limit to how long a localized area of chronic bursitis may last —certainly many years. Examination discloses a full range of movement, with sometimes discomfort at the extremes of range. A painful arc is present. No resisted movement causes any pain.

If a small patch of bursa is found tender, the diagnosis is confirmed or disproved by the induction of local anaesthesia at this point. Disappearance of the painful arc shows that the right spot was chosen. If no tenderness at the accessible area of bursa can be detected the subacromial part must be at fault, and local anaesthesia is induced diagnostically there.

Patient's Posture—In acute bursitis the patient is given an injection of morphine before the infiltration. A 5 ml syringe is filled with steroid suspension and a fine needle 2 cm long is fitted. The whole affected extent of the bursa is reached by a multiple series of little infiltrations. Another 5 ml syringe is now filled and fitted with a needle 5 cm long. The part of the bursa lying under the acromion is now infiltrated by a horizontal approach (illustrated).

In chronic bursitis the diagnostic injection of local anaesthetic solution often proves curative, and if the patient is much better when seen a week later, local anaesthesia should be repeated at exactly the same spot. If the diagnosis was confirmed but no lasting benefit ensued, steroid is substituted.

After-treatment—In acute bursitis the patient is seen two days later in case some small area of bursa escaped infiltration and requires treatment.

Results—In acute bursitis the shoulder is sore next day, but mobile, and the patient can go about his business with some discomfort. A second attack is likely within five years. In chronic bursitis relief should be permanent after one to three injections.

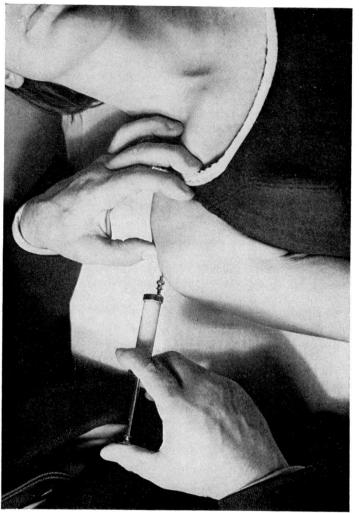

PLATE 34

BICEPS MUSCLE: TENDON OF LONG HEAD

Massage Technique

Lesion—As elsewhere, tendinitis here is the result of overuse or of one severe strain. The mid-part of the tendon of the long head is usually at fault.

Physical Signs—A full and painless range of passive movement is present at the shoulder-joint and no resisted movement hurts. Resisted flexion and supination of the elbow hurt at the uppermost part of the arm.

Patient's Posture—The patient adopts the half-lying position on the couch, his arm by his side and his pronated hand lying on the front of his thigh. This position brings the bicipital groove to lie directly anteriorly.

Technique—The physiotherapist sits at his side, facing him. She identifies the biceps tendon lying in the groove on the humerus, if necessary by feeling it become taut on an elbow flexion movement resisted at his forearm. She presses her whole thumb flat on the tendon, applying counter-pressure by her fingers at the back of his arm. She now gives the friction by adducting and abducting her thumb to and fro over the tendon. Alternatively, she can leave her thumb pressing on the tendon and rotate the patient's humerus to and fro under it, using his flexed forearm as a lever.

Duration of Treatment—Twenty minutes on alternate days.

Results—In my experience every case of tendinitis here recovers fully after two or three weeks' massage given in this way, even if the disorder has lasted many years. Hence steroid infiltration is not required.

Caution—Neither the lower part of the anterior edge of the deltoid muscle nor the short head of biceps must be mistaken for the tendon.

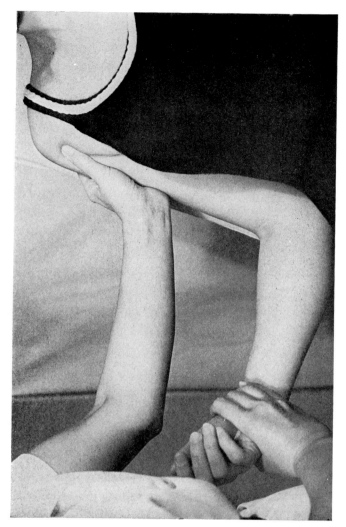

PLATE 35

BICEPS MUSCLE: BELLY

Massage Technique

Lesion—This nearly always lies at the deep aspect of the lower half of the muscle belly. It results from a single excessive strain during, say, heavy lifting, and a painful scar forms which is apt to go on hurting indefinitely every time the muscle contracts.

Physical Signs—The pain is felt at the mid-arm and is evoked by resisted flexion and supination of the elbow. The shoulder-joint and the muscles about it are found normal.

Patient's Posture—The patient adopts the half-lying position. His arm and forearm are supported by the couch, and the elbow is thus held in about 45° of flexion.

Technique—The physiotherapist sits facing the patient and grasps the affected area of muscle between her fingers and thumb, the interphalangeal joints of which are held well flexed. While maintaining this grip, she pulls her whole hand bodily towards herself, thereby imparting the friction.

Duration of Treatment—This should last fifteen or twenty minutes. More than a few weeks' treatment on alternate days is seldom required except in very chronic cases.

Results—Full relief is to be expected. Only very chronic cases, lasting five years or more, may prove intractable.

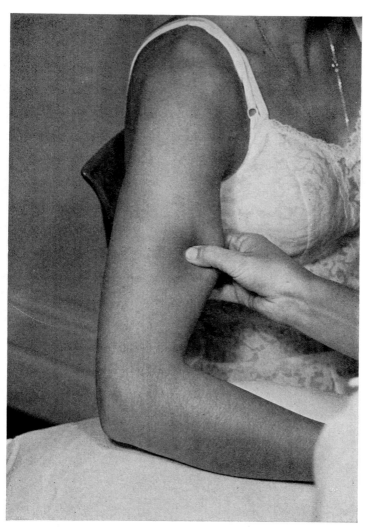

PLATE 36

BICEPS TENDON: INSERTION AT RADIAL
TUBEROSITY

Massage Technique

Lesion—Strain at the teno-periosteal junction, i.e. between the lower tendon of the biceps muscle and the tuberosity of the radius.

Physical Signs—The pain is felt at the front of the elbow and radiates along the front of the forearm to the wrist. Passive flexion, extension and supination at the elbow are full and painless, but the extreme of pronation hurts, since the tender tendon is then squeezed between the shaft of the ulna and the projecting tuberosity. Resisted flexion and supination at the elbow evoke the pain in the forearm; resisted extension and pronation do not hurt.

Patient's Posture—The patient adopts the half-lying position on the couch and places his fully supinated forearm on a pillow on the physiotherapist's lap.

Technique—The physiotherapist sits at right-angles to the patient, facing his forearm. She flexes her thumb at the interphalangeal joint so as to apply its tip to the radial tuberosity anteriorly. Counter-pressure is applied by her fingers at the back of his forearm. Friction is then imparted to the tendon at the tuberosity by means of the other hand which, grasping the patient's hand, alternately pronates and supinates his forearm. At each rotation, full supination should be achieved, but it is unnecessary to go any farther than half pronation, for beyond this point the tuberosity will have swung out of reach of the operative thumb.

Result—Full relief is to be expected in four to six sessions of friction.

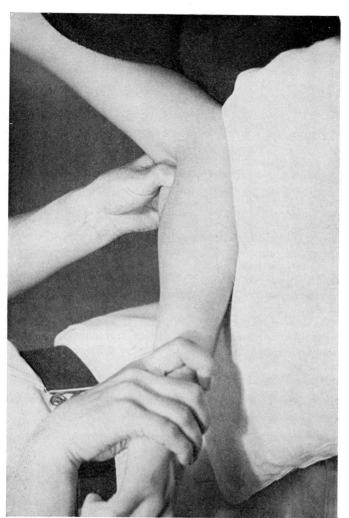

PLATE 37

BICEPS TENDON: INSERTION AT RADIAL TUBEROSITY

Injection Technique

Lesion—A painful scar lying at the insertion of the biceps tendon into the tuberosity of the radius.

Physical Signs—The pain is felt at the flexure of the elbow, radiating to the front of the wrist. A full range of movement is present at the elbow-joint but full passive pronation is painful, since the tendon is then pinched against the upper shaft of the ulna. Resisted flexion and supination at the elbow cause pain, resisted extension and pronation are painless. The resisted wrist movements do not hurt. No tenderness can be elicted by digital probing.

Patient's Posture—The patient lies prone on the couch, his arm by his side and his elbow held in full extension. His forearm is now fully pronated, so as to bring the tuberosity of the radius round to face posteriorly. The groove formed by the joint between the head of the radius and the capitellum is identified posteriorly. A point is taken 2 cm below the joint line. This will not be found tender. A 2 ml syringe is filled with steroid suspension and a thin needle 2 cm long is fitted. The shaft of the radius is identified and the needle inserted vertically downwards until it touches either bone directly or tendon then bone. In the former event, the needle is partly withdrawn and a search made with the point of the needle for tendinous resistance. When it is encountered, a series of droplets is injected in the region of the tuberosity.

After-treatment—Exertion is avoided for a week. After two weeks the elbow is tried out.

Result—One to three injections are required, since it is difficult to infiltrate the entire scar accurately in the absence of tenderness.

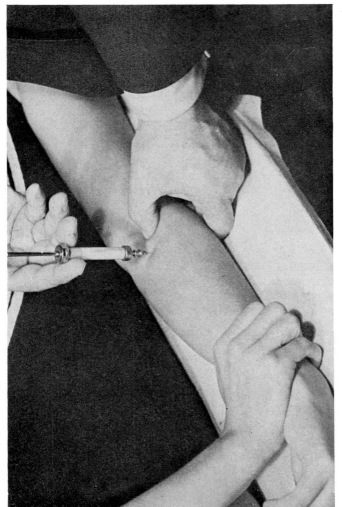

PLATE 38

TENNIS ELBOW: COMMON EXTENSOR TENDON

Premanipulative Friction

The term 'tennis elbow' is used to cover all non-specific lesions affecting the wrist-extensor group of muscles near the elbow.

Lesion—In nine out of ten cases the painful scar lies at the teno-periosteal junction, where the common extensor tendon takes origin from the lateral epicondyle, anteriorly.

Physical Signs—The pain is felt at the outer side of the elbow, radiating along the dorsum of the forearm to the wrist. The passive and resisted movements at the elbow are found painless. Resisted extension and radial deviation of the wrist hurt at the elbow whereas resisted flexion and ulnar deviation prove painless. When tenderness is sought along the upper extent of the extensores carpi radialis the tendon is found affected at its epicondylar attachment.

Indication—Massage to the affected fibres at the epicondyle has two effects: it produces reactive hyperaemia at the scar that is to be ruptured, thus acting as a local analgesic; it also softens it. Massage alone is valueless for this type of tennis elbow; it is merely the preliminary to the manipulation, which is rendered less painful and more likely to succeed.

Patient's Posture—The patient sits with his elbow bent to a right-angle and fully supinated. This brings the lateral epicondyle into prominence. The physiotherapist sits on the same couch, facing the patient's arm, i.e. at right-angles to him.

Technique—The physiotherapist must find the right spot by using her knowledge of anatomy rather than by asking the patient, for most places in this region are tender in normal persons. In particular, pressure exerted from in front over the head of the radius is always painful. Since the tear lies at the origin of the common extensor tendon from the bone, i.e. at the *front* of the lateral epicondyle, it is here, not at the apex of the epicondyle, that friction is required.

The physiotherapist places one hand at his wrist and holds his forearm fully supinated. She then bends the distal joint of the thumb of her other hand to a right-angle and presses deeply on the front of his epicondyle. Counter-pressure is applied by the fingers lying against the inner side of his elbow. The thumb is used facing towards the olecranon. She keeps the tip of her thumb pressing against the tip of the epicondyle and then flexes her fingers and thumb synchronously. The thumb is drawn across the epicondyle by flexion of the fingers and she ensures that her thumb-tip remains on the epicondyle by the further flexion of her thumb.

The massage is kept up for fifteen minutes whereupon the manipulation (Plate 40) follows at once.

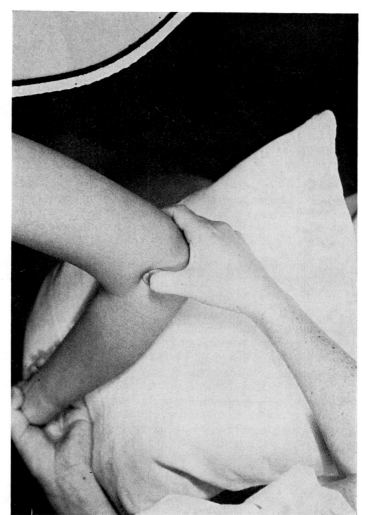

PLATE 39

TENNIS ELBOW

Mill's Manipulation

Lesion—The teno-periosteal variety of tennis elbow. The only movements found to hurt the elbow are resisted extension and resisted radial deviation at the wrist. This manipulation is called for only when the site of tenderness shows that the lesion lies at the humeral epicondyle.

Contra-indication—If a full range of extension is not obtainable at the elbow-joint, the manipulation cannot succeed and may well provoke instead a traumatic arthritis at the joint.

Intention—To pull apart the two surfaces joined by the painful scar. If full separation is attained, permanent lengthening results of that part of the common tendon relevant to the extensor carpi radialis brevis muscle. The rest of the tendon now takes the strain; fibrous tissue under no tension fills the gap; cure results with freedom from liability to recurrence.

Patient's Posture—The patient sits upright with her arm abducted to the horizontal and so far medially rotated that the olecranon faces upwards.

Technique—The operator stands behind her, level with her trunk (not level with her elbow). At the moment of the manipulation it is vital that her wrist should be kept fully flexed. This is almost impossible unless the operator stands well away from the arm.

The patient's forearm must be fully pronated and the wrist flexed. This posture stretches the common extensor tendon, so the patient eases the tension by flexing her elbow a little. If the right elbow is at fault, he grasps her hand with his right hand and forces these two movements to their extreme, his thumb on her palm, his fingers at the dorsum.

The operator now places his left hand on the olecranon, thus extending the elbow somewhat. He now focuses his attention on his right hand at her wrist, so as not for a moment to relax the pressure maintaining full pronation of her forearm and full flexion of her wrist. While this tension is strongly maintained, he suddenly forces full extension at the elbow with his left hand with a smart jerk, taking the patient unawares. This manipulation is very painful at the instant of its performance, since it applies the maximum stretch to the painful scar. It is carried out once each visit, immediately after friction, while the hyperaemia lasts. Four to twelve sessions are required and not every teno-periosteal tennis elbow responds well.

Caution—Before manipulating, the operator must satisfy himself that the case is suitable by ascertaining three facts:

(a) Is there a full range of extension at the elbow-joint? Limited extension contra-indicates any attempt at Mill's manipulation.

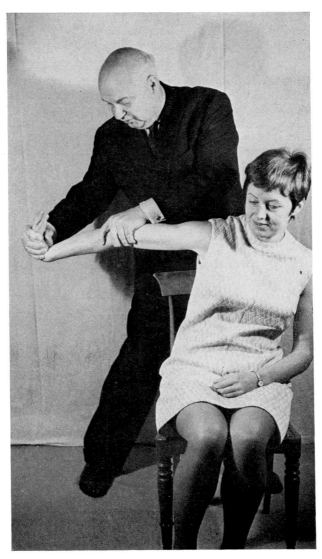

PLATE 40

(*b*) Is a tennis elbow present? If so, resisted extension of the wrist is the movement that elicits the pain at the elbow.

(*c*) Is it of the teno-periosteal variety? If so, the epicondyle is tender.

Hence, before the first manipulation, and at each subsequent visit the operator satisfies himself that these criteria remain fulfilled. If Mill's manipulation is badly performed, especially if full flexion at the wrist is not maintained, the brunt of the thrust towards extension is borne by the elbow-joint, and a traumatic arthritis is apt to supervene. It is for this reason that the elbow is examined at each attendance, so that any elbow-joint which has been forced too hard can be singled out at once. Further manipulation is then postponed for a week or two until the joint has recovered; were it to be repeated notwithstanding, quite a severe arthritis could be provoked.

TENNIS ELBOW: COMMON EXTENSOR TENDON

Injection Technique

Lesion—A painful scar at the origin of the common extensor tendon from the lateral epicondyle of the humerus.

Physical Signs—A full range of passive movement at the elbow-joint. No resisted elbow movement hurts. Resisted extension of the wrist hurts at the elbow. Tenderness lies at the teno-periosteal junction.

N.B. The other types of tennis elbow do not benefit from steroid injections.

Intention—To leave the painful scar in situ, but to stop the persistent inflammatory reaction to the long-past injury. To this end the area is infiltrated with steroid suspension, since this abolishes the cells' capacity to sustain inflammation. This then ceases and when the steroid has disappeared at the end of a fortnight the effect continues. Most patients recover completely after one or two injections. A few relapse after some months, because the scar has been left in being, and repeated tension on it reactivated the lesion. A very few derive no benefit. These must be treated by going back to the massage and manipulation that we employed before hydrocortisone was found effective in 1953.

Patient's Posture—She sits with her elbow supported on a desk, the elbow at a right-angle and fully supinated. In this position the lateral epicondyle is at its most prominent.

Injection Technique—The operator now applies his thumb to the anterior aspect of the epicondyle with his fingers on the ulnar side of the elbow (see Plate 39) and ascertains the boundaries of the tender spot—how far it extends towards the apex, the base and the superior and inferior edges of the epicondyle. Within this small ambit there is considerable variation.

He fills a 1 ml tuberculin syringe with a suspension of triamcinolone (as effective as hydrocortisone but provoking a much less painful reaction) and fitted with a very fine needle not more than 2 cm long. He thrusts it vertically through the skin until he feels the needle touch bone. He injects a droplet here, keeping his thumb on the spot, and feels where the tiny bulge appears. He must now remember the confines of the lesion, and also that it is cubic, not just along a plane surface. He therefore injects twenty or so droplets into the area of tenderness, near the surface of the tendon no less than down on the bone, feeling exactly where each droplet appears under his thumb. Great precision is required, for the entire lesion must be infiltrated with a series of tiny neighbouring punctures, by a half-withdrawal of the needle and its reinsertion at a slightly different angle. Multiple punctures avoid the many failures that are encountered today. Patients are frequently encountered in whom a number of injections have failed, but this method succeeds.

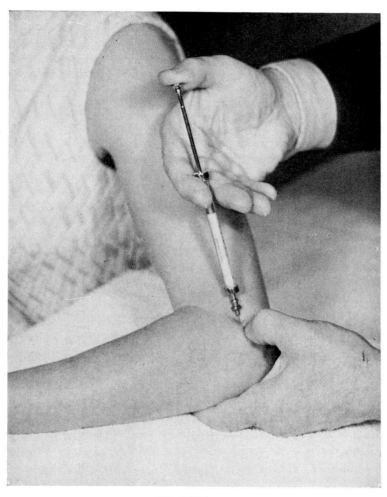

PLATE 41

After-treatment—If triamcinolone is employed the patient will suffer considerable discomfort at the time of the injection and until next morning. If hydrocortisone is used, the pain is quite severe for two days and an analgesic at night will be required. She must not use her hand much for a week afterwards, but at the end of a fortnight should be able to play tennis and so forth. She should be seen again after a day or two's normal activities and resisted extension at the wrist tested again. If it is wholly painless, no more need be done. If it aches slightly, so little that the patient declares herself to be quite happy to put up with such minor discomfort, the injection *must* be repeated, or full relapse within a month or two is a certainty. If two adequate injections fail to cure, a third is seldom helpful.

Results—Two-thirds of all teno-periosteal tennis elbows get well with one or two injections and stay well. The remaining third remain well for two to six months and then relapse at regular intervals. This can go on for several years, since the steroid infiltrations inhibit the tendency to spontaneous cure that otherwise takes place after a year.

The failures require (*a*) massage and Mill's manipulation; (*b*) sclerosant injections; or (*c*) tenotomy (see Volume I).

PLATE 42

TENNIS ELBOW: BODY OF TENDON

Massage Technique

Lesion—The physical signs indicate that the lesion lies in the extensores carpi radialis muscles (see Plate 39), but the tenderness is found in the body of the tendon, 5 to 10 mm below the epicondyle. Scarring at this site is uncommon.

Indication—Friction is in my experience more successful than steroid suspension when the substance of the tendon is affected.

Patient's Posture—The patient sits and holds his forearm 45° short of full extension and in nearly full pronation at the elbow-joint. The affected part of the muscle then overlies the head anteriorly.

Technique—The physiotherapist sits facing the patient, holding his forearm in the above position by one hand at his wrist. She grasps the patient's forearm with the fingers and thumb of her other hand. With the flexed thumb she identifies the antero-medial edge of the muscles and finds the affected area. Tenderness here is universal and careful comparison of the two sides is therefore essential. The physiotherapist imparts the friction by drawing her thumb outwards by alternate flexion and extension movements of her wrist. By using the fingers as a fulcrum, her thumb catches the edge of the tendon; at each stroke this is felt to slip under her thumb. Twenty minutes twice weekly suffices. Manipulation or exercises do not follow.

Result—Six sessions of this treatment usually afford lasting relief.

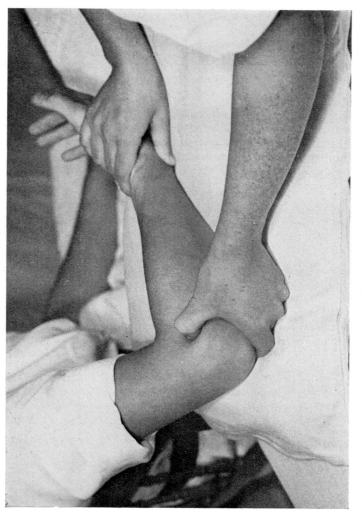

PLATE 42

TENNIS ELBOW: BELLY OF EXTENSOR MUSCLES

Injection Technique

Lesion—When the lesion lies at the upper part of the belly of the extensor carpi radialis muscle, the pain is usually less severe than in teno-periosteal scarring.

Physical Signs—The elbow is normal; a full and painless range of passive movement is present and no resisted elbow movement hurts either. When resisted extension of the wrist is tested, pain at the upper forearm is provoked; resisted flexion and both deviations prove painless. Palpation shows the epicondyle not to be tender. One possibility is then a lesion in the belly and palpation reveals its site.

Patient's Posture—The patient sits, her forearm supported on a table. Her elbow is flexed to a right-angle and held supinated. The lesion is now sought by deep palpation avoiding the brachio-radialis muscle, which takes no part in extending the wrist, but is deceptively tender.

Technique—A 10 ml syringe is filled with 0·5% procaine solution and a 5 cm thin needle is fitted. The lesion is now held pinched up by the physician's left thumb and index finger and the needle inserted obliquely through the belly of the brachio-radialis muscle until the point lies between his fingertips. While the 10 ml are being injected the needle is kept moving so as to infiltrate all over the area of the lesion. Five minutes later resisted wrist extension is tested again. If the right spot has been dealt with, this movement no longer hurts.

Result—Two or three weekly injections afford lasting relief in almost every case. Massage is extremely painful and seldom successful.

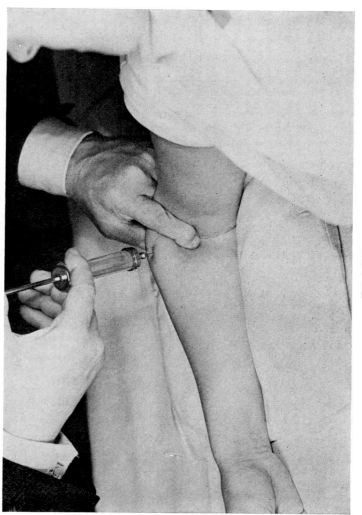

PLATE 43

TENNIS ELBOW: ORIGIN OF EXTENSOR CARPI RADIALIS LONGUS MUSCLE

Massage Technique

Frequency—It is unfortunate that this is so rare a type of tennis elbow, only one or two in a hundred cases, since it is the easiest to cure.

Indication—Lesion of the extensor carpi radialis muscle at its origin from the supracondylar ridge of the humerus. Massage is extremely effective in this variety of tennis elbow; steroid suspension is not.

Patient's Posture—The patient sits with his elbow held at a right-angle and fully supinated.

Technique—The physiotherapist sits facing the patient and places the tip of her thumb on the antero-lateral aspect of the humerus, just above the epicondyle. Her fingers apply counter-pressure at the back of the elbow. She imparts the friction by drawing her thumb backwards and forwards over the area of muscular origin, bending her thumb a little more at the interphalangeal joint during the movement towards herself.

Duration of Treatment—Twenty minutes two or three times a week. Manipulation and exercises do not follow.

Result—Full relief may be confidently expected in three to six treatments.

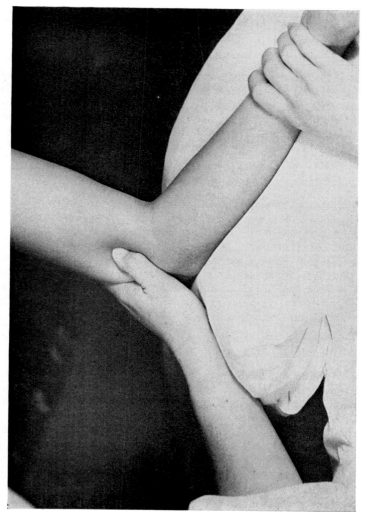

PLATE 44

GOLFER'S ELBOW: COMMON FLEXOR TENDON AT MEDIAL HUMERAL EPICONDYLE

Massage Technique

Lesion—A painful scar at the origin of the common flexor tendon from the medial humeral epicondyle. It results from repeated overstrain chiefly in patients aged 40 to 60. A strong forehand drive at tennis is apt to cause a golfer's elbow, and a patient may give himself a golfer's elbow on his right side and a tennis elbow on his left side by playing golf. The two names do not have aetiological significance, they merely designate the common cause.

Intention—To break up the fibrous scar by friction.

Physical Signs—The pain is felt at the inner side of the elbow and is not referred far down the forearm. The passive elbow movements are of full range and flexion, extension and supination against resistance are painless. Resisted pronation often hurts since the pronator muscle takes origin partly from the common flexor tendon. Resisted flexion at the wrist, but not resisted extension, provokes pain at the elbow. The tender area is found directly on the anterior aspect of the medial epicondyle of the humerus at the origin of the flexor tendon; occasionally it lies a little farther down at the inferior edge of the epicondyle.

Patient's Posture—The patient sits on a high couch, the physiotherapist standing behind him level with his elbow.

Technique—The physiotherapist holds his elbow in extension by pressing upwards on his upper forearm and downwards on his wrist. Her other hand spans the front of his elbow, the thumb at the outer side for counter-pressure, the index, supported by the long finger-tip, applied to the front of the epicondyle. The movement of her finger must not be vertical (this enables her merely to give massage to the apex) but almost horizontal, as it follows the surface of the epicondyle. The motive force to the finger is alternating flexion and extension of the wrist. The very strongest friction is scarcely powerful enough.

The massage is very painful and lasts some fifteen minutes. It is continued two or three times a week till the patient is well. Six to twelve sessions are often required.

After-treatment—The patient should avoid doing anything that hurts until recovery is complete.

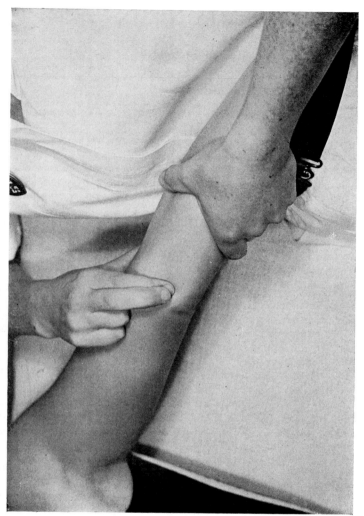

PLATE 45

GOLFER'S ELBOW: COMMON FLEXOR TENDON

Injection Technique

Lesion—A painful scar exists at the origin of the common flexor tendon at the medial epicondyle of the humerus.

Physical Signs—A full range of passive movement is present at the elbow without pain at any extreme. The resisted elbow movements do not hurt, except for pronation, but resisted flexion of the wrist tested with an extended elbow hurts, whereas resisted extension does not.

The tender point is found at the anterior aspect of the medial humeral epicondyle. If the musculo-tendinous junction is at fault 5 mm farther down, the treatment is massage; hydrocortisone is no longer effective.

Intention—To transform a painful scar in the tendon into a painless one, devoid of inflammation.

Patient's Posture—The patient sits with her forearm supported on a table and the elbow held fully supinated and in slight flexion.

Technique—The four edges of the tender area of tendon are carefully ascertained and the physician places his thumb on the most tender point. Triamcinolone is the steroid of choice; it is just as effective as hydrocortisone and provokes much less after-pain (for twelve rather than forty-eight hours). A 1 ml tuberculin syringe is filled with the suspension and fitted with a fine needle 2 cm long. It is thrust vertically downwards until the resistance of the tendon is felt and a droplet injected there. The needle is pushed on until its tip reaches bone, and a further droplet is injected at the teno-periosteal junction. By means of a series of withdrawals and reinsertions the whole affected area is infiltrated. The physician's thumb feels the exact site as each droplet goes in. He can thus be sure of covering the whole area.

After-treatment—The hand is used as little as possible for a week and after a fortnight the patient tries her elbow out. She is seen again after a day or two's full use and resisted flexion of the wrist is tested anew. If it causes any discomfort at all, the injection must be repeated or full relapse is inevitable.

Result—Nearly all golfer's elbows of the teno-periosteal variety get well with one or two steroid injections. Recurrence after some months is rare. If this does happen, deep friction to the scar must be substituted.

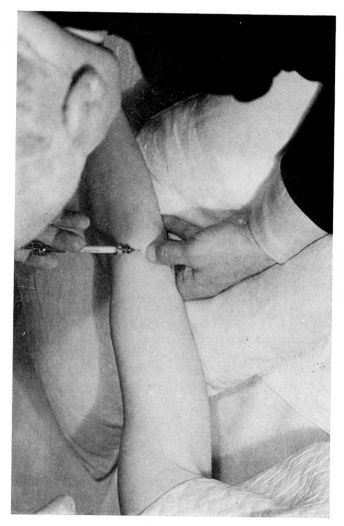

PLATE 46

GOLFER'S ELBOW: MUSCULO-TENDINOUS JUNCTION

Massage Technique

Lesion—Strain occurs at the musculo-tendinous junction as well as at the teno-periosteal junction. It follows a series of repeated often occupational strains rather than a single injury. The affected fibres lie level with the inferior edge of the medial epicondyle. The treatment is massage; hydrocortisone is ineffective.

Physical Signs—See Plate 45.

Patient's Posture—The patient adopts the half-lying position on the couch, his arm stretched out horizontally and supported. His arm is laterally rotated so as to bring the medial epicondyle to face forwards.

Technique—The physiotherapist stands behind his elbow and holds his forearm supinated and his elbow extended with one hand; this maintains the medial epicondyle in an accessible position. With the index finger of her other hand, reinforced by the middle finger, she identifies the medial epicondyle and then shifts her hand a quarter of an inch distally; this brings the ulnar border of her index finger to lie against the lower border of the epicondyle. Her thumb applies counter-pressure at the outer aspect of the elbow. By keeping her finger pressing, and by flexing and extending her wrist, her whole hand is made to rotate to and fro round the forearm. As a result, the physiotherapist's index finger is drawn backwards and forwards over the musculo-tendinous junction. Considerable pain is provoked.

Result—Recovery is to be expected in from four to eight sessions.

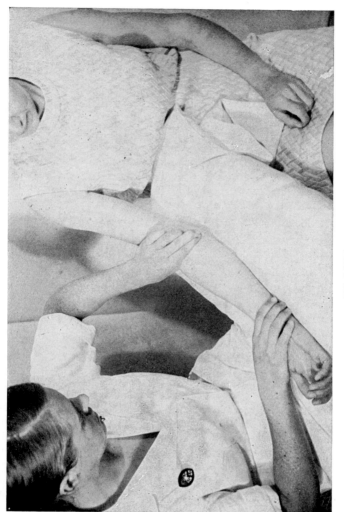

PLATE 47

ELBOW-JOINT: REDUCTION OF DISPLACED LOOSE BODY

Lesion—A loose body in the elbow-joint may form as the result of an injury which chips off a piece of cartilage—in such a case the radiograph does not reveal its existence. In osteochondrosis dissecans the fragment consists of bone and is visible on the X-ray plate. In marked osteoarthrosis, several bony loose bodies may form and give rise to attacks of internal derangement.

Physical Signs—The non-capsular pattern is present. If the loose body lies in the triangle formed by capitellum, head of radius and the base of the coronoid process, extension is limited, flexion not. In such cases manipulative reduction is often successful. If the loose body lies anteriorly, catching between the surface of the humerus and the tip of the coronoid process, flexion alone is limited and manipulative reduction is not possible.

Indication for Manipulation—Displacement of a loose body causing limitation of extension.

Patient's Posture—The patient adopts the half-lying position; keeping her trunk at the far side of the couch she abducts her affected arm to the horizontal and bends her elbow to a right-angle. An assistant, standing at her head, supplies counter-traction by grasping her arm just above the elbow with both hands. Another assistant steadies the thorax with her hand, so that it does not move towards the manipulator when he pulls. Her other hand holds the shoulder on to the couch, so that it does not shift forwards at the moment when he extends the elbow.

Technique—Traction must be maintained while rotation is forced and the elbow-joint gradually extended meanwhile. The manipulator therefore grasps the patient's wrist with both hands and pulls hard. He pivots on his foot while rotating her forearm quickly to and fro, and, at the last moment, by bending his trunk away from the couch, extends the patient's elbow as far as it will go and then forces it a little farther. No endeavour must be made to achieve full extension at first. He and the patient may feel a click during one of the attempts, the range of movement being afterwards found to have increased. However, since the elbow remains the site of traumatic arthritis consequent upon the original subluxation of the loose body, the joint does not regain its full range of movement immediately, even after successful reduction. Experience alone teaches the manipulator when reduction has probably been obtained and how long to go on trying at any one session.

After-treatment—If the displacement has persisted for some months before reduction is carried out, a traumatic arthritis that may take some weeks to subside may delay recovery. If so, an intra-articular injection of hydrocortisone is required when the patient is seen a day or two later.

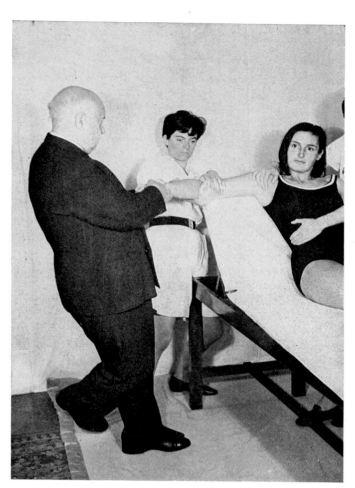

PLATE 48

ELBOW-JOINT: INTRA-ARTICULAR INJECTION

Lesion—Traumatic or rheumatoid arthritis.

Physical Signs—The capsular pattern of limited movement. In the early stage, these proportions are slightly more restriction of flexion than of extension, with full and painless passive rotation. Only in advanced arthritis is rotation limited as well.

Patient's Posture—The patient lies prone, her arm by her side, the elbow straight and the forearm fully supinated. In this position the crack between the capitellum and the head of the radius is easily felt.

Technique—A 2 ml syringe is filled with steroid suspension and a thin needle 2 cm long is fitted. The interval between the humerus and the head of the radius is identified and the needle inserted vertically downwards to its full length.

Results—In traumatic arthritis two, possibly three, injections at weekly intervals restore full range; this otherwise takes some three months with the elbow held flexed, first in a collar-and-cuff bandage, later in a sling.

When rheumatoid arthritis of some standing has led to organic change, a full range can never be restored but even so pain ceases, usually for many months. Thereupon the injection can be repeated. There need be no fear of steroid arthropathy, since the elbow is not a weight-bearing joint.

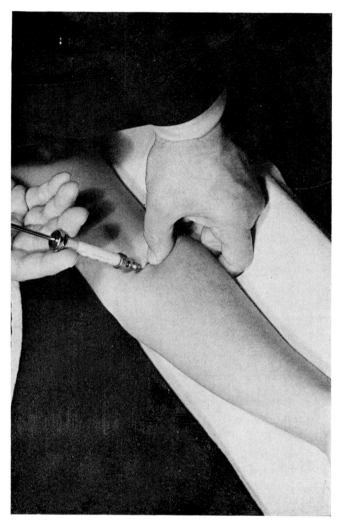

PLATE 49

PLATE 50

SUPINATOR MUSCLE

Massage Technique

Lesion—The strain in the muscle fibres of the supinator (brevis) muscle appears always to lie in that part of the belly palpable between the upper ends of the shafts of radius and ulna posteriorly. It is rare and always mistaken for a tennis elbow. The only effective treatment is deep massage.

Physical Signs—Unlocalized pain is felt in the elbow region. A full range of painless passive movement is found at the elbow-joint. Resisted supination hurts, particularly when it is tested with the elbow held voluntarily in extension, so as to prevent assistance from the biceps muscle. Resisted flexion of the elbow does not hurt, thus exculpating the biceps muscle. The resisted movements at the wrist are painless. The supinator muscle is not found particularly tender.

Patient's Posture—The patient's forearm is supported in full pronation. In this position the muscle belly is at its most accessible.

Technique—The physiotherapist places her thumb over the affected area of muscle and presses in deeply, slightly flexing her interphalangeal joint. Her fingers supply counter-pressure at the back of the patient's elbow. Alternate abduction and adduction of her thumb supply the deep friction.

Duration of Treatment—Fifteen minutes two or three times a week.

Results—Cure takes four to eight sessions.

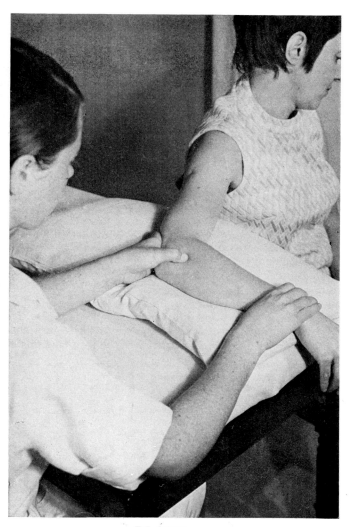

PLATE 50

LOWER RADIO-ULNAR JOINT

Injection Technique

Lesion—Isolated arthritis of the lower radio-ulnar joint is apt to come on for no apparent reason; a few cases are traumatic. In either event, forcing movement and massage both increase symptoms. The only effective conservative treatment is intra-articular injection of steroid suspension.

Physical Signs—Pain at the wrist brought on at the extreme of both passive rotations of the forearm. The passive movements at the wrist prove painless and no resisted movement hurts. The lower radio-ulnar joint is seldom appreciably tender.

Patient's Posture—The patient sits with her pronated hand supported on a table.

Injection Technique—A 1 ml syringe is filled with steroid suspension and fitted with a needle 2 cm long. The head of the ulna is easily seen and felt. By moving the ulna backwards and forwards on the radius the line of cleavage between them can be identified. A point is chosen on this line, 5 mm proximal to the sharp lower edge of the ulna. The joint is not much more than 1 cm long, hence the insertion is made level with its midpoint. The needle is thrust down till it hits bone at about 1·5 cm. It is then manoeuvred about until it is felt to slip beyond, without resistance. The needle is too short to emerge on the far side of the joint, and the injection is carried out.

Results—Uniformly good.

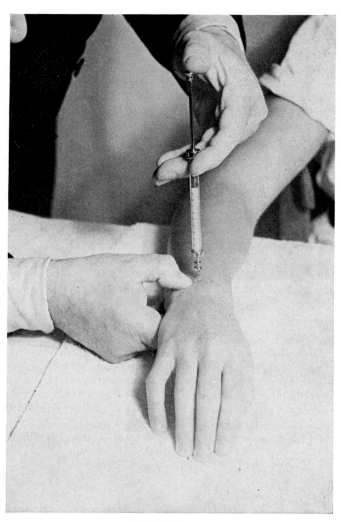

PLATE 51

CARPAL TUNNEL

Injection Technique

Lesion—Compression of the trunk of the median nerve under the transverse carpal ligament. This may be idiopathic or frictional, i.e. caused by to-and-fro movements of the wrist while it is kept extended or by disorders causing thickening of the tendons, e.g. a trigger, rheumatoid arthritis, acromegaly or myxoedema.

Physical Signs—Paraesthesia felt at the palmar aspect of all four digits but not the little finger. Keeping the wrist flexed for a minute and suddenly extending it causes a shower of pins and needles.

Patient's Posture—The patient sits, her forearm supported in full supination on a table with the wrist slightly extended.

Injection Technique—A 2 ml syringe is filled with steroid suspension and fitted with a needle 5 cm long. A point is chosen 4 cm above the wrist on its dorsal surface. The needle is thrust in almost horizontally and is passed its full length into the carpal tunnel. Since the needle runs nearly parallel to tendons and nerve, it does not pierce them but comes to lie between them. The entire syringeful is injected under the transverse ligament.

Result—This is both diagnostic and therapeutic. Many diagnoses of pressure on the median nerve in the carpal tunnel are tentative, since differentiation from the thoracic outlet syndrome and from acroparaesthesia of cervical origin is often difficult. If the pins and needles cease for some weeks after the injection, the right spot was clearly injected. If they stay away for months or years, all that is needed is another injection. If they come back quickly, division of the ligament is called for. If they do not cease at all, the diagnosis is mistaken.

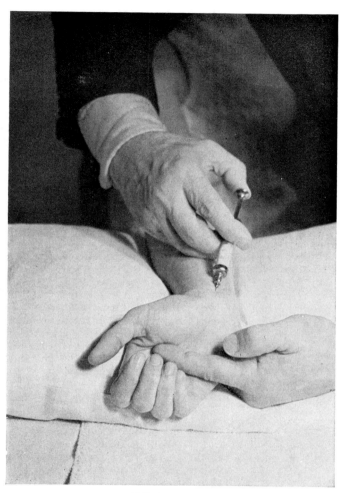

PLATE 52

EXTENSORES CARPI RADIALIS TENDONS

Massage Technique

Lesion—Teno-synovitis here results from overuse. The lesion lies at the distal half-inch of the tendons and at the teno-periosteal junction at the dorsal aspect of the base of the second and third metacarpal bones.

Physical Signs—The pain is acutely felt at the dorsum of the wrist. A full and painless range of movement is present at the joint; resisted extension and radial deviation hurt and the other two resisted movements do not. The tender spot is easy to find. Deep friction is the treatment of choice.

Patient's Posture—The patient sits on a pillow, and his wrist flexed over the edge of the couch.

Technique—The physiotherapist sits beside the patient, half-facing him. With one hand she holds his wrist flexed, so as to stretch the tendons. With the middle finger-tip of the other hand she identifies the affected stretch of tendon. Usually both radial extensor tendons are affected. She reinforces with the index finger. Friction is imparted to the tendons by means of a horizontal to-and-fro movement of her whole forearm and hand.

Duration of Treatment—Twenty minutes three times a week. Neither exercises nor passive movements should follow. For the duration of treatment, the patient should avoid such exertion as causes pain. Splintage is quite unnecessary.

Result—Recovery should be complete in two weeks.

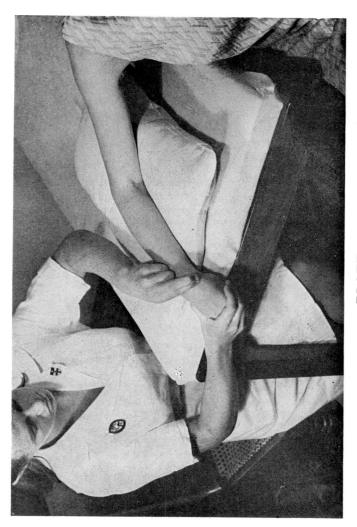

PLATE 53

LIGAMENTS ABOUT CAPITATE BONE

Massage Technique

Lesion—Adhesions form dorsally at these ligaments after a flexion sprain of the wrist, with or without actual subluxation of the capitate bone. If a subluxation has existed for months, manipulation restores alignment but residual symptoms may continue owing to persistence of the consequent chronic ligamentous strain. The ligament between the capitate and either the lunate or the metacarpal bone—sometimes both—is that commonly affected. No ligament at the dorsum of the wrist is immune, however, and search for tenderness must go on until all the affected ligaments have been identified. In general ligamentous adhesions require manipulative rupture. At the wrist, however, this generalization does not hold and manipulation of the usual sort causes aggravation, whereas massage is quickly curative. Splintage is quite useless.

Physical Signs—The pain is felt at the dorsum of the wrist and is elicited by full passive flexion of the joint. The other passive and resisted movements do not hurt. The tender spots lie superficially and are easily found if the wrist is kept flexed.

Patient's Posture—His wrist is held fully flexed so as to make each ligament as accessible as possible.

Technique—The physiotherapist sits at the patient's side, facing him. She maintains flexion of his wrist by the pressure of one hand, and places the tip of her thumb on the ligament. To this end she has to push the digital extensor tendons aside and get the tip of her thumb between them directly on to the ligament. Pressure is maintained by her fingers at the front of the wrist. The frictional movement is imparted by alternate radial and ulnar deviation of her wrist.

Alternative Technique—See Plate 54a.

Duration of Treatment—Each affected ligament receives some ten minutes' transverse friction.

Result—No matter whether the sprain is recent or of many years' standing, full recovery is established after two to six sessions.

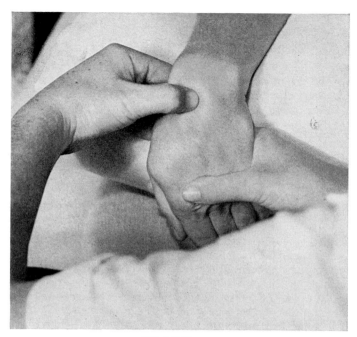

PLATE 54

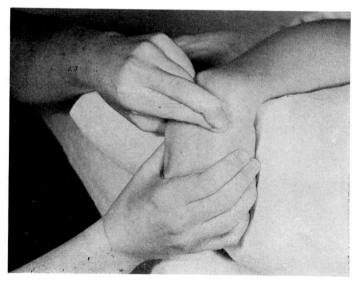

PLATE 54a

EXTENSOR CARPI ULNARIS TENDON

Massage Technique

Lesion—Teno-synovitis here usually follows over-use. The lesion usually occurs at the part of tendon between the metacarpal and cuneiform bones, but may occur between the latter and the head of the ulna, or rarely at the groove on the ulna.

Physical Signs—The pain is felt at the ulnar side of the wrist and is evoked by resisted extension and ulnar deviation. The passive wrist movements are of full range but radial deviation may hurt by stretching the tendon. While the wrist is held in full radial deviation, the tender spot in the tendon is sought.

Patient's Posture—The patient sits with his forearm placed pronated on a high couch.

Technique—The physiotherapist stands facing him. With one hand she grasps his fingers and maintains full radial deviation at the wrist. This position separates the base of the metacarpal bone from the cuneiform bone and the head of the ulna, thus enabling the physiotherapist's finger to obtain adequate access at each site. She grasps the patient's wrist with her hand in such a way that her long and index fingers lie on the affected stretch of tendon, and her thumb on the side of the wrist. The friction is imparted by a to-and-fro movement of her fingers across the tendon; this is attained by alternate flexion and extension movements at her wrist. The thumb is used as a fulcrum and to supply counter-pressure.

Duration of Treatment—Twenty minutes three times a week. No exercises follow. Until well, the patient should avoid any painful exertion. Splintage does not hasten recovery.

Result—Full relief is obtainable in two weeks.

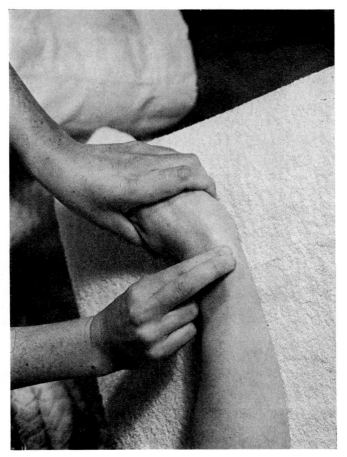

PLATE 55

ABDUCTOR LONGUS AND BOTH EXTENSOR POLLICIS TENDONS IN LOWER FOREARM

Massage Technique

Lesion—Teno-synovitis here is always the result of occupational over-use and is common at hay-making time. All three tendons are affected together. In recent cases crepitus is common, but has been encountered even after several months' immobilization.

Indication for Massage—Teno-synovitis, acute or chronic. Neither crepitus, swelling nor an effusion contra-indicates massage.

Physical Signs—The pain is felt at the radial side of the lower forearm and is evoked by resisted extension and abduction of the thumb. Moving the thumb may set up crepitus.

Patient's Posture—The patient sits and places his forearm on a pillow on a high couch, letting his wrist flex over the edge.

Technique—The physiotherapist sits facing the patient's forearm, facing him. With one hand she holds his wrist flexed, her thumb and fingers at the front of the wrist and her thumb along the affected tendons where they cross the dorsal aspect of the lower end of the radius. She imparts the friction by alternately adducting and abducting her thumb while maintaining pressure. The tendons are clearly palpable as her thumb rides over them.

Duration of Treatment—Twenty minutes three times a week. No exercises follow. Splintage affords no added advantage.

Result—Full relief is achieved in a fortnight.

N.B.—When the abductor longus and extensor brevis tendons are affected at their carpal extent (de Quervain's disease, styloiditis radii, tenovaginitis stenosans) massage is very painful and takes three months to succeed. Since one injection of steroid suspension is curative, both massage and operative slitting of the tendon sheath are obsolete.

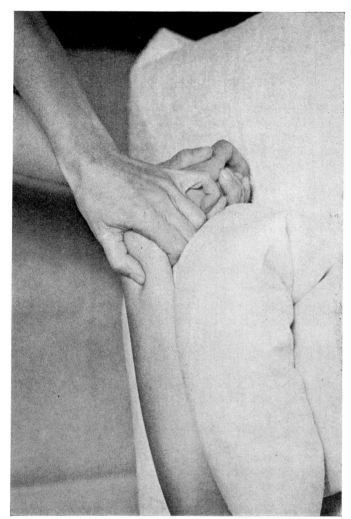

PLATE 56

ABDUCTOR LONGUS AND EXTENSOR BREVIS POLLICIS TENDONS AT CARPUS

Injection Technique

Lesion—The lesion is a teno-vaginitis but often comes on without the repeated overuse that causes tendon trouble elsewhere. It is known as de Quervain's disease, teno-vaginitis stenosans and styloiditis radii. The outstanding finding is the misleading tenderness of the styloid process of the radius; hence the name. Untreated, it continues for several years. The disorder used to be treated by slitting the tendon sheath at operation, or by three months' deep massage. Both are now out of date.

Physical Signs—The pain is felt at the radial side of the wrist, radiating up the forearm and down the thumb. A full range of movement is present at the wrist, but full passive ulnar deviation often hurts, since this stretches the tendons. Resisted radial deviation of the wrist may hurt too, since the thumb tendons assist this movement. Resisted extension and abduction of the thumb hurt. The tendons are tender at their carpal extent but not so markedly as at the styloid process itself, where no lesion lies. There is usually a visible swelling here.

Patient's Posture—The patient sits at a table, her forearm supported on a cushion. An assistant holds her thumb fully flexed and the wrist in full ulnar deviation and slight extension. This stretches the tendons which can be seen and felt.

Injection Technique—A 1 ml syringe is filled with steroid suspension and fitted with a thin needle 2 cm long. A point is chosen level with the base of the first metacarpal bone and the needle thrust in horizontally a short way. The operator pinches the tendon between his thumb and index fingers and passes the needle along, almost parallel to the tendon, piercing the sheath. The needle tends to run along the surface between tendon and sheath, no resistance being encountered. A small amount is now injected and, if the tip lies correctly, a small sausage shape can be felt to form along the course of the tendon, extending to the groove on the radius. If so, the syringeful is injected here.

After-treatment—The patient uses her hand as little as possible for a week, then she does what she likes.

Result—Consistent success is obtainable with one injection; occasionally two are required.

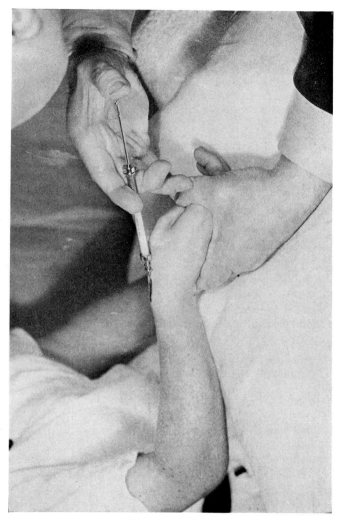

PLATE 57

PLATE 58

DIGITAL FLEXOR TENDONS IN LOWER FOREARM

Massage Technique

Lesion—This is an over-use teno-synovitis. It occurs well above the level of the carpus. Physiotherapists are liable to this lesion.

Massage is effective; so is steroid suspension injected between the tendons.

Contra-indication—Rheumatoid teno-synovitis of these tendons, identified by local warmth and/or the development of nodules along the tendons. In these cases only hydrocortisone is effective.

Physical Signs—The pain is felt at the anterior aspect of the lower forearm and is brought on only by resisted flexion of the fingers.

Patient's Posture—The patient sits with his forearm supinated and supported on a high couch.

Technique—The physiotherapist sits facing the patient. With one hand she holds his fingers and wrist extended so as to stretch the digital flexor tendons. She places three fingers of the other hand on the affected length of tendon. Friction is imparted by her drawing her whole forearm to and fro so that the fingers ride over the tendon from side to side.

Duration of Treatment—This should last twenty minutes on alternate days. Exercises do not follow and the patient should avoid such movements as cause pain until well. Splintage is unnecessary.

Results—Lasting relief is secured in a fortnight.

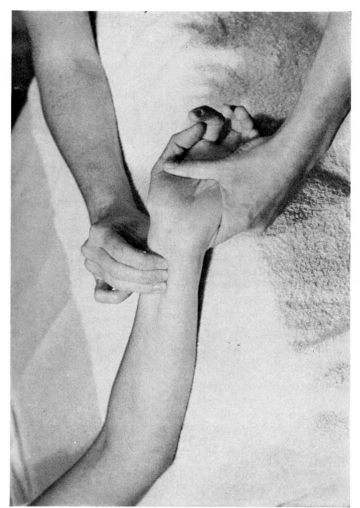

PLATE 58

FLEXOR CARPI ULNARIS TENDON

Massage Technique

Lesion—A single overstrain causes a painful scar to form at the teno-periosteal junction between the tendon and the base of the fifth metacarpal bone, beyond the pisiform bone. Both deep friction and injection of a steroid suspension are effective.

Physical Signs—The pain is localized and is provoked by resisted flexion and ulnar deviation at the wrist.

Patient's Posture—The patient sits with his forearm held horizontally and the wrist extended.

Technique—Only an exceptionally strong physiotherapist can give effective friction here. She sits by the patient's side facing him. Her one hand grasps his palm, thus holding his hand in extension. The patient's little finger stays loosely flexed so as to relax the hypothenar muscles. The physiotherapist presses her thumb with all her might on the affected point, applying her fingers at the dorsum of his wrist for counter-pressure. By alternately pronating and supinating her forearm, the thumb is drawn to and fro over the teno-periosteal junction. This friction hurts the physio-therapist far more than the patient.

Duration of Treatment—As long as the physiotherapist can manage. Ten minutes, followed by ten minutes' rest, then another ten minutes once a week is enough.

Results—Four to six treatments suffice.

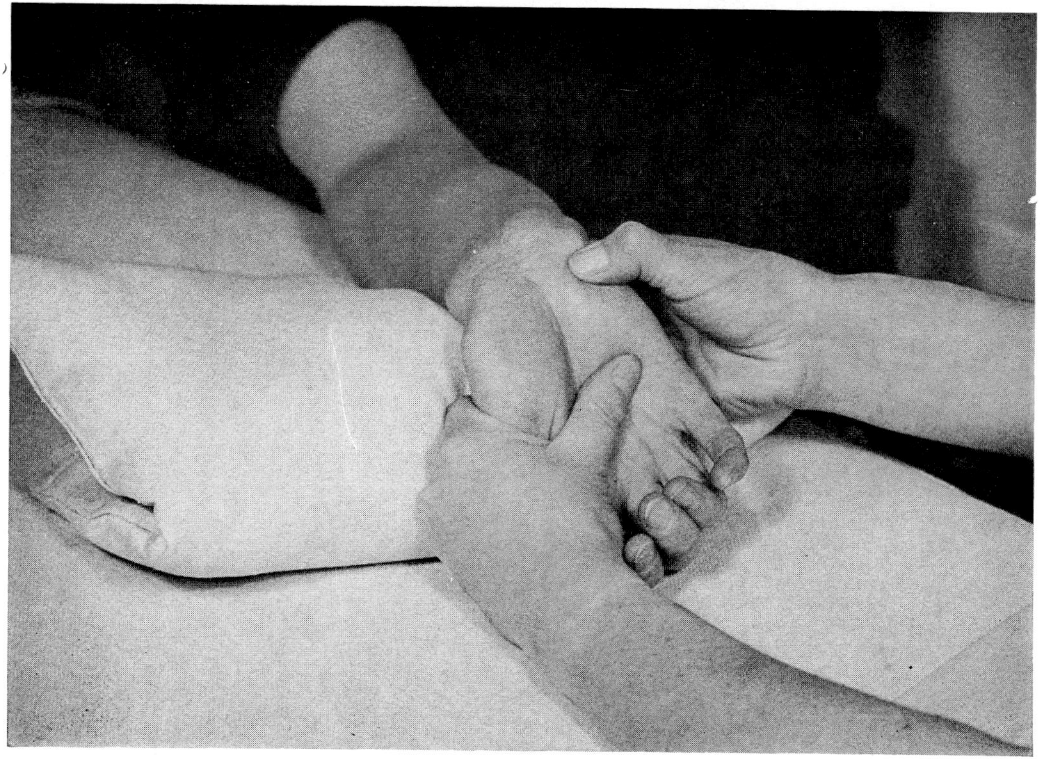

PLATE 59

WRIST-JOINT: REDUCTION OF CARPAL
SUBLUXATION I

Lesion—Persistent subluxation between the capitate and lunate bones.

Physical Signs—The pain is localized to the dorsum of the wrist. Passive flexion is full and painful; extension is 5° or 10° limited and also hurts. The passive deviations are painless, as are the resisted movements. The ligaments about the capitate bone are tender.

Patient's Posture—The patient lies on a high couch and bends her elbow to a right-angle. An assistant stands behind her, her fingers locked about the front of the patient's arm just above the elbow. The arm is thus held against the back of the couch.

Technique—The manipulator stands level with the patient's hips, his foot against the assistant's foot, placed forwards for his benefit. He leans backwards and grasps the patient's forearm and hand, one of his thumbs lying just above, the other just below, her wrist. He pulls only with the hand grasping the patient's hand. During traction, his two hands are moved vertically up and down in opposite directions while his little finger presses up against her palm to ensure an antero-posterior glide devoid of flexion-extension element. (The photograph shows the extreme of downward movement of the manipulator's distally placed hand.) This manoeuvre is not painful and is repeated until a full range of movement has been restored to the wrist.

N.B.—Traction on the wrist is lost if the manipulator pulls with the hand holding the patient's forearm.

Results—Reduction is easy and immediate relief follows even in cases that have persisted for years. Symptoms due to secondary ligamentous strain occasionally remain after reduction, but disappear at once following one or two sessions of deep massage. If the ligament between the capitate and the third metacarpal bone has ruptured the reduction cannot last.

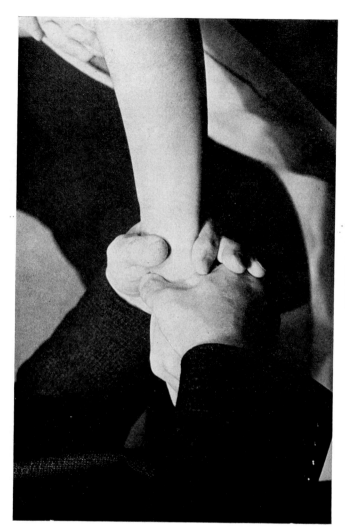

PLATE 60

WRIST-JOINT: REDUCTION OF CARPAL SUBLUXATION II

Indication—If the first manipulation has not secured full painless range at the wrist and repetition makes no further difference, the final minor adjustment should be attempted by this method.

Patient's Posture—Unchanged.

Technique—The manipulator grasps the patient's hand as before and leans backwards, applying strong traction to the wrist. His right thumb and index encircle the joint and, when he has pulled for a few seconds, he squeezes the wrist as hard as he can. This applies further traction and presses the bones together at the same time. A little click is felt when reduction is achieved.

Duration of Treatment—Once or twice is enough.

Note—It is not possible to maintain reduction if the capitate—third-metocarpal ligament has actually ruptured. Ligamentous sclerosis is then indicated.

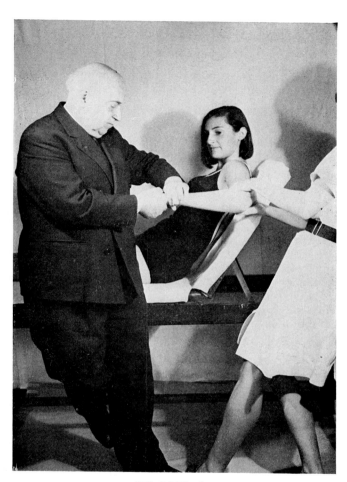

PLATE 61

TRAPEZIO-FIRST-METACARPAL JOINT

Massage Technique

Lesion—Osteoarthrosis or traumatic arthritis. The anterior aspect of the joint capsule is usually that chiefly affected.

Physical Signs—The pain is felt in the thenar area and is brought on by passive backwards stretching of the thumb in abduction. The resisted thumb movements are painless as are the passive and resisted wrist movements. The trapezio-first-metacarpal joint is found tender anteriorly.

Patient's Posture—The patient sits and puts his hand, palm facing upwards, on a high couch.

Technique—The physiotherapist sits by the patient's side, facing him. She holds his thumb with one hand, hyperabducting it in extension so as to bring the front of the joint into prominence. The thumb of her other hand is well flexed at the terminal joint and placed on the joint line. Her fingers apply counter-pressure dorsally. She imparts the friction by alternately pronating and supinating her forearm. This moves the thumb to and fro over the joint capsule.

The physiotherapist now flexes the patient's thumb and brings his forearm more into pronation. Using the same technique as before, she now applies friction to the outer aspect of the joint (not illustrated).

Duration of Treatment—Fifteen minutes twice a week.

Results—Traumatic arthritis responds well; recovery is secured in two or three weeks. The effect is good in early osteoarthrosis but in the advanced case intra-articular silicone is to be preferred and largely obviates the necessity for operation.

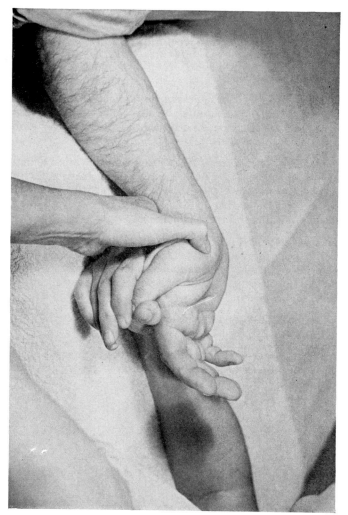

PLATE 62

TRAPEZIO-FIRST-METACARPAL JOINT

Injection Technique

Lesion—Traumatic or rheumatoid arthritis or osteoarthrosis of the trapezio-first-metacarpal joint.

Physical Signs—In early cases the pain is brought on by pressing the thumb backwards while it is held in abduction. Later the first metacarpal bone becomes fixed in adduction. In osteoarthrosis, crepitus is present and osteophytes are palpable anteriorly.

Patient's Posture—The patient sits, her supinated forearm resting on a table. An assistant distracts the joint surfaces pulling hard on the thumb and exerting counter-pressure with her other hand at the upper forearm. The base of the first metacarpal bone is identified dorsally, with the assistance of the gap resulting from the distraction.

Injection Technique—A 1 ml syringe is filled with steroid suspension and fitted with a thin needle 2 cm long. The needle is directed at the gap at an angle of 60°. If it hits bone at about 1 cm it does not lie intra-articularly and the tip must be moved until no resistance is felt at 1·5 cm. The injection is now given.

After-treatment—The patient avoids exertion for a few days.

Result—In rheumatoid or traumatic arthritis success is to be expected. In osteoarthrosis intra-articular silicone (12 000 centistoke) is often effective. For this reason arthroplasty and arthrodesis are required less often than formerly.

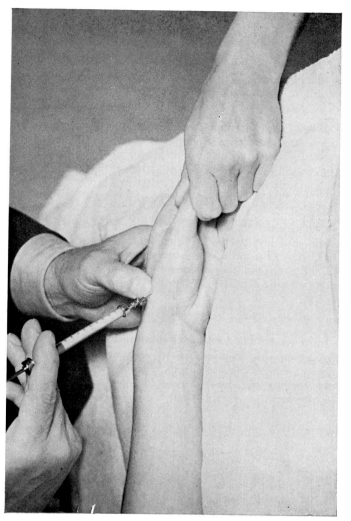

PLATE 63

DORSAL INTEROSSEOUS MUSCLE OF HAND

Massage Technique

Lesion—This is nearly always traumatic, either as the direct result of a blow or secondary to a metacarpal fracture. Strain from over-use occurs in players of stringed instruments. It is a remarkable condition for it goes on unchanged for years, resisting every treatment except massage.

Physical Signs—The pain is felt at the back of the hand. On examination, vague discomfort may be elicited at the extremes of passive movement at one metacarpo-phalangeal joint, but the pain is not felt at the joint itself. Resisted abduction brings on the pain, and tenderness is easily detected between the metacarpal shafts, usually distally.

Patient's Posture—The patient rests his hand on a high couch.

Technique—The physiotherapist sits opposite him, steadying his forearm with one hand. She lays the tip of the middle finger of her other hand between the shafts of the metacarpal bones on the affected area of muscle. The index finger may reinforce the dorsum of the long finger. She imparts the friction by rotating her forearm.

Duration of Treatment—Fifteen minutes is enough. Two or three treatments are all that is required.

Results—In my experience, success follows invariably and quickly, no matter how long the symptoms have lasted. A musician can confidently be told that he will be able to play again more or less without symptoms on the day after the first session of massage, even if he has been wholly incapacitated for months.

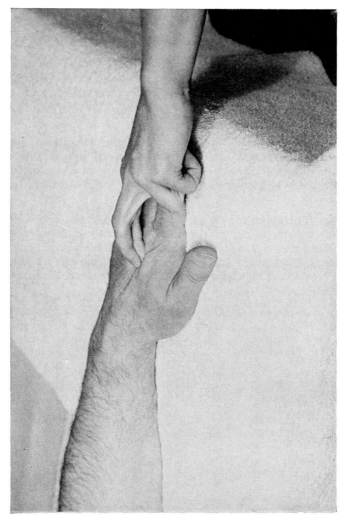

PLATE 64

DORSAL INTEROSSEOUS TENDON OF HAND

Massage Technique

Lesion—Strain of the tendon of the interosseous muscle usually follows sprain of the finger but also occurs in musicians from repeated overstrain. The disorder is often thought to be incurable, since it may go on unchanged for many years and responds to no other treatment except accurate deep friction.

Physical Signs—The pain is accurately felt at one side of one knuckle. Passive stretching of the phalanx away from the painful side hurts, as does resisted movement towards the painful side. The interosseous tendon is found tender either at its insertion into the base of the phalanx or where it crosses the joint.

Technique—The difficulty is to get the other knuckle out of the way, so that the physiotherapist can get the tip of her thumb on to the tendon. To this end, she uses one hand to abduct and depress the adjacent knuckle, while flexing the unaffected finger. She can now get the tip of her flexed thumb on to the tendon and give the massage by a small adduction–abduction movement.

Duration of Treatment—Fifteen minutes twice a week for two or three weeks suffice to bring lasting relief, however long the trouble has lasted.

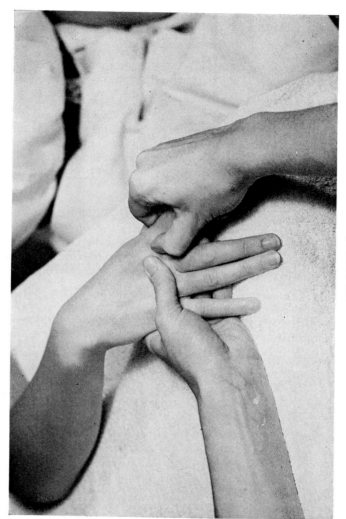

PLATE 65

PLATE 66

INTERCOSTAL MUSCLE

Massage Technique

Lesion—Scarring in this muscle occurs as the result of direct injury, often secondary to fracture of a rib, occasionally for no apparent reason.

Physical Signs—These are largely negative. The pain is so localized that visceral disease or root pressure from a thoracic disc lesion is ruled out. Examination of the active thoracic movements is negative and the resisted movements of the scapula and abdomen do not hurt either. When tenderness is sought, it is found on the muscle rather than the rib itself.

Patient's Posture—The patient adopts the half-lying position on the couch.

Technique—The physiotherapist sits by his side and puts the tip of the middle finger of one hand in the sulcus between two ribs. She may reinforce this finger with the index. The nether finger should be moved to and fro over the affected area in line with the ribs. The movement is imparted by alternately flexing and extending the elbow- and shoulder-joints.

Duration of Treatment—Ten to fifteen minutes on alternate days. Two or three adjacent intercostal muscles are often affected together; each spot should receive not less than ten minutes' friction. One to three sessions suffice to afford lasting relief.

Results—No matter how long-standing the condition, or whether it is of traumatic or apparently spontaneous onset, quick success is invariable.

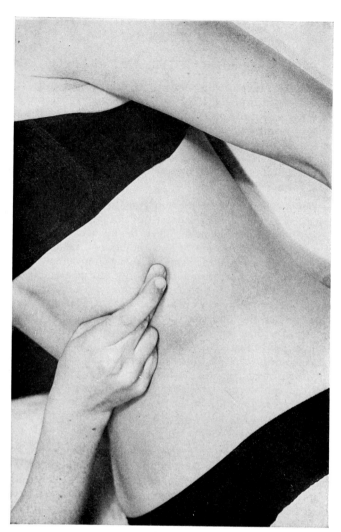

PLATE 66

THORACIC SPINE: EXTENSION DURING TRACTION I

First Manipulation for Thoracic Disc Lesion

Lesion—Formerly, thoracic disc lesions were called 'fibrositis', 'inter-costal neuritis' or 'pleurodynia', the latter presumably because a deep breath or a cough is apt to hurt. Central disc protrusion impinges against the dura mater causing pain at the centre or to one side of the back of the chest. The impact of a postero-lateral displacement is on the intercostal nerve root, causing pain felt radiating within the relevant dermatome, most often along one costal margin, but occasionally to one side of the sternum or to the iliac fossa.

Physical Signs—These relate to the joint, the dura mater, the nerve root and the spinal cord. The *joint signs* consist of the partial articular pattern characterizing internal derangement. When the six active thoracic move-ments are tested, some are found to hurt, others not (flexion, extension, side-flexion each way, rotation each way). The same movements hurt more when tested passively; the resisted movements are painless. The *dural symptoms* are pain on a deep breath and coughing; the *dural signs* are pain brought on or aggravated by neck flexion and/or scapular approximation, both of which stretch the dura mater against the protrusion. Though root pain is common, *root signs* are rare; pins and needles, cutaneous analgesia, or a weak intercostal muscle very seldom appear. *Cord signs* comprise a spastic gait, inco-ordination of the lower limbs, weakness of the bladder and an extensor plantar response. Any evidence of interference with the function of the spinal cord provides an absolute contra-indication to manipulation. Pins and needles in the toes without any organic pyramidal signs call for great caution and suggest a tentative trial of traction rather than of manipulation.

Patient's Posture—The patient lies prone on a low couch, one assistant holding her feet. If, as is usual, the lesion lies at a level between the sixth and the twelfth joint, the other assistant pulls on the arms; they grasp each other's wrists (see Plate 67a). If an upper thoracic disc lesion is present or if the patient has a stiff shoulder the assistant holds the head (see Plate 67b). The patient is asked to relax when she feels the assistants pull. The physiotherapist's traction not only makes success much more likely, but provides an essential safeguard for the integrity of the spinal cord. Since centripetal force is acting on the contents of the joint at the moment of the manipulative thrust, the fragment, if it moves at all, moves towards the centre of the joint. This is an important precaution, since damage to the spinal cord may prove irreparable.

The other safeguard is the avoidance of general anaesthesia. This is contra-indicated since it is impossible to tell on an unconscious patient if manipulation is making her better or worse. Nearly all the cases of damage

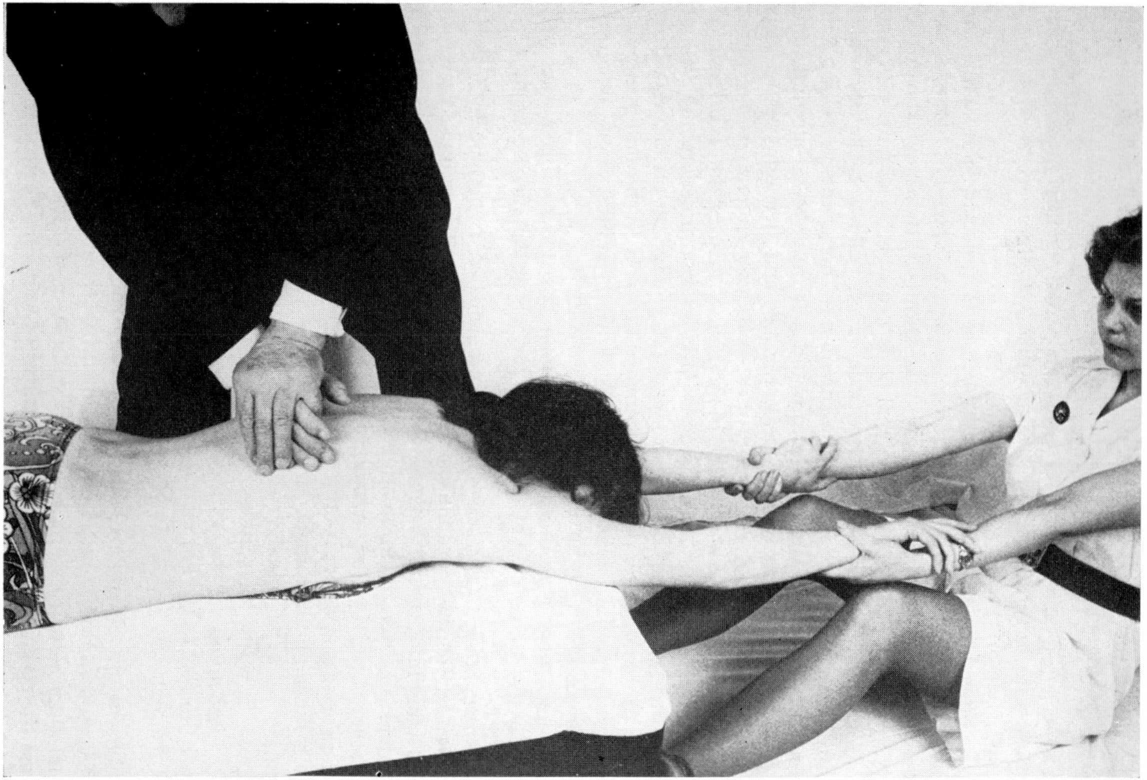

PLATE 67

sustained to the spinal cord during manipulation result either from an attempt during anaesthesia or from chiropractice.

Technique—The correct level is ascertained by gently extending each thoracic joint in turn until the level at which symptoms are most strongly elicited is discovered.

The ulnar border of the palm is applied at the selected joint so that the centre of the fifth metacarpal bone presses on the spinous process at the affected joint. Reinforcement is now given with the other hand, the operator's thumb applied to this metacarpal bone. Now both assistants pull and, after a couple of seconds to let the stretch become effective, the manipulation thrust is given (see Plate 67). At the lower thorax this is a sharp jerk towards extension of very small amplitude; it requires no strength and causes no pain. At the upper thorax, the ribs and sternum greatly limit spinal mobility; here considerably more force is required. At the lower thoracic joints a click is always felt, but its significance (or not) is discovered only at the subsequent examination. After each manoeuvre the patient stands and reports any change in symptoms, including on taking a deep breath; the manipulator notes any change in the signs. If this first manipulation has helped—it usually has—it is repeated several times until re-examination shows no further benefit has accrued.

The next move is to repeat the same manoeuvre as has been employed centrally just to one side of the spinous process at the affected level.

Maintenance of Reduction—The maintenance of a thoracic lordosis is impossible, for the sternum cannot stretch. The patient must therefore avoid combining trunk flexion with rotation during weight-bearing. In practice, however, mainipulative reduction at whatever intervals prove necessary is the simplest measure.

If a corset is ordered, it must not restrict movement at the lumbar spine, which must be encouraged to move instead of the thoracic spine. The ordinary corset supplied in these cases with steels from gluteal folds to scapulae is worse than useless. The steels must start at an upper lumbar level (depending on the level of the thoracic lesion) and continue to an upper thoracic level. The cloth part of the corset can be continued down in the ordinary way (see Plate 87).

Caution—In elderly patients, particularly those with emphysema and stiff costovertebral joints, it is not difficult to fracture a rib at the lower costal margin during a prone thrust. Even a layer of thick foam rubber put across the couch is not always an effective precaution. The patient should be warned of this tiresome but not important possibility and as far as possible only the rotary manoeuvres should be employed.

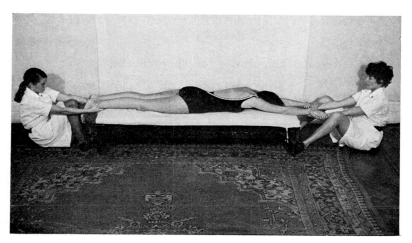

PLATE 67a

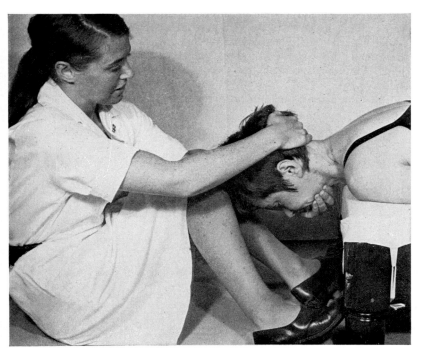

PLATE 67b

THORACIC SPINE: EXTENSION DURING TRACTION II

Second Manipulation for Thoracic Disc Lesion

See general remarks on p. 242

Indication—The first measure has not achieved full reduction.

Patient's Posture—The patient lies, as before, prone on a low couch. The fact that the couch is low enables the manipulator to balance his body weight directly above her thorax and to keep his elbows straight, thus avoiding any buffering of the jerk such as occurs if his elbows bend. Admittedly, this is not very important in lower thoracic disc lesions, since so little force is required. But it is a great help at the upper levels, where strong pressure may well be needed.

Technique—This manoeuvre rotates the two vertebrae forming the affected joint simultaneously in opposite directions—a movement impossible of voluntary performance.

The manipulator extends his wrist, thus bringing his pisiform bone into prominence. He abducts the thumb of his other hand and draws it backwards. This makes the trapezio-first-metacarpal joint prominent. He applies these two bony projections to the patient's thorax, to either side of the spinous process, one just above and the other just below the affected joint. Traction is applied by the assistants and the extension force applied suddenly.

If re-examination shows improvement, the manoeuvre is repeated.

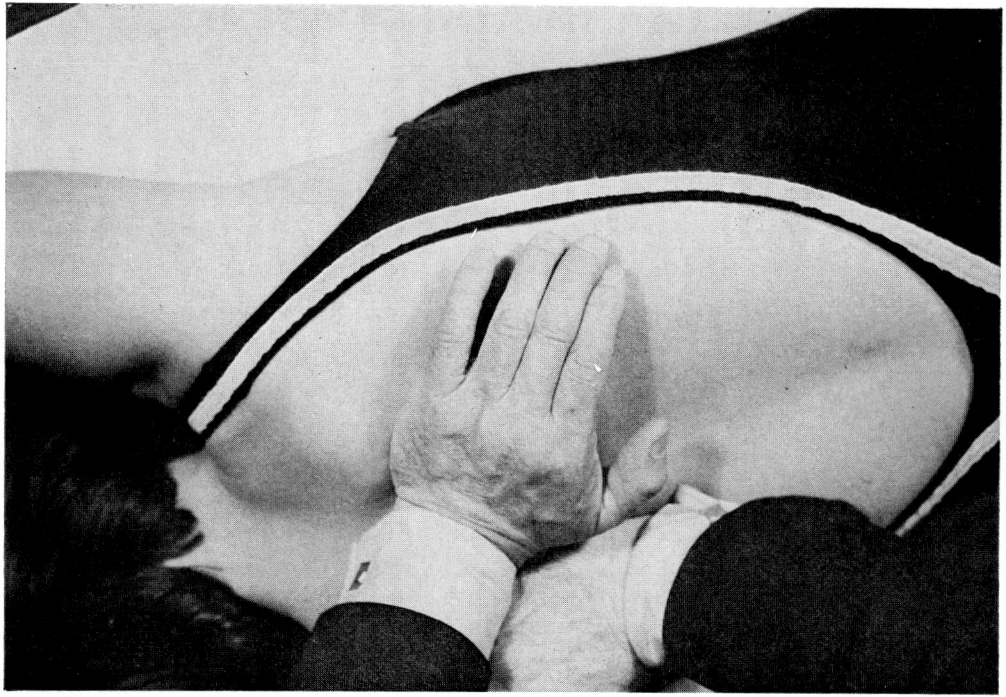

PLATE 68

THORACIC SPINE: ROTATION DURING TRACTION I

Third Manipulation for Thoracic Disc Lesions

See general remarks on p 242

Indication—

1. If the first two manipulations have had good effect but have ceased, on being repeated, to bring about further improvement, the rotational manipulations should follow.

2. If the first two manipulations have had no effect on the patient's symptoms, rotation during traction is indicated.

3. If gentle forcing of even a small degree of extension at the affected thoracic spinal joint causes considerable pain, it is clear that the patient will not be able to tolerate the first two manipulations at all. In such a case, rotation during traction may be cautiously attempted.

*Patient's Posture—*The patient lies on her side on a low couch and stretches her arms above her head. When the traction is applied she must relax her spinal muscles as much as possible, so that the joints bear the stress.

*Assistants—*Two are required. They sit on the floor facing the patient and each other, their feet steadied against the legs of the couch. One assistant grasps the patient's ankle, leaving the other leg free. The second assistant and the patient grasp each other's wrists. The traction is applied with due regard to the movement about to be forced by the manipulator, so that he is aided by the way in which his assistants direct their pull. They can pull their strongest for only a few seconds. The patient's trunk is therefore fully rotated in the desired direction before they apply their traction. After a couple of seconds, the thrust is made.

*Technique—*If examination has shown that only one passive rotation hurts, or that one hurts more than the other, the more comfortable direction is chosen first. The manipulator places his one hand on the patient's buttock, the other against the prominent border of her scapula. Since her arm is in full elevation and strongly held, this bone serves admirably as a shelf against which to press. He twists the thorax as far as possible before the traction starts. The assistants pull and he pauses long enough for the traction to exert its full effect, and uses his body weight to press the patient's thorax towards, and her pelvis away, from himself with a strong jerk. This is not a pure movement of the arms; it is rather a forcing of his arms in opposite directions by the momentum imparted by the downward thrust of his trunk.

When re-examination after each repetition, first in the painless then in the painful direction, shows that no further progress is being made, the manipulator passes on to the stronger measures. In fact most thoracic disc displacements do not get beyond the prone pressures and this technique of rotation, for reduction carried out during traction seldom proves difficult and one or two sessions usually suffice.

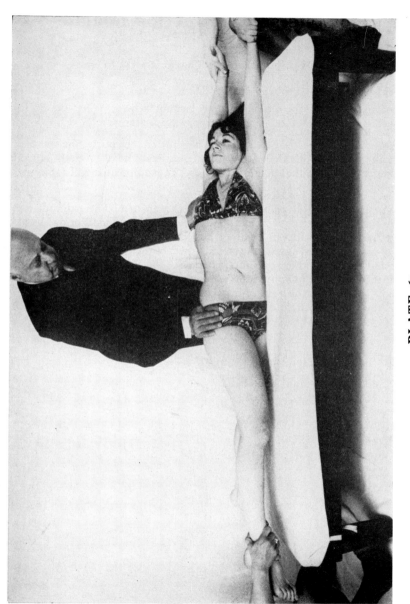

PLATE 69

THORACIC SPINE: ROTATION DURING TRACTION II

Fourth Manipulation for Thoracic Disc Lesion

See general remarks at p. 242

Indication—If the third manipulation has not helped, or has ceased to help, this different method of forcing rotation is called for.

Patient's Posture—The patient lies on her side on the couch. She and one assistant grasp each other's wrists; the other assistant holds on to the ankle. She pulls the leg in the same direction as the manipulator will force the pelvis.

Technique—The less painful rotation is chosen first. The manipulator stands facing the patient's lumbar region. He hooks the fingers of one hand about the anterior superior spine of her left ilium, and presses with the heel of his other hand against the lateral aspect of the thorax at the required level and twists the thorax on the pelvis until the tissue resistance is felt. Then the assistants pull and after a couple of seconds further rotation is forced. To this end he rotates his thorax, thus pulling his hand on the pelvis towards himself, and pushing the thoracic hand sharply away.

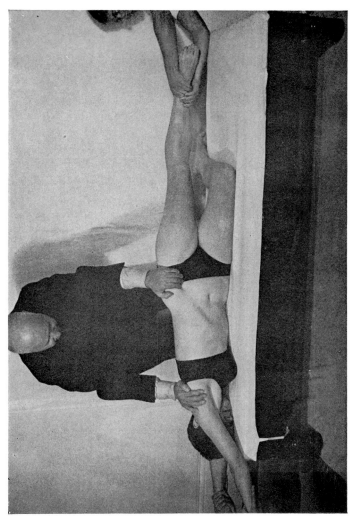

PLATE 70

THORACIC SPINE: ROTATION DURING TRACTION III

Fifth Manipulation for Thoracic Disc Lesion

See general remarks at p. 242

Indication—This manoeuvre is suited only to *upper* thoracic disc protrusions.

Patient's Posture—She lies prone on a low couch, her feet grasped by one assistant, her head by another. Her head is held turned slightly in the direction in which her thorax is to be rotated. She puts her forearm behind her back; this brings the shoulder forwards, thus providing a better prop for the manipulator's elbow.

Technique—The manipulator stands level with the patient's thorax and crooks his elbow about her shoulder. He places his other hand on the ribs at the sixth to eighth levels. He clasps his hands. He raises the elbow applied to her shoulder, taking up slack, and presses with the hand on the ribs. The assistants then pull. By a side-flexion movement of his thorax, he increases his pull with his elbow and his pressure with the heel of the other hand, applied just to one side of the thoracic spine at the requisite level. The upper thoracic spinal joint is thus simultaneously rotated and extended during traction.

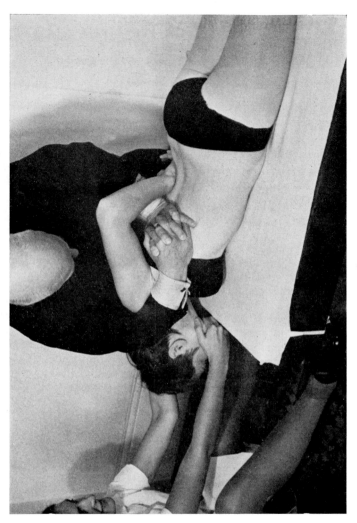

PLATE 71

THORACIC SPINE: ROTATION DURING TRACTION IV

Sixth Manipulation for Thoracic Disc Lesion

See general remarks at p. 242

Indication—This manoeuvre is seldom required, but may be employed if one rotation remains obstinately painful. The method involves rotation using the leverage supplied by the patient's thigh.

Patient's Posture—The patient lies prone on the couch. Her ankle is held by one assistant while the other assistant and the patient grasp each other's wrists. Strong traction is applied after the thorax has been rotated fully by the manipulator.

Technique—The manipulator stands facing the patient's waist. He flexes the patient's hip until her thigh is at right-angles to her body and curves his hand about her knee, holding it off the couch. His other hand, placed palm downwards at the side of the lower thorax farther from himself, holds the patient's upper trunk flat on the couch. When the patient relaxes and the assistants are pulling well, he draws her knee towards himself without letting her thorax move. The pelvis is thus strongly rotated by means of the leverage afforded by the length of the patient's femur added to the width of the half-pelvis. Since the thoracic lever is so much the shorter, he uses his body weight to reinforce there, while the upward pull on the thigh is effected only by the strength of his arm. A balance is thus achieved. Great purchase is obtained in this way; this method is especially called for when a small physiotherapist has to deal with a large strong patient.

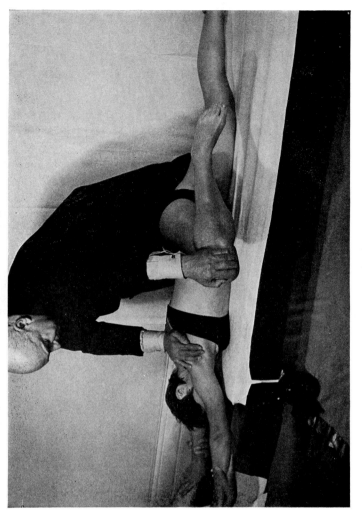

PLATE 72

THORACIC SPINE: ROTATION DURING TRACTION V

Seventh Manipulation for Thoracic Disc Lesion

See general remarks at p. 242

Indication—If rotation remains obstinately painful, this manoeuvre is called for. This method ensures that both the thoracic and the pelvic levers afford added strength to the rotary force.

Patient's Posture—The patient lies face upwards on the couch. She and one assistant grasp each other's wrists and the other assistant holds her ankle.

Technique—The manipulator stands at the patient's waist facing towards her hips. He flexes the hip on the side away from himself to a right-angle and applies his palm to the outer aspect of her knee. His fingers overlie her patella; his forearm is almost fully supinated. The heel of his other hand engages against the outer border of the patient's scapula, which is fixed in relation to her thorax by the traction which holds her arms fully elevated. He rotates the thorax fully until he feels tissue tension mounting. The assistants now pull and he rotates her pelvis further by pressing her knee smartly towards the floor while keeping her thorax still on the couch with his other hand.

Results—Manipulation for a thoracic disc displacement seldom fails. One to three sessions are required. The real trouble is the maintenance of reduction, since to keep the thoracic spine in lordosis is impossible. Hence patients usually have to return at intervals for repetition.

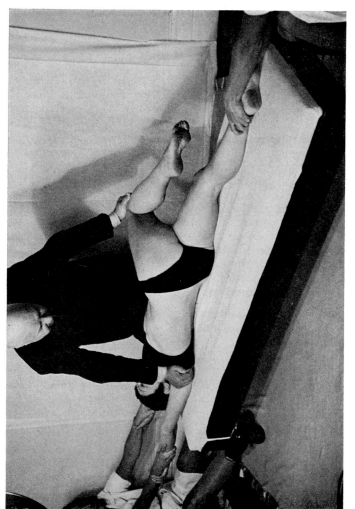

PLATE 73

LUMBAR SPINE: FORCED EXTENSION
(CENTRAL)

First Manipulation for Lumbar Disc Lesion

Lesion—Disc lesions are almost unknown at the first and second lumbar levels; some 5% occur at the third level. The remainder lie at the fourth and fifth levels, slightly more often at the fourth. They cause internal derangement at the lumbar joint and examination discloses the partial articular pattern. In other words, part of the joint is blocked, part not. A small central protrusion gives rise to backache only, with articular signs only. A large central protrusion gives rise to more severe articular signs with signs of impaired dural mobility as well. A postero-lateral displacement impinges on the nerve root. The signs are therefore articular, dural and those indicating impaired mobility and/or conduction along the compressed root.

Disc protrusions consist of cartilage or nucleus or both. Nuclear protrusions are rare at cervical and thoracic levels, where manipulation is therefore always the first thought, but quite common at the lower lumbar joints. Hence the distinction must always be drawn between the cartilaginous displacements for which manipulation is required and the nuclear displacements that necessitate traction.

Indications—The cartilaginous displacement that (if small) causes backache or (if large) causes lumbago is nearly always best treated by manipulation. Hence all such disc lesions should be treated thus unless some contra-indication exists. They cause the partial articular pattern of internal derangement; there may be a painful arc, usually on trunk flexion. They may impinge against the dura mater, limiting its mobility; in consequence straight-leg raising becomes bilaterally limited.

Manipulation, then, is carried out at once unless there is a good reason against this measure.

Contra-indications—This is first and foremost when the pain in the back is not caused by a displaced fragment of disc. Though most backache results from disc trouble, not all does; these cases must be sorted out.

Unsuitable disc lesions also exist. They are dealt with in detail in Volume I and will therefore be merely listed here.

1. Danger to the fourth sacral root. Sacro-perineal numbness and weakness of the bladder or anus are reported.
2. Hyperacute lumbago. Epidural local anaesthesia or oscillations are required.
3. The last month of pregnancy.
4. Spinal claudication.
5. Too large a protrusion. Sciatica with gross lumbar deformity or with neurological deficit in the lower limb.
6. Too soft a protrusion. Small nuclear protrusions require traction.

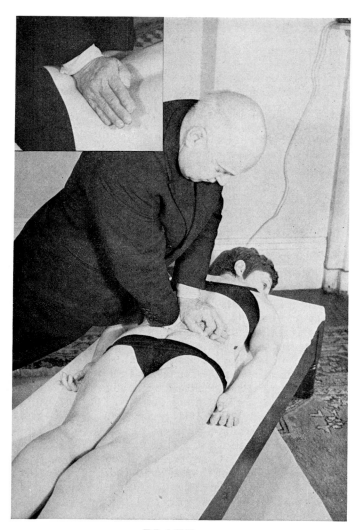

PLATE 74

7. Root pain lasting longer than six months in a patient under sixty years old.
8. Compression phenomena. The pain results from the joint bearing the patient's weight.
9. Post-laminectomy. Not dangerous but seldom successful.
10. Neurosis. If the patient will allege aggravation whether he is helped or not, he is best left untreated.

Lumbago with deviation provides an indication that the prone pressures will almost certainly fail, whereas the rotations are likely to succeed. Hence such deviation invites manipulation but not by the method illustrated in this Plate.

Patient's Posture—The patient lies face downwards on a low couch. A couch of the height ordinarily found in physiotherapy departments cannot be used, for the manipulator's body weight must be poised right over the patient's trunk. The maximum height for the couch is 50 cm, and it must be firm. It is not possible to perform any of these manipulations on a sprung couch or on the bed in a patient's house; a mattress on the floor is quite suitable, however.

Technique—The manipulator stands level with the patient's waist, facing towards her. He places one hand across her lumbar region without pronating the forearm fully, so that the mid-shaft of his fifth metacarpal bone engages against the prominence formed by the spinous process of the relevant lumbar vertebra. He reinforces with his other hand, his thumb pressing on the ulnar side of the lower hand (see Plate 74 *inset*). The whole width of the palm of the nether hand must not be used for the manipulator's strength is then dissipated by the attempt of force movement at several joints at once; it is by tilting this hand a little so that the ulnar border is applied to only one spinous process at a time that an effective movement can be imparted at the appropriate level.

Each upper limb is kept rigid, so that it acts as a stiff rod communicating the thrust of the manipulator's trunk as he bends his head and thorax abruptly forwards. He leans on the patient's back for a few seconds, taking up the slack. When he feels the patient relax and has secured some extension, he gives the final downward jerk. Only minor discomfort is caused, unless acute lumbago is present, when a more gentle start is often necessary. If pressure towards extension sets up pain felt in the lower limb, *the prone pressures must cease*. If rotation is now tried and this also shoots a pain down the limb, the manipulative attempt is abandoned forthwith.

Assessment of Progress—If straight-leg raising was limited, this is tested afresh. If a cough hurt, the patient is asked to cough and state if it still hurts. If only the standing lumbar movements caused pain, the patient is asked to stand and bend backwards and sideways to judge if there is any change in the degree of pain; the operator watches to observe any alteration in the range of movement. If the patient or the manipulator—usually

PLATE 74 (continued)   261

both—feels a thud at the lumbar spine as extension is forced, no more is done until the effect has been assessed when the patient stands and tries her trunk movements. If the patient has considerably less pain and the range of movement has markedly increased, it is probably unnecessary and it may be unwise to go on. If she has improved only slightly, manipulation continues and, in the end, trunk flexion has to be tested before the operator can be sure that full reduction has been secured. But if trunk extension still hurts there is no point in testing trunk flexion which is, after all, the way to increase any displacement. If she is worse, the question arises whether the case is in fact suitable for manipulative treatment. Since decision on this point is often difficult to arrive at, and manipulation is by no means free from danger if persisted in spite of warning signals, the operator—whether physiotherapist, bonesetter or osteopath—would be most unwise to proceed further without reporting the facts to the doctor in charge of the case. It is only by starting gently, paying attention to the patient's statements while being manipulated, and by re-examination after each manoeuvre that mistakes—perhaps irretrievable—can be avoided.

Anaesthesia—Anaesthesia leaves the manipulator in the dark. Has any particular manoeuvre proved successful? Is one technique helping more than another? Is the displacement getting larger or smaller? Which manipulation offers the best chance of success? Shall he go on or stop? Anaesthesia deprives the operator of all the information that he requires for proper selection of method and the exercise of due care; it is therefore strongly contra-indicated. Moreover, in my experience, recurrent intra-articular subluxations that have been previously reduced under general anaesthesia prove quite easy to reduce without anaesthesia; conversely, those that cannot be reduced while the patient is conscious nearly always defy attempts at reduction under anaesthesia.

Traction—In contradistinction to cervical and thoracic disc lesions, traction by assistants does not facilitate the reduction of a lumbar protrusion. The joints are so large and strong that manual traction has no effect on them. Mechanical traction does separate the joint surfaces (see Volume I), but so stretches the spinal ligaments that, if manipulation during mechanical traction is attempted, the joint can be felt, when forced, not to move at all.

Occasional help is afforded by giving a patient twenty minutes' traction and then removing the harness. While he still lies on the couch, he is manipulated.

LUMBAR SPINE: FORCED EXTENSION
(LATERAL I)

Second Manipulation for Lumbar Disc Lesion

See general remarks at p. 258

Indication—If the attempt at reduction by the method shown on the previous plate has neither fully relieved the patient nor made him worse, this manipulation follows at once.

Technique—If the pain is central, no indication is afforded whether to start on the left side or the right. If the patient's pain is unilateral, or more severe on one side than the other, the less painful side is manipulated first. The manipulator stands level with the patient's waist, facing it. He puts one hand, reinforced by the other, on her back in such a way that his pisiform bone just clears the vertebral spinous process. He keeps his forearm just short of full pronation and the wrist extended, so that the bony projection overlies the base of the spinous process at the fourth or fifth lumbar level. The prominent pisiform gives rise to localized pressure; hence the major pressure falls on only one joint at a time. He swings his body weight above the patient's lumbar region and lets his hand stay pressing for several seconds until all the play has been taken out of the joint. He then jerks his head and thorax downwards, and communicates the downward thrust by keeping his arms rigid. By leaning well over the patient, he exerts a strong rotational stress at the same time as extension is forced. This manipulation is particularly successful in the elderly. Osteopaths seldom use this technique, since it smacks to them of chiropractice; here lies the explanation, I think, why our physiotherapists may succeed after laymen have failed.

Result—The manipulator's hand is on the patient's back and reduction can often be felt to occur as a palpable thud, nearly always felt by the patient, and sometimes even audible to an onlooker. By contrast with the cervical and thoracic spinal joints which click repeatedly when manipulated whether any lesion is present or not, the lumbar joints do not give rise to these thuds during manipulation, or during that depicted in the previous plate, unless the intra-articular cartilage is damaged and a loose fragment moves.

Straight-leg raising or coughing is now tested; alternatively the patient rises and the lumbar movements are examined, objectively and subjectively, after each pressure. If a thud followed by considerable improvement is noted, no more is done until the following day.

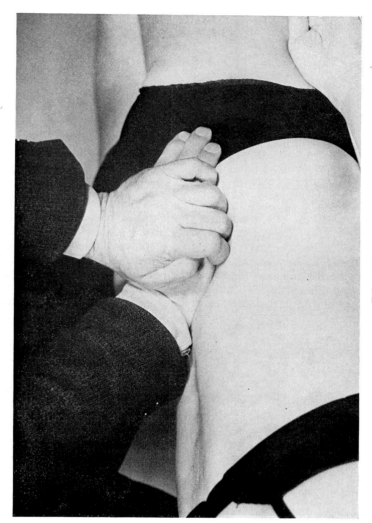

PLATE 75

LUMBAR SPINE: FORCED EXTENSION (LATERAL II)

Third Manipulation for Lumbar Disc Lesion

See general remarks at p. 258

Indications—If the previous methods of attempted reduction have helped, but their repetition affords no further benefit, this manipulation follows. If the previous manipulations have not helped at all, it is unwise to proceed to this and to the fourth manipulation.

Patient's Posture—He lies prone on a low couch, his head supported on a small pillow.

Technique—The operator stands on the side away from the patient's pain, level with his hips. One hand grasps the patient's knee round its lateral aspect; the ulnar border of the other presses just above the posterior spine of the ilium. The hip is now extended and then strongly adducted; this opens the lumbar joint on the side of the joint where the displacement lies. The manipulator now leans heavily towards the patient's head; this presses the lumbar hand down and pulls the knee hand up. Hyperextension of the lumbar joint during side-flexion away from the painful side results.

Result—A loose fragment of disc nearly in place may be fully reduced.

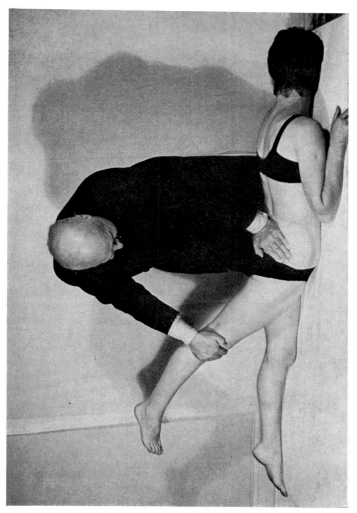

PLATE 76

LUMBAR SPINE: FORCED EXTENSION
(LATERAL III)

Fourth Manipulation for Lumbar Disc Lesion

See general remarks at p. 258

Indication—If the patient is very strongly built, the manipulator may feel that an unusual degree of pressure is required. In such a case, great force can be exerted by employing the knee. It is suitable when a small physiotherapist is faced with treating a large man.

Patient's Posture—The patient lies face downwards on a low couch.

Technique—The operator stands facing the patient's waist on the same side as her pain. He grasps the front of her near knee with one hand and extends her hip to the utmost, until her pelvis just rises off the couch. He places the palm of his other hand, after fully supinating his forearm, on the sacrospinalis muscle covering the fourth and fifth lumbar levels on the painful side. He places his knee on his hand. While maintaining extension at the hip with one hand, he adducts the thigh, thus tilting the pelvis away from the painful side and opening the joint on that side. He now forces his other hand downwards by pressing on it with his knee. The patient's lower lumbar joints are thus forcibly extended during unilateral pressure towards rotation.

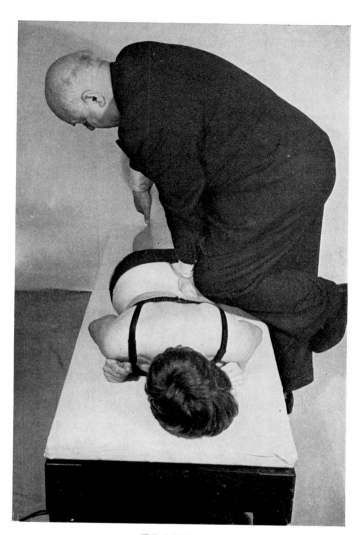

PLATE 77

LUMBAR SPINE: FORCED
EXTENSION WITH DISTRACTION (LATERAL IV)

Fifth Manipulation for Lumbar Disc Lesion

See general remarks at p. 258

Indication—The previous manoeuvres towards extension have helped but full reduction has not been secured.

Patient's Posture—The patient lies prone on a wide couch and side-flexes her trunk towards the painless side as far as possible, thus widening the joint space on the affected side. This gives the displaced fragment room to move.

Technique—The operator stands on the patient's good side and bends his elbows almost to a right-angle. He crosses his forearms and places the heel of his nether hand against her iliac crest on the bad side, applying it just lateral to the edge of the sacrospinalis muscle. The whole palm of his upper hand indents the upper lumbar area, so that the heel of his hand can push upwards under her lowest ribs.

He exerts traction by leaning his trunk forwards, so that his hands are forced apart. He now jerks his thorax downwards, keeping his elbows rigid. This applies a sudden extension thrust at the fourth lumbar level together with momentary further distraction.

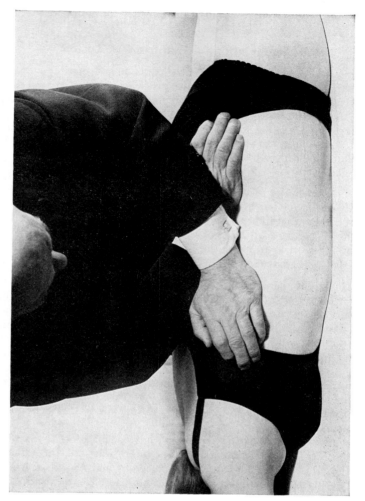

PLATE 78

LUMBAR SPINE: ROTATION STRAIN I

Sixth Manipulation for Lumbar Disc Lesion

Indication—Strictly speaking the lumbar joints do not rotate appreciably owing to the engagement of the articular processes meeting at each facet joint. Only at the fifth level is there enough obliquity to allow some rotation, and here the ilio-lumbar ligament proves a bar to much movement. Nevertheless applying a rotation strain is a very effective way of securing reduction at a low lumbar level. This technique is particularly indicated in cases of lumbago with marked lateral deviation of the lumbar spine.

Patient's Posture—The patient lies on the painless side, since the manipulator wishes to bring the joint surfaces apart on the side where the displacement lies. Her pelvis is rotated on the thorax as far as it will go. She lies in such a way that the backward angle her thorax makes to the vertical is the same as the forward angle of her pelvis. The upper thigh is flexed to a right-angle, so as to bring the femoral trochanter into prominence. The nether leg lies extended.

Technique—The manipulator stands behind her, level with her waist, and puts the heel of his hand against her greater trochanter. Application of pressure here secures the maximum length of pelvic lever. His other palm rests on the front of her shoulder. He now uses his body weight to force the thorax upwards and pelvis downwards, thus obtaining considerable distraction at the lumbar joints. He stays so for a few seconds, meanwhile, increasing the pressure towards rotation. During the strong distraction, he jerks his body forwards thus increasing this stress at the same moment as he forces full rotation. A snap or two is nearly always heard but these are of the ligamentous type and do not necessarily herald any improvement.

If this manoeuvre is carried out on a high couch, such as most lay manipulators possess, distraction becomes impossible and the rotation has to be carried out with the arms only, unaided by body weight, since the operator's arms are used almost horizontally instead of vertically. It then becomes a weak manipulation, much less likely to succeed.

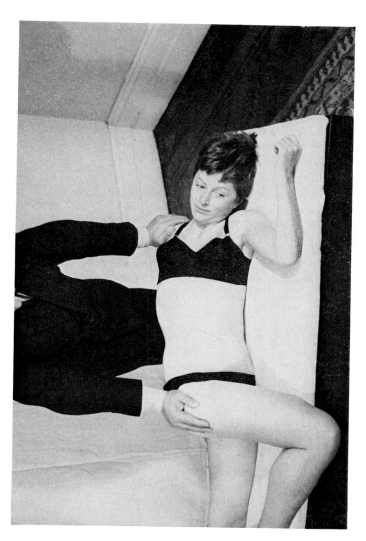

PLATE 79

LUMBAR SPINE: ROTATION STRAIN II

Seventh Manipulation for Lumbar Disc Lesion

Indication—This is the reverse of the manipulation illustrated in the previous plate.

Patient's Posture—The patient lies on her good side since the manipulator wishes to separate the joint surfaces on the side where the displacement lies. Her thorax is rotated forwards and her pelvis backwards in equal degree. Her upper thigh lies in extension at the hip.

Technique—The manipulator stands at her back, level with her waist. He puts one hand on the anterior part of her iliac crest and presses downwards. He lays his other palm on her upper thorax, steadying the heel of his hand against the spine of the scapula close to the acromion, and presses upwards. Strong distraction now results as his body weight is brought vertically above the patient. While stretching her thorax and pelvis apart in this way, he gradually increases rotation until the tissue tension mounts. With a downward jerk of his body, he forces his arms simultaneously farther apart and into further rotation. Little ligamentous snaps are felt and heard, and mean nothing, but a thud is significant, as the subsequent examination will show.

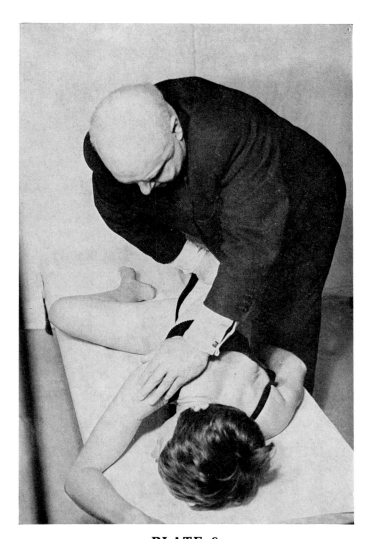

PLATE 80

LUMBAR SPINE: ROTATION STRAIN III

Eighth Manipulation for Lumbar Disc Lesion

Indication—If the manipulation illustrated on the previous plate has helped, but not enough, this method is used to increase the rotation thrust.

Patient's Posture—The patient lies with her thorax flat on a low couch, twisting the pelvis so that it is rotated towards the painful side, i.e. the lower part of her trunk is lying on the painless side.

Technique—The manipulator stands at the patient's back, facing her waist. He puts a hand as laterally as he can on her shoulder, and holds her thorax to the couch by pressing with his body weight via the short lever. He grasps her knee with the other hand and flexes her hip joint through about 45° and then abducts it fully. This is the long lever. He now puts his knee against her nether buttock. While maintaining pressure on her right shoulder, he rotates his thorax sharply to the left. This forces his right hand down even more, thus keeping her thorax on the couch at the same time as it jerks her pelvis backwards via the lever provided by the femur. A stronger rotation results than can be afforded by the previous manoeuvre, in which the levers are of almost equal length.

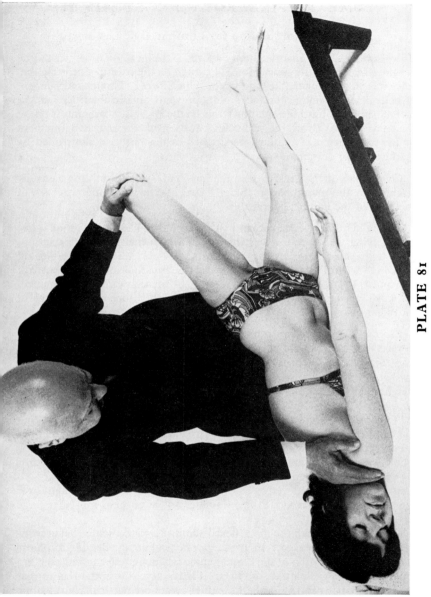

PLATE 81

LUMBAR SPINE: ROTATION STRAIN IV

Ninth Manipulation for Lumbar Disc Lesion

Indication—This manipulation affords stronger rotation than the previous two, but little distraction. The thigh on the painful side is chosen, since it is on this side that the joint gapes when forced. Though engagement of bone against bone at the facet joints prevents appreciable rotation, the fact remains that putting a rotation strain on the lower lumbar joints is one of the most effective ways of securing reduction of a subluxated fragment of the intra-articular annulus, particularly when this is accompanied by marked lateral deviation.

Contra-indications—Arthritis at the hip-joint, which would be painfully strained by the manipulation. Elderly patients, in whom the strength of the neck of the femur is unreliable.

Patient's Posture—The patient assumes the half-lying position on a low couch, lying well over towards the side at which the manipulator stands, so that his knee supports her hip. This prevents her from slipping off the couch when the movement is forced. She must not lie in the centre of the couch, for in this position the extreme of rotation cannot be obtained, her knee engaging against the edge of the couch before the full range of movement is reached.

Technique—The manipulator stands level with the patient's waist, facing towards her feet and on the side away from the pain. By facing her feet, he uses the width of his body to enable his arms to drop almost vertically from his shoulders. The more obliquely his arms lie, the less force his body weight exerts at the moment of the final quick thrust. He flexes the thigh on the side farther from him and adducts it across her body. He supinates his forearm, and applies his palm to the outer side of her knee. By pressing this knee strongly towards the floor, the manipulator forces rotation of the pelvis with the mechanical advantage of the extra leverage afforded by the whole length of her femur. His other hand, pressing firmly at the patient's far shoulder, keeps her thorax flat on the couch. Since the pelvic lever is so long and the thoracic lever so short, he concentrates his body weight over the arm applying pressure to her shoulder and uses mere muscular force to move the knee.

The degree to which the hip is flexed should be varied somewhat according to the lesion present. In patients who show considerable kyphosis and/or lateral deviation of the lumbar spine when viewed standing, the hip must usually be well flexed—up to 60° if necessary. It is in these cases that the manipulations shown in the next three plates are particularly valuable. In patients who hold the lumbar spine vertical, it is often best to start with the thigh brought up rather less than a right-angle.

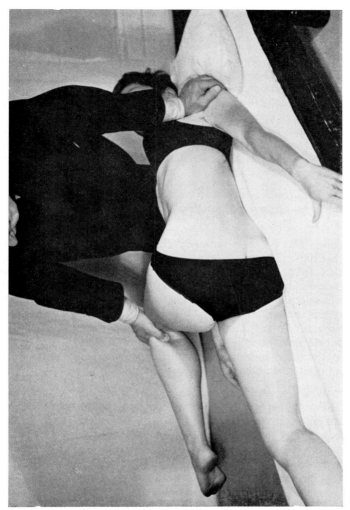

PLATE 82

LUMBAR SPINE: ROTATION STRAIN V

Tenth Manipulation for Lumbar Disc Lesion

Indication—This manipulation, devised by Miss J. Hickling, is a variant of that illustrated at Plate 82. It secures rather more flexion and side-flexion at the lumbar joint and may be called for in patients with a marked lumbar kyphosis, or considerable lateral deviation, or if the previous manipulation has helped, but not enough.

This technique has the virtue that the manipulator, by drawing the patient's lower knee towards himself, and keeping her pelvis in position with his knee applied at her iliac crest, can side-flex the lumbar spine strongly away from the painful side, thus opening the joint.

Patient's Posture—The patient lies on her back on a low couch with hips flexed and knees crossed; the thigh on which the operator will press lies underneath.

Technique—The operator stands level with the patient's waist, facing towards her hips. If the symptoms or signs are unilateral, he stands on the side remote from the pain. He twists both her knees towards himself, thereby side-flexing the pelvis on the lumbar spine and opening the lumbar joint on the affected side. He now applies one hand to her shoulder, which is thereby kept down on the couch. He grasps her lower thigh with the other hand, drawing it towards himself until her free knee lies supported against his thigh. He now presses both hands downwards with extra pressure applied as the tissue resistance to further rotation is felt. Rotation is thus forced during lumbar side-flexion.

Results—Only one-half of all patients with disc lesions respond to manipulation. In backache, some two-thirds of cases are reducible by manipulation, being cartilaginous; the remainder respond to traction, being nuclear. Few prove entirely irreducible; they need epidural local anaesthesia or peripheral nerve blocks. In lumbago almost every case proves reducible by manipulation in one to four sessions. Hyperacute lumbago calls for epidural local anaesthesia or sustained traction in bed; traction is contra-indicated. When root pain has supervened, only one-third of all cases benefit from manipulation. The remainder require traction, epidural local anaesthesia, sinu-vertebral block or laminectomy.

Prevention of Recurrence—Further attacks must be prevented as far as possible by explanation to the patient that she must maintain her lordosis at all times by:

1. An effort of memory. This involves her maintaining a constant postural tone in her sacrospinalis muscles, using them to keep the joint still in the good position.

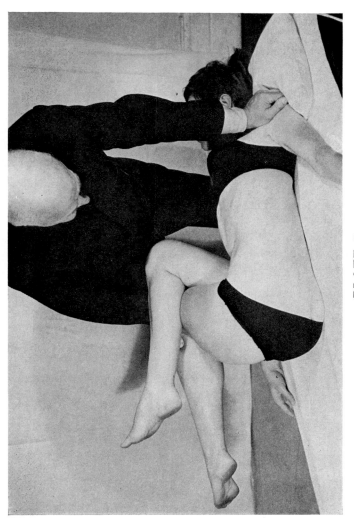

PLATE 83

2. Means of a corset.
3. Sclerosing injections into the posterior spinal ligaments.

She makes her choice, and in severe instability may opt for all three. She must realize that the disc consists of cartilage, an avascular structure, which cannot regenerate or unite. In backache and lumbago there is a strong tendency to recurrence (44% in three years) which she must be taught to avoid. In root pain which has recovered after the development of neurological deficit either by the passage of time or after the induction of epidural local anaesthesia, the patient need not take more than slight care of her back and need not wear a corset, for the tendency to recurrence is slight. In these cases, recovery is mediated by shrinkage of the protruded fragment. It is lying beyond the edge of the joint and appears thus to lose its synovial nutrient fluid and gradually shrivel away. There is thus no loose fragment ready to emerge again. It is only when root pain has recovered by reduction that the patient needs to be so careful.

CORRECTION OF LATERAL DEVIATION I

Indication—Lumbago with marked lumbar deviation. If the rotary manipulations have failed to restore a symmetrical posture or a full range of side-flexion in the restricted direction has not been achieved, this manipulation and the next (see Plate 85) are called for.

Patient's Posture—The patient lies on her side, the convex curve nethermost. She twists her trunk, the upper side of her thorax backwards and her pelvis forwards. She now flexes her upper thigh and puts that foot on her other knee. She puts the hand of the upper limb at her waist.

Technique—The manipulator stands facing the patient's head and clasps her bent knee between his knees. Both his hands are now laid flat on her upper thorax, his one palm engaging against her far shoulder. He now rotates her thorax and pelvis in opposite directions, using his knees against hers for the femoral lever. At the same time, he applies strong traction by upward pressure on her thorax. The lumbar joints are now pulled apart and side-flexed in the direction that tends to correct the lateral list. Further rotation is forced simultaneously, with the operator's entire body weight supported above the patient by his two hands and knees. He stays so for as long as possible, exerting a sustained correcting force.

The patient stands for re-examination and the manoeuvre is repeated until the deformity has been corrected and a full range of side-flexion is restored; or until repetition affords no further benefit.

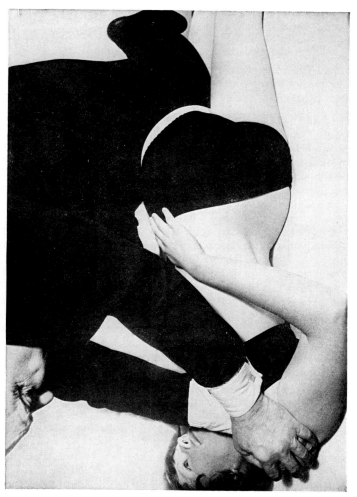

PLATE 84

CORRECTION OF LATERAL DEVIATION II

This method was devised by R. McKenzie, M.N.Z.S.P., of New Zealand, who has supplied the text and the photograph.

Indication—Providing that the onset of symptoms is no longer than twelve weeks prior to the commencement of treatment, and providing no paresis is evident, all patients with this common deformity are suitable.

Patient's Posture—The patient must stand with feet about one foot apart, to provide as wide and as stable a base as possible.

Manipulation Technique—Having established the nature of the deformity by observation and the level of the lesion by passive testing, the operator stands to the side of the patient to which the trunk is deviating. The patient's elbow is placed at right-angles by his waist and is used to increase pressure laterally against the lower rib cage.

The operator presses his own shoulder against the patient's elbow in order to give counter-pressure against the force exerted from the other side by the therapist's arms encircling the patient's trunk, simultaneously pulling the pelvis from the far side towards himself. It is essential that this pressure be maintained for at least one and a half to two minutes. During this time the trunk can be felt to move or slide towards the midline. This movement takes place slowly, is desirable, and must be maintained. Slight overcorrection should be aimed at. It is necessary to repeat the above several times so that the movement becomes more fluid and more easily accomplished with each correction. It is essential that side-gliding, and *not* side-bending, movement is produced when correction is made.

This is the easiest part of the correction to make and in order to stabilize the correction it is now necessary to restore the lordosis. Holding the patient in the corrected position the operator assists the patient to extend the lumbar spine. Still in the standing position, this extension movement is repeated again and again until the range of lumbar extension is freely restored.

Having manipulated the patient to the point where passive correction is possible it is now essential to teach the patient self-correction. This is best taught in front of a full-length mirror. The hand on the side of the deviation must be placed against the lower lateral rib cage and the other hand on the opposite lateral iliac crest. Using the hands as a guide the patient performs a 'hula' action, correcting the deformity a little at a time until he can control the lateral deviation. Once this is achieved the patient must then actively maintain it and at the same time commence extending the lumbar spine by bending backwards. This is repeated perhaps thirty or forty times. In order to maintain this correction after leaving the therapist, the patient must repeat the correction hourly. Providing the patient maintains his lordosis and practises correction actively, most symptoms will have disappeared after forty-eight hours. Repeat corrections should be performed by the therapist for at least three or four consecutive daily sessions.

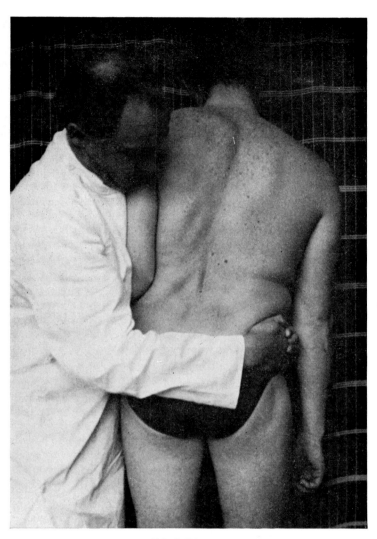

PLATE 85

TRACTION COUCH FOR REDUCTION OF NUCLEAR PROTRUSION

Traction is the treatment of choice for a small nuclear protrusion. A fragment of cartilage can be clicked back; the nucleus is soft and can be influenced by suction only. Hence these are the cases that lay manipulators cannot benefit. Traction provides the only method of improving on recumbency—the only effective treatment before traction was devised (Cyriax, 1950). The intention is to achieve rapid reduction by distracting the joint surfaces mechanically—a positive purpose—instead of merely avoiding the compression of the upright posture by putting the patient to bed and leaving him there. Recumbency is usually successful in the end but, even when it is, wastes an endless amount of the patient's time and the nation's money. Moreover, traction carries the further advantage of enabling the patient to be up and about, attending to his business, during treatment. Obviously traction brings the joint surfaces much farther apart than just lying in bed, in consequence a much greater centripetal force acts on the protruded part of the nucleus.

History—The first traction couch for disc lesions was made in Scotland for me in 1949. My two physiotherapists then, Miss J. Hickling and (as she was then) Miss S. Dandridge, worked out for me how to use it. It was a rediscovery of a method in use in Europe 500 years ago.

Effects of Traction—Traction has three beneficial effects:
1. Suction. A sub-atmospheric pressure is induced when the bones move apart, with centripetal effect on the contents.
2. Distraction. The increase in distance between the articular edges may disengage a protrusion that was just too large to shift during mere avoidance of compression during recumbency. X-rays have shown an increase in width of the joint of 2·5 mm.
3. Ligamentous tautening. Movement apart of the vertebrae tautens the posterior longitudinal ligament, which then exerts centripetal force on a central protrusion.

The Couch—This is 2 m long, 60 cm high and 50 cm wide. Near the head of the couch is an opening 8 × 30 cm through which the patient breathes when treated prone. An upright bearing a hook stands at each end of the couch; to the post at the feet is attached a spring balance. At this end the post moves along a horizontal screw-threaded bar when the wheel is turned. Both uprights are 30 cm high so that the straps can clear the patient's trunk when applied above it.

The Harness—
1. *The Thoracic Harness*: A belt with shoulder-straps is tightened outside a layer of thick foam-rubber, put on outside the patient's ordinary clothes (see Figs 1, 2 and 3). The two straps can lie both posteriorly, both anteriorly; or one above, one below. The harness is applied as low down on

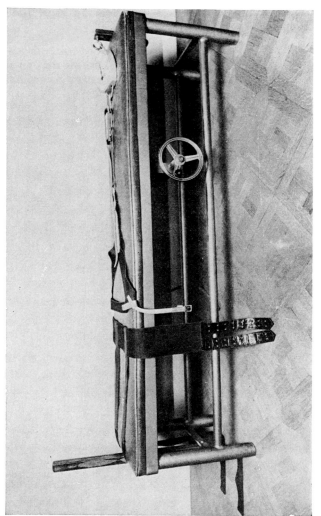

PLATE 86

the thorax as possible, partly so as to confine the pull to the lumbar spine, parly to allow him to breathe easily.

2. *The Pelvic Harness:* This consists of a Y-shaped band; the two arms join to form one strap that passes via the spring balance to the moving post. The arms of the Y encircle the pelvis and meet level with the sacrum or the symphysis pubis, depending which technique is adopted. This harness is prevented from slipping downwards by a transverse band ending in loops through which the arms of the Y pass. These are applied so as to take their

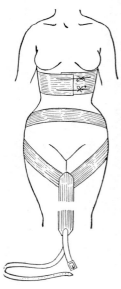 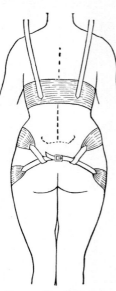

FIG. 1. Anterior view of the harness.   FIG. 2. Posterior view of the harness.

bearing either from the iliac crests or, lower down, from the greater trochanter of each femur. The whole harness is put over a thick sheet of foam-rubber encircling the entire pelvis. The strap is tightened before the wheel is turned.

3. *The Spring Balance:* This should register up to 100 kg. It serves two purposes: first, to measure the amount of traction applied, so that uniform treatment can be given; and second, to ensure an even degree of traction: this is the more important purpose. If the belt slips slightly, traction ceases almost completely unless a buffer mechanism intervenes to take up the slack. The spring balance has exactly this action and, by showing how much traction has been lost, enables the physiotherapist to restore the optimum strength again.

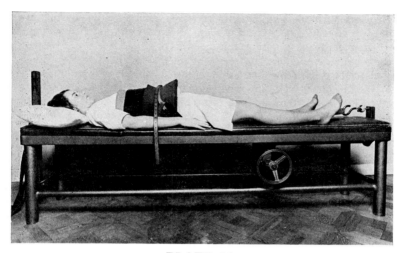

PLATE 86a

Traction: Arrangement of harness I

Distraction mainly at the anterior part of the joint, i.e. during the extension of the lumbar spine. The patient is treated supine. A small pillow may be inserted beneath the lumbar spine.

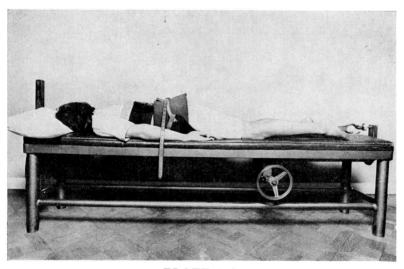

PLATE 86b

Traction: Arrangement of harness II

Distraction mainly at the anterior part of the joint, i.e. during the extension of the lumbar spine. The patient is treated prone. The thoracic harness is applied so that the straps run beneath the patient.

Patient's Posture—The patient lies prone or supine, whichever in due course proves effective. Some useful guides exist. Of these, the position that the patient finds most comfortable in bed (provided it is prone or supine) is the best guide for a first treatment. If this is little help, an assessment of the degree of pain and/or limitation of lumbar movement can be helpful.

1. If extension is pain-free and flexion hurts, traction will be comfortable if given in slight extension. The distraction will then occur chiefly at the anterior part of the joint. This can be achieved in two ways: (*a*) the patient lying supine with or without a small pillow supporting the lumbar spine (Plate 86a) or, (*b*) in prone lying with both straps beneath him (Plate 86b).

2. If both flexion and extension are painful (or neither) distraction of the joints with the articular surfaces parallel may be tried. The patient lies prone with the straps of the thoracic harness passing over his head, and the lumbar harness underneath him (Plate 86c).

3. When extension is painful and flexion pain-free, the distraction should-fall mainly on the posterior part of the joint. The lumbar spine needs to be in a slight degree of flexion to achieve this. (*a*) The patient lies prone with the straps from both harnesses above him (Plate 86d). (*b*) Supine, with both straps underneath (Plate 86a), but with both knees bent up and well supported by pillows. This position has been found particularly useful in third lumbar disc lesions when flexion is painless and extension painful.

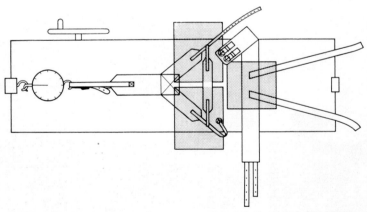

Fig. 3. The arrangement of the harness before the patient lies down.

The thoracic harness fastens the patient to the stationary hook at the head of the couch. The traction is now applied through the pelvic harness attached via the spring balance to the moving hook at the foot of the couch. The four photographs show the different ways of arranging the harness. These variations are important, since, in a difficult case, trial of several techniques may well be required before the physiotherapist finds the one best suited to any one individual.

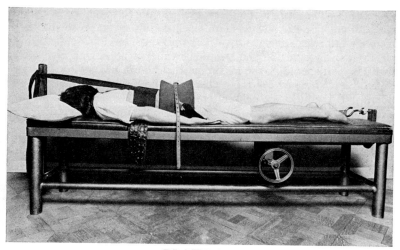

PLATE 86c

Traction: Arrangement of harness III

Distraction of the joint with the articular surfaces held parallel. The patient is treated prone. The thoracic harness is applied so that the straps pass behind the patient's head.

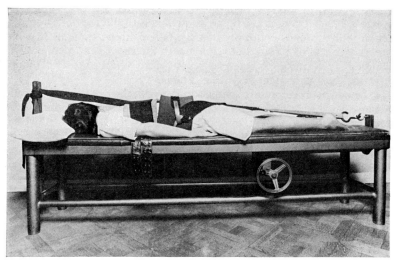

PLATE 86d

Traction: Arrangement of harness IV

Distraction mainly at the posterior part of the joint. The patient is treated prone. The pelvis harness is applied so that the Y-shaped strap passes over the patient's buttocks. The thoracic harness is arranged so that the straps pass behind the patient's head.

Technique—The harness should be applied smoothly and firmly with the minimum amount of adjustment of the patient's position, so that he is encouraged to relax from the first. The traction should be applied slowly with the explanation that the treatment will last approximately half an hour. The pull should be the maximum that he can tolerate for that time but *must never increase the pain*. This will allay fears engendered by the similarity to 'the rack' and help him to feel that he has some control of the situation. He is told to report any discomfort to the physiotherapist at once.

Traction must be sustained throughout the session of treatment, since it becomes effective (i.e. begins to move the joint surfaces apart) only after two minutes' continuous tension. This is how long it takes for the muscles to fatigue, only then letting the distracting force fall on the ligaments. The intermittent traction so often preferred by laymen—an electrical device is more impressive—defeats its own object. This method merely invokes the involuntary contraction induced by any short-lived pull on a muscle (the stretch reflex); for the muscles have not been given time to relax. Hence the vertebrae have not begun to move apart before the pull ceases again.

Since the effectiveness of traction depends on the muscles relaxing and allowing the stress to fall on the joints, pain leading the patient to stee himself renders the method useless. Traction in the order of 40 to 90 kg is applied, ultimately as strongly and for as long as the patient can bear it. The first treatment is cautious, particularly in a case of nuclear lumbago that has only recently lost its twinges. The physiotherapist is within call throughout the treatment. The pain often ceases after a few minutes' traction, but this does not imply that the pull is strong enough. It is not temporary relief from pain, but reduction of the protrusion, that is being attempted. The criterion is not symptomatic relief, but the greatest amount of traction that the patient finds comfortable.

As the patient becomes accustomed to the pull, the traction can usually be increased considerably at intervals of two or three minutes during the first ten minutes of treatment, by which time the maximum has usually been reached. This is only possible with a manually operated machine. The amount of sustained traction given on an electric couch has to be pre-set and cannot be adjusted to the patient's tolerance once the switch is turned. If traction, however applied, hurts, the case is unsuited to this treatment.

The patient should not eat a large meal before the session and should be encouraged to keep as relaxed and as still as possible during the stretch. He must avoid coughing.

Particular care is exercised while the tension is being released and the harness loosened, at the end of the session, since this is the time when twinges are most likely to occur. The patient is reminded to remain quite still and resist the temptation to take a very deep breath the moment he is free of the confines of the thoracic harness.

Five minutes' rest on the couch after the treatment gives the patient a chance to 'regain his normal length' before compressing the joint again by

PLATE 86 (continued)

293

standing. He should be shown how to get off the couch keeping his back straight by rolling on to one side, putting his feet over the edge of the couch and rising sideways to a sitting position.

If traction has not begun to prove effective after a few days, the question of a different posture on the couch arises, or of a different position for the straps. If these alterations are made and the patient has not begun to improve after two weeks, treatment should be abandoned. The physiotherapist should not despair too soon, however, as many patients begin to get better only during the second week. Obviously, if a patient is much better but not well after a fortnight, a third week's daily treatment is justified.

Before each session, symptoms and physical signs are noted afresh and any alteration given due weight. However, it is no use examining a patient immediately after a session of traction. Ephemeral changes for better or for worse detected at that moment mean very little; the patient must be re-examined before traction starts each day.

Interval between Treatments—Treatment must be given daily, for the attempt is to secure more reduction in half an hour than the patient, by bearing weight on the joint for the rest of the day, can reverse. It is remarkable that this should in fact prove quite possible. However, daily treatment is essential otherwise the protrusion is apt to have returned to the same size by each attendance. In cases of urgency traction can be given twice a day, but three times has not proved tolerable. Alternatively, in such cases, one long stretch of up to an hour has proved effective.

Results—In the course of a week or two, many protrusions that would otherwise have had to be treated by prolonged rest in bed recede while the patient is ambulant. The pain eases; straight-leg raising gradually becomes of full range; lastly the trunk movements cease to hurt. When the patient is nearly well, a painful arc on straight-leg raising often appears. Traction is not always successful, however, even when it is reserved for nuclear protrusions, since once they have become large enough to impair conduction along a nerve root it is too late.

After-treatment—Pulpy protrusions ooze out gradually. They start bulging backwards if the patient sits badly, or stands bent forwards for some time, the lower back in kyphosis. They are apt to appear some hours or even the day after exertion involving trunk flexion. Gradual nuclear protrusion is the explanation for waking with acute lumbago after, say, digging the previous afternoon. Hence the mechanism of his disorder must be explained to the patient, who must be careful thenceforth to maintain his lumbar lordosis while holding any position for some while, especially seated. He need not avoid stooping and coming up again quickly; thus he can, for example, play tennis safely. A belt may be required in forgetful patients.

Indications—

1. *Nuclear protrusion:* Protrusion of the soft nucleus at a lower thoracic

or any lumbar level calls for immediate daily traction. By contrast, hard cartilaginous displacements require manipulation. Differentiation is not always easy and is set out in Volume I. In general a slow onset of pain some time after stooping or on remaining seated a long while suggests the slow ooze of pulpy material. Side-flexion towards the painful side hurting in the back, or any movement other than trunk flexion setting up the root pain, carries the same suggestion.

Traction acts in the same way as rest in bed but much more strongly. It does not merely avoid compression; it provides positive decompression. Hence sustained traction often achieves as much or more after a few hours' treatment as rest in bed for weeks. Moreover, it enables the patient to be up and about the whole time.

The result of traction is the same whether the protrusion (as long as it is small) lies postero-centrally setting up local pain only or postero-laterally setting up pain in the lower limb, or both.

2. *Failure of manipulation:* Cases occur in which the consistency of the displacement cannot be determined. If so, manipulation is tried first, since it is the more direct approach and supplies a quick answer. If it fails, traction is substituted; but several hours should elapse between the manipulative attempt and traction, since painful twinges may occur as the traction is released if the second treatment succeeds the first too quickly (see Contra-indications).

3. *Primary postero-lateral root pain:* When root pain starts in the limb without previous backache, the protrusion appears alway to consist of nuclear material. Hence manipulation always fails and traction is regularly successful in cases that have lasted not more than some months, but there is a considerable liability to recurrence.

4. *Recurrence after laminectomy:* Manipulation seldom avails, but can be safely attempted in suitable cases. By contrast, traction is often successful both when laminectomy has failed and after recurrence.

5. *Upper lumbar disc lesions:* These are very uncommon. At the first and second lumbar levels manipulation rarely helps but traction usually succeeds.

6. *Bilateral long-standing limitation of straight-leg raising:* Young adults with months or years of backache associated with marked bilateral limitation of straight-leg raising need to be treated by daily traction for about three months. If they have not begun to get better after a week or two, there is no need to despair; it may take a good month before any improvement is noted.

7. *Lower thoracic disc lesions:* If manipulation unexpectedly fails, traction is substituted.

8. *Bone to bone:* Patients with marked kyphosis, whether postural, due to old osteochondrosis, or after fracture of a vertebral body, may develop

PLATE 86 (continued) 295

pain caused by erosion of the anterior aspect of the intervertebral disc and consequent impingement of bone against bone anteriorly. Considerable improvement lasting many months may result from a course of sustained traction.

The same applies to the lateral erosion of disc substance at thoracic or lumbar levels on the concave side of a scoliosis. Bone eventually engages painfully against bone and traction may well afford long periods of relief.

Contra-indications—

1. *Displacement of a fragment of annulus:* Not only does sustained traction usually fail to bring about reduction, but, even if it should eventually, it is a far slower and more cumbersome method than manipulation.

2. *Lumbago with twinges:* Patients whose lumbago gives rise to severe twinges on movement are made *much worse* by traction—to such an extent that when the tension begins to be released the slightest reduction is agonizing. The patient cannot get off the couch for some hours, twinging each time the traction is eased off a little. The ordeal leaves the patient, at best, unimproved. Any patient, therefore, who has had acute lumbago due to a nuclear protrusion must be treated very cautiously when he has recently lost his twinges and is first given traction.

The best way to deal with this emergency, should it arise, is to leave him on the couch for a good fifteen minutes until neck flexion has ceased to hurt and the range of straight-leg raising begins to rise. If that does not suffice, the rotation manipulation using the leverage of one thigh should be carried out several times, gently at first. If all this fails (which is very unusual) epidural local anaesthesia must be induced without delay.

3. *Respiratory embarrassment:* Patients with gross emphysema, heart disease, a thoracoplasty or any severe respiratory disorder may not be able to stand the band about the thorax. The same applies to elderly patients.

4. *Root pain with loss of conduction:* Once signs of neurological deficit have appeared—weak muscle, absent reflex, analgesic skin—reduction by any means is no longer possible whether the displacement consists of nuclear material, cartilage or both. The protrusion is larger than the aperture whence it emerged, and cannot be sucked or manipulated back. Epidural local anaesthesia is the method of notice in nearly all such cases.

5. *Long-standing root pain:* Sciatica that has lasted longer than six months is seldom affected by traction.

6. *Elderly patients:* Since the nucleus disappears and is replaced by cartilage between the ages of fifty and sixty, elderly patients cannot have a nuclear protrusion. If reduction is to be attempted, manipulation is the treatment of choice.

7. *Sciatica with deformity:* Gross lumbar deformity in a case of sciatica shows that traction will fail. Indeed, the attempt is so painful that the intention has to be abandoned. If the patient's lumbar spine is fixed in

flexion or side-flexion by such pain felt down the limb that he cannot even reach the vertical, it is most unlikely that any treatment but laminectomy will avail.

Too-swift Release—One of the reasons for traction having a bad name in the U.S.A. is the fact that on many couches the tension is applied by turning a wheel held by a rachet. For release, this has to be disengaged, whereupon the wheel whizzes round, all the distraction ceasing instantaneously. This is most unnerving for the patient and often causes severe twinges of pain. Two minutes' gradually diminishing tension is the least that is safe and in a patient who had lumbago recently five minutes is not too long. An ordinary wooden couch can be converted to a traction couch merely by screwing a vertical post with a hook on it to one end and a similar post at the other traversed by a screw-threaded bar turned by a wheel. This has a hook which does not turn as the bar revolves. The traction can thus be applied and released as slowly as circumstances dictate.

The sketch (Fig. 4) should enable any small engineering firm to make the traction pillar. Each upright is removeable at the turn of a screw, so that the couch can be converted instantly for ordinary purposes. Alternatively, any reader who wants these two attachments, with or without the harnesses, has only to write to my secretary at 32 Wimpole Street, London W1.

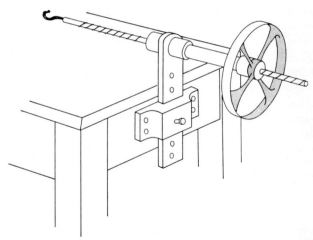

FIG. 4. A mechanism to convert an ordinary wooden couch into a traction couch.

MAINTENANCE OF REDUCTION: CORSETRY

Low Lumbar Levels

Corset—The aim of the corset is twofold: to maintain the patient's lumbar spine in lordosis and to prevent all movement as far as is possible. Hence the steels must fit the lumbar spine and buttocks exactly. Anteriorly, the corset projects over the lower ribs just enough to catch there if the patient bends forwards. The middle of the corset must lie at the level of the lesion; in other words, its centre is level with the iliac crests (Spencer: Banbury).

The simple test to decide whether a corset fits or not is to kneel behind the standing patient. The examiner's fingers encircle her flanks anteriorly; his thumbs are applied to the steels at each side of the spine, at the fourth or fifth lumbar level. Squeezing with his hands, he presses the steels forwards against her lumbar lordosis with his thumbs. If a gap exists and the steels can be bent farther forwards to touch the trunk, they cannot maintain the lordosis properly. Flat steels against a curved back are worse than useless, for their lower extent follows the curve of the upper buttock, the upper part forcing the unfortunate patient's lumbar spine into flexion.

Plastic Support—If a cloth corset with two posterior steels does not suffice, or a lower thoracic disc lesion is present, a stiffer support is indicated. A plastic corset is moulded to a plaster cast of the patient's trunk, and makes an exact and rigid fit. The sternal projection hinders all flexion movement. Yet it is light, hygienic, pleasant to wear, removable at night, adjustable for meals, and can be worn indefinitely—all the advantages not provided by plaster casts. These I regard as entirely out of date.

Caution—A very common error today is to apply a corset or a cast without reducing the displacement first, and patients suffer much hardship thereby.

Low Thoracic Levels

When a lower thoracic joint has to be supported it is important to allow free range at the lumbar spinal joints which have to move instead. The steels of the corset must therefore start at an upper lumbar level, leaving merely the cloth part of the belt covering buttocks and lumbar spine. At upper thoracic levels, no corset is effective.

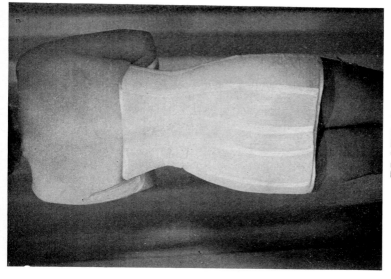

PLATE 87a

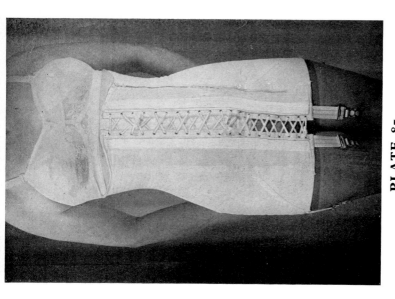

PLATE 87

LUMBAR FACET JOINT: INTRACAPSULAR INJECTION

Lesion—When a patient suffering from ankylosing spondylitis develops unilateral lumbar pain, the cause is inflammation of a zygo-apophyseal joint. This takes place more often at an upper than a low lumbar facet joint.

The common reason for injecting a facet joint is not a lesion of the joint at all but the endeavour to cause capsular sclerosis. After reduction is complete in many cases the fragment of disc, or the nuclear bulge, proves unstable. Ligamentous sclerosis is then indicated in order to stabilize the joint as much as possible. The supraspinous, interspinous and ilio-lumbar ligaments are therefore infiltrated with a sclerosing solution (see p. 302); so are the ligaments of the facet joints.

Patient's Posture—The patient lies prone on a low couch and relaxes his sacrospinalis muscles, so as to enable the interval between each spinous process to be identified. A horizontal line is drawn joining the upper edge of each iliac crest (the long line in the photograph). This crosses the division between the fourth and the fifth lumbar vertebrae. Other lines are drawn horizontally from the supraspinous ligaments above and below. A spot is marked on the line 1·5 cm from the midline at the fourth and 2 cm at the fifth level; here are the surface markings of the joints.

Injection Technique—The operator sits facing the patient. A 5 ml syringe is filled with 40 ml of sclerosant solution (P2G) and 1 ml of 2% procaine and fitted with a thin needle 5 cm long. The needle is thrust in vertically downwards. If it meets bone, the point lies against the lamina. If it is felt to traverse a tough ligament and then hit bone, the point of the needle lies within the ligament and just over 1 ml in all is infiltrated in various adjacent positions.

The same is repeated at the other three facet joints at one sitting, i.e. the fourth and fifth lumbar joints on each side are infiltrated.

The injections are painful at the time of the injection; for it takes the local anaesthetic a couple of minutes to act. The patient is then comfortable for an hour, then sore for the rest of the day.

After-treatment—The patient should avoid bending forwards and must sit with his lumbar spine held in lordosis, otherwise he stretches out the very ligaments in which contracture is to be provoked.

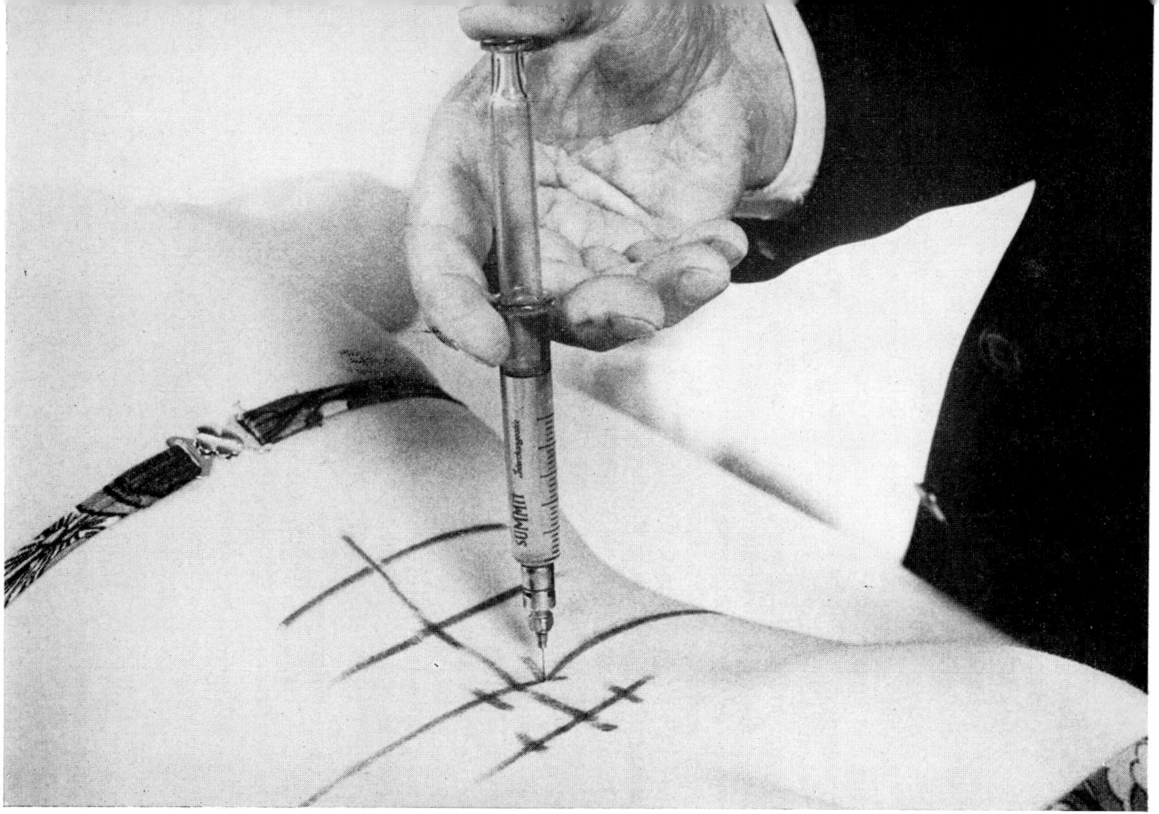

PLATE 88

SCLEROSANT THERAPY
BY R. BARBOR

Indications
1. Prevention of recurrent disc protrusion.
2. Stabilization of the sacro-iliac joint.
3. Pure ligamentous strain.
4. Stabilization of a spondylolisthetic joint.

1. When a fragment of disc has been reduced but proves unstable, stabilization by ligamentous sclerosis is indicated. To this end a chemical irritant is injected into the ligamento-periosteal junction of the ligaments supporting the affected joint. The main ligaments are the supraspinous, attached to the spinous processes above and below the joint. If the lesion is in the lumbo-sacral joint, then, in addition, the ilio-lumbar ligaments should also be infiltrated at both ends and on both sides.

2. In recurrent subluxation of the sacro-iliac joint stabilization of the joint is attempted by the injection of a dextrose sclerosant solution into all the supporting ligaments. The ligaments to be infiltrated are the short and long posterior sacro-iliac, the interosseous, and the ilio-lumbar ligaments. It is advisable to treat all those not only on the painful side, but on the other side too, since I found that, when the bad side was treated alone, pain was apt to appear later on the good side.

3. Chronic ache in the back or buttock may result from strained ligaments. This may arise as the aftermath of a displacement but not necessarily so. In these cases all the affected ligaments require infiltration with a sclerosant solution.

4. The instability of a spondylolisthetic joint can be reduced by the sclerosant injection of both the supporting ligaments and the ligaments at the lateral facets above and below the affected joint.

Contra-indications
1. Disc displacement still in being.
2. Subluxation of the sacro-iliac joint still in being.

The Solution—The dextrose sclerosant solution consists of:

Phenol 2·0–2·5%
Dextrose 20–25%
Glycerine 20–25%
Pyrogen-free water to 100%

This is mixed in the syringe with 1:2 procaine solution in saline in the proportion of 4 ml sclerosant to 6 ml procaine.

The Syringe and Needle—A 10 ml Luer-lock syringe is used because of the considerable pressure that has sometimes to be exerted to force the sclerosant fluid into a tough ligamentous attachment. If the plunger will not move, the tip of the needle lies subperiosteally. It should be slightly withdrawn until flow starts. The needle is 6·35 cm long and gauge 20 (see Plate 89).

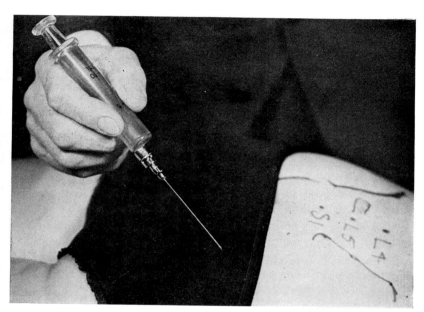

PLATE 89

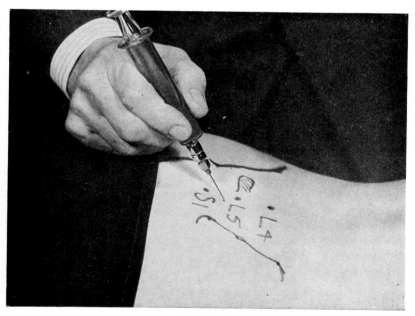

PLATE 89a

Ligaments requiring Infiltration—The ligaments to be dealt with are:

1. The supraspinous ligaments at the fourth and fifth lumbar levels.
2. The ilio-lumbar ligaments.
3. The posterior sacro-iliac and interosseous ligaments.
4. The sacral extent of the sacro-tuberous and the sacro-spinous ligaments.

These ligaments are treated, not along their entire length, but at each ligamento-periosteal junction.

This may seem an extensive infiltration, but I have tried injecting small groups of ligaments or even one individual only, and found that the more were dealt with the better the result. If there is no pain felt radiating to the lower limb, the sacro-tuberous and sacro-spinous ligaments can be omitted. If, as would seem reasonable, the painful side is treated alone, a lesser pain is apt to appear on the other side as the original symptom improves. Hence it is best always to infiltrate symmetrically.

Technique of Injections—All ligaments are infiltrated at their point of insertion to periosteum, and no fluid is introduced unless the tip of the needles is felt impinging against bone. One skin puncture only is made, the needle being half-withdrawn and then reinserted in another direction to reach each separate ligament.

The lumbo-sacral supraspinous ligament : The tip of the needle is directed first to one end then the other, 0·5 ml being injected along each insertion (see Plate 89a).

The fourth lumbar supraspinous ligament : The needle is largely withdrawn and the skin drawn well upwards until the needle lies at the fourth–fifth interspace. The attachments to the fourth and fifth spinous processes are now infiltrated in the same way.

The ilio-lumbar ligaments : This ligament runs horizontally, joining the fifth lumbar transverse process to the adjacent ilium. The needle is largely withdrawn again, and then aimed at the tip of the fifth lumbar transverse process. The needle is directed 30° from the vertical and 30° towards the head and touches bone at a depth of some 5 cm 0·5 ml is injected on each side, only when the tip is felt to touch bone (see Plate 89b). The needle is again withdrawn and the angle altered so that it points towards the iliac insertion of the ligament. The physician places his thumb on the crest of the ilium and aims his needle at that point, but 1 to 2 cm deeply, depending on the armount of subcutaneous fat present (see Plate 89c) and 0·5 ml is injected there.

The posterior sacro-iliac ligaments : Again the needle is partly withdrawn and reinserted at an angle of 30° from the skin and thrust forwards until bone is reached. Three or four little injections are made along the posterior aspect of the sacro-iliac joint, especially at the ligamentous attachments to the posterior superior spine (see Plate 89d).

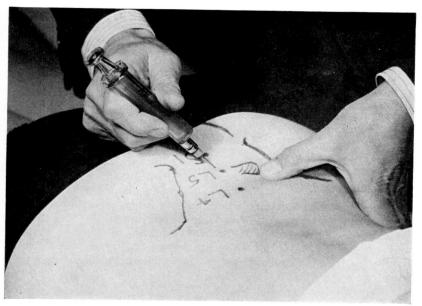

PLATE 89b

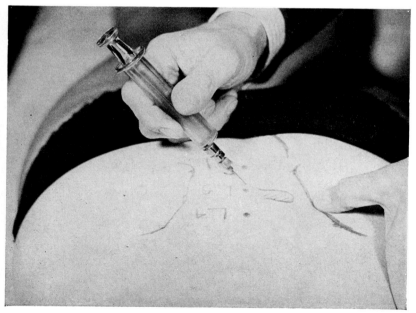

PLATE 89c

Interosseous sacro-iliac ligaments: The angle of the needle is changed to 45° and aimed just above the posterior superior spine (see Plate 89e).

The sacro-tuberous and sacro-spinous ligaments: The medial end of each ligament is attached to the side of the sacrum at the lower three levels. The needle is largely withdrawn once more and the skin drawn down towards the coccyx as far as possible. The needle is now pushed forward at about 20° away from the midline and 20° downwards from the horizontal (see Plate 89f) and 0·5 ml is injected at each side.

Interval between Injections—The injections smart as the solution goes in. Then the local anaesthetic takes effect and all ache ceases for an hour or so. That afternoon and evening the back is sore. By the next day the patient feels little or nothing. Rarely a more prolonged and severe reaction is experienced and indicates a strong reaction of the tissues to the chemical solution. Though disagreeable at the time it presages a good result. The infiltrations are given three times in all, at weekly intervals, and the patient must wait for three weeks after the final session for the sclerosis to have made good headway. He then walks two miles a day for two weeks before he tries his back out carefully. Relapse or insufficient relief indicates the need for another injection.

For statistical survey of results see Volume I.

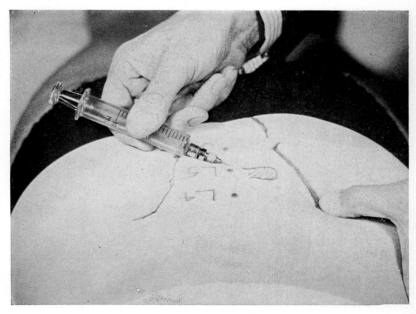

PLATE 89d

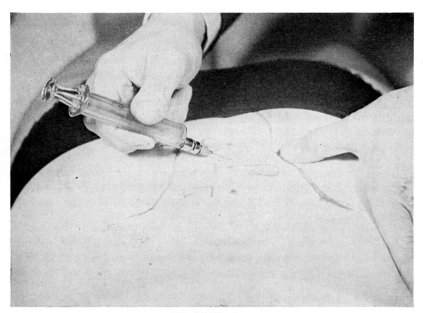

PLATE 89e

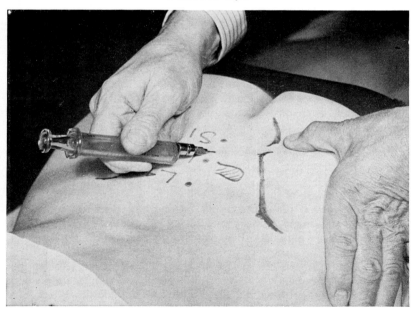

PLATE 89f

SINU-VERTICAL BLOCK

Indications—This injection is required in many different situations all difficult to deal with, in which the everyday treatments either have failed or are clearly not applicable.

1. *Failure of Epidural Injection.* It may happen that a case appears entirely suitable for epidural local anaesthesia, but the injection affords no lasting benefit. A second injection with the addition of a steroid suspension likewise fails. Unless the symptoms are severe, thus calling for laminectomy, the next approach is via the intervertebral foramen.

2. *After Laminectomy.* Manipulation is quite safe but is successful only occasionally, usually if there is a new displacement at an adjacent joint. Traction is much more often successful in recurrence at the same level. Epidural local anaesthesia has its successes but scarring may prevent the solution reaching the right spot. A good approach now is the sinu-vertebral block.

3. *Compression Phenomenon.* When this causes backache arthrodesis is required. A mushroom phenomenon causing root pain is very often abolished, even for years on end, by identification of the right root by means of sinu-vertebral blocks and then using the identical approach to inject a steroid suspension round the affected root. Often one infiltration suffices for semi-permanent relief, surprisingly enough.

4. *Before Arthrodesis.* It is not always clear at which level arthrodesis is required. If root pain is present, a sinu-vertebral block can be induced at the fourth and fifth foramina to see at which level the symptoms cease for the duration of the anaesthesia.

Patient's Posture—The patient lies prone on a low couch and relaxes his muscles so as to facilitate palpation of the intervals between each two spinous processes. A horizontal line is drawn at the level of the iliac crests, identifying the level of the fourth–fifth intervertebral joint. The supraspinous ligaments are marked and a spot chosen 3 or 4 cm from the midline between two lines at the level deemed to be appropriate.

Technique—The operator sits facing the patient on the painful side. A syringe is filled with 2 ml of 2% procaine and fitted with the thinnest possible needle, 9 cm long. The needle is thrust in at 45° to the vertical, aiming at the centre of the vertebral body. The spot chosen is where the lamina is narrowest. If the needle hits bone after passing 2–3 cm, it has encountered the lamina. If so, it must be largely withdrawn and thrust in again a little more obliquely. If it passes to its full length and then hits bone, the posterior aspect of the vertebral body has been attained. If it meets hardish resistance that can be penetrated, the needle is piercing the disc and should be slightly withdrawn. It is possible to enter the theca and aspiration is now carefully watched, to make sure no fluid flows back into the syringe. If this precaution shows the needle sited extradurally, the solution is injected. No discomfort is felt in the back or down the limb.

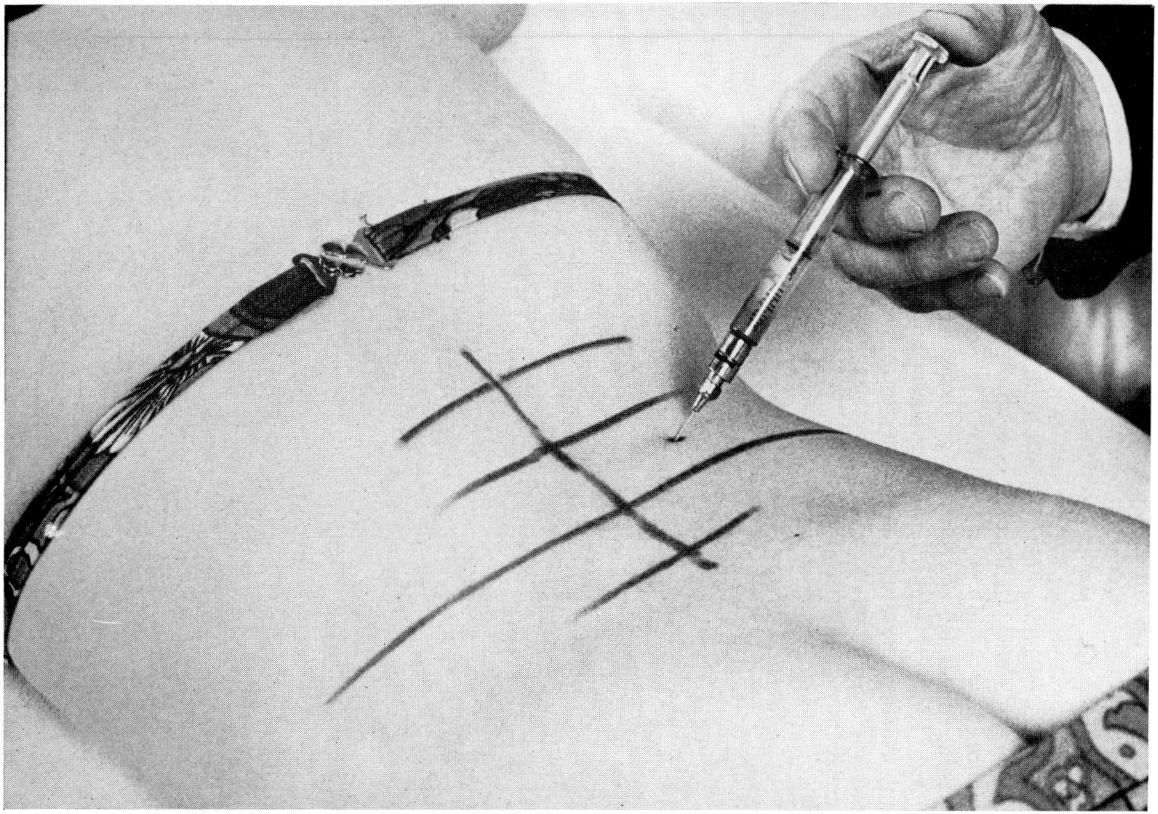

PLATE 90

Result—After the lapse of two minutes, the patient reports on his pain and, if straight-leg raising was limited, it is tested afresh. If no improvement is noted, the injection is repeated, either the same day or at the next attendance, at the other low lumbar level. It may well happen that neither induction is effective; then the third lumbar and the first sacral foramina must be infiltrated. If no result is obtained then either, this approach is abandoned.

In the mushroom phenomenon and after laminectomy, once the right foramen has been singled out by temporary relief due to local anaesthesia, 2 ml of a steroid suspension are injected at the next attendance. In compression causing root pain the result is almost always excellent; after laminectomy quite often satisfactory.

SACRO-ILIAC JOINT: FACET JOINT

Sacro-iliac Joint

Readers must not be disappointed that in this book no mention is made of
reducing displacements of the sacrum on the ilium. I have come slowly to
the conclusion that they do not occur. Years ago I believed them to be
common, then rare; now I regard them as a misdiagnosis. Naturally, if a
small low lumbar disc lesion causes pain in the buttock and is on that
grounds called sacro-iliac strain, 'manipulating the sacro-iliac joint' may
well afford instant relief, since these manipulations also affect the lumbar
joints. But in these cases the examiner will find that some of the lumbar
movements set up the pain in the buttock and springing the sacro-iliac
joints does not. Hence, the gluteal symptoms are clearly referred from a
lumbar lesion. Were the sacro-iliac joint to subluxate, no muscle exists
that, by its contraction, could maintain the displacement. The fibres of
the sacrospinalis muscle overlie the joint longitudinally, it is true, but do
not span it transversely and thus cannot fix the ilium on the sacrum.
Apologists have put forward the alternative of spasm of the pyriformis
muscle, but if this actually happened, the hip would be fixed in full
abduction, and it is not.

Facet Joint

The same applies to the facet joints. Osteopaths used to reduce a subluxated
vertebra, then it became a sacro-iliac displacement. Then, unwillingly,
they adopted the disc lesion, but this was a medical discovery and thus
basically unwelcome. Now they are tending more and more to manipulate
the facet joint. When asked—and I have asked repeatedly—for the evidence
on which these changes in pathology have been based, I have so far received
no reasonable answer, though I must admit to having made enquiries only
from medical men practising osteopathy, not from laymen. Stoddard
admits that the attribution of symptoms to a facet lesion is based on
assumption. Until some evidence is put forward, so unlikely an hypothesis
cannot be seriously entertained.

Factors against Acceptance—In the first place, how do two parallel
cartilaginous surfaces 'bind'? This phenomenon does not occur at any
other joint in the body.

In the second place, how do symptoms and physical signs fit in with
this theory? When the decision has to be reached in any one case whether
it is possible for a facet lesion to be responsible, all cases of central pain, or
of symptoms that started centrally and then became unilateral, would have
to be discarded, since a tissue lying unilaterally cannot give rise to central
pain. If a cough hurts, neck flexion hurts or straight-leg raising is limited,
the facet joint would be exculpated since a lesion there cannot interfere
with the mobility of the dura mater. If a joint fixes suddenly, the only

cause at all the other joints in the body is internal derangement. The alternative theory, a pinched synovial fringe, is untenable, for synovial membrane is devoid of nerves and pinching it is painless. If a loose body becomes displaced on bending forwards, presumably trunk flexion or side-flexion towards the painless side would disengage it and stop the pain. Yet the very movement a patient with lumbago cannot perform is bending forwards. Hence, those patients in whom these two movements do not cause relief must be excluded. Again, those who later develop root pain with neurological deficit must also be retrospectively omitted. Those cases in which epidural local anaesthesia stops the pain for the time being also have to be discarded, since none of the solution gets inside any joint. If these criteria are observed, I doubt if in more than one in a hundred cases of backache can the lesion be ascribed to a facet joint. We all agree that the gross deviation of a lumbar joint which occurs in lumbago results in an asymmetrical posture. When a patient bends sideways, one facet moves up and the other down, of course; this naturally takes place also if a disc protrusion causes the intervertebral joint to be held with a list to one side. But this does not imply that the facet joint is at fault; on the contrary, it is behaving with perfect normality. It is often alleged that the articular derangement, whatever it may be, at the facet joint sets up muscle spasm and that this is the cause of the pain. However the deviation of the lumbar spine is often *away* from the painful side. This phenomenon disproves the notion of painful spasm. It must not be thought that the possibility of locking the facet joints for manipulative purposes implies that the fault lies with the facet joints. Joint surfaces engage when pushed as far as they will go, and in the case of the spine this fact provides a handy lever for the operator who wishes to manipulate in the osteopathic or chiropractic manner.

COCCYGODYNIA

Massage Technique

Lesion—In many cases of coccygodynia the pain is referred from the lumbar region. Other cases are psychogenic. Since only local coccygodynia benefits from treatment to the coccyx, these other two types must be sorted out.

Pain arising from the coccyx nearly always affects women and is nearly always traumatic, e.g. a fall seated, less often childbirth. The lesion may lie at (*a*) the posterior sacro-coccygeal ligament; (*b*) the intercoccygeal ligaments; (*c*) the origin of the gluteus maximus muscle from the sides of the sacrum; and (*d*) the tip of the coccyx. The exact site of tenderness must be determined.

Patient's Posture—The patient lies prone on the couch and relaxes the gluteal muscles.

Technique—The physiotherapist sits at the patient's side, facing towards his feet. She places her thumb, reinforced by the middle finger, on the affected spot. If the lesion is at the sacro-coccygeal or intercoccygeal ligaments she imparts the friction by alternate small adduction–abduction movements of her thumb. If the gluteal fibres of origin are involved, she pressures deeply inwards and forwards at the side of the coccyx and draws her finger up and down the edge of the bone by a supination–pronation movement of her forearm. When the tissues at the tip of the coccyx are affected, the friction may have to be given vertically or horizontally, depending on which particular strand of fibrous tissue there is involved.

Duration of Treatment—Twenty minutes twice a week are required. Four to six sessions should suffice. Steroid suspension is also very effective in local coccygodynia.

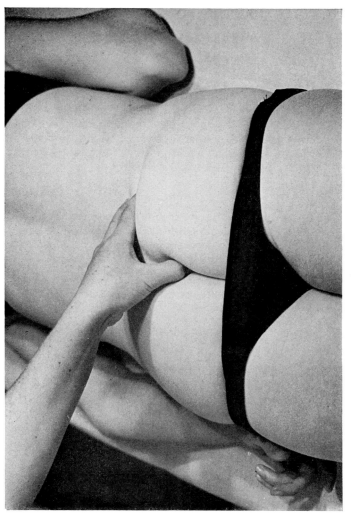

PLATE 92

PLATE 93

HIP-JOINT

Forced Flexion

Lesion—Osteoarthrosis of the hip-joint in a reasonably early stage. The cases that do best have little erosion of articular cartilage superiorly but a ring of osteophytes projecting towards the femoral neck.

Physical Signs—Restricted movement in the capsular pattern. At the hip the proportions are: little or no range of medial rotation and of abduction, full range of adduction and lateral rotation, corresponding with 90° limitation of flexion and 15° limitation of extension. The resisted movements are painless. The more elastic the end-feel the better the result of stretching.

Indications—Osteoarthrosis of the hip-joint in the first or second stage. Pain at night associated with osteoarthrosis can often be completely abolished by forcing. Movement is little altered; most patients achieve no increase in range, but the pain on walking is much decreased. The benefit is not permanent, but some years' relief can often be secured.

Contra-indications—Osteoarthrosis in the third stage; spondylitic arthritis during a flare; rheumatoid arthritis; traumatic arthritis, especially in children or adolescents, which is best treated by recumbency.

Patient's Posture—The patient assumes the half-lying position on the couch.

Technique—The physiotherapist stands at the side of the couch facing the patient's head and level with his knees. She flexes the thigh at the hip-joint as far as it will comfortably go; his knee flexes automatically when this is done. She then forces the thigh towards further flexion by steadily increasing pressure applied at the knee. No jerk is given. This continues, with pauses, for some five or ten minutes.

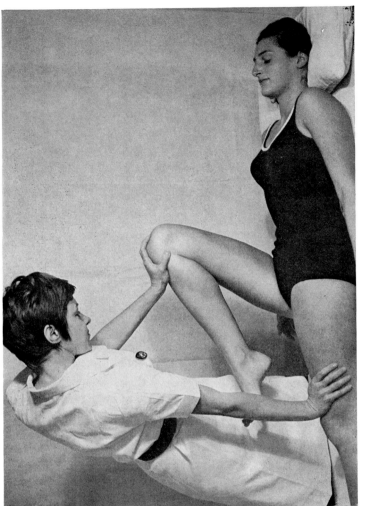

PLATE 93

PLATE 94

HIP-JOINT

Forced Extension

Indications—See page 316. In addition, children are occasionally encountered in whom an excessive forward tilt of the pelvis is the result of a small amount of congenital limitation of extension at the hip-joints.

Patient's Posture—The patient lies face downwards on the couch and relaxes the flexor muscles of her hip-joint.

Technique—The extension movement must be confined to the hip-joint by preventing any stress from reaching the lumbar spinal joints. The physiotherapist, standing level with the patient's thigh, must therefore keep the pelvis on the couch by strong pressure with one hand applied at the mid-buttock. The other grasps the front of the thigh just above the patella, and she gradually pulls upwards with all her strength. This stretching is continued for five to ten minutes, with intervals for resting both the patient and herself.

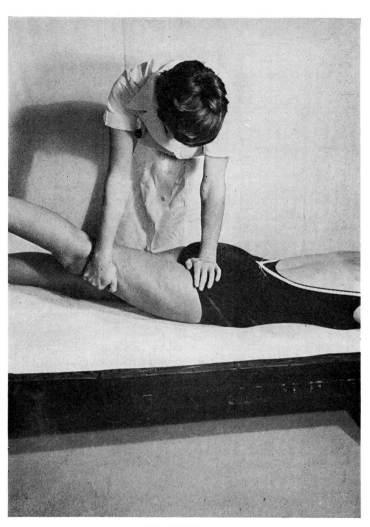

PLATE 94

PLATE 95

HIP-JOINT

Forced Rotation

Forcing Medial Rotation

Patient's Posture—The patient lies prone on the couch and flexes the knee on the affected side to a right-angle.

Technique—The physiotherapist stands level with the patient's hips. She must not allow the pelvis to tilt during the manipulation; to this end she must hold down the buttock on the far side by strong pressure with one hand. Her other hand grasps the patient's ankle and forces his leg outwards. This leverage enables rotation of the thigh at the hip to be strongly forced without much effort; too much pressure must not be exerted for fear of fracturing the neck of the femur.

Forcing Lateral Rotation

This is required only in dancers, who may find themselves handicapped in certain steps by a range of lateral rotation too small for their purposes, though it would be ample for ordinary persons.

The movement is forced in the reverse way. The physiotherapist stands level with the patient's hips facing his feet. She applies one hand to his buttock, while her other hand forces the leg medially. It is immaterial on which side of the couch the physiotherapist stands, though better purchase is obtained by standing on the side distant from the affected hip-joint. (Not illustrated.)

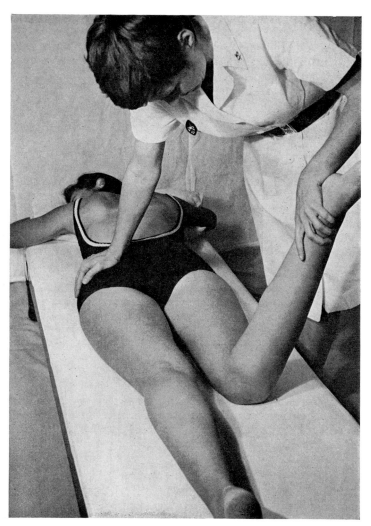

PLATE 95

HIP-JOINT: REDUCTION OF LOOSE BODY I

Lesion—A loose body forms in the hip-joint more often than is generally realized. Usually the hip-joint is already osteoarthrotic, and in my experience the loose body hardly ever shows on the radiograph, i.e. it consists of cartilage only. However, the patient's complaint is of sudden twinges with giving way of the limb, punctuating a minor ache from the osteoarthrosis that scarcely troubles her at all. If there is no arthrosis, the only complaint is of being let down by sudden twinges at the front of the thigh.

Physical Signs—The history of sudden twinges and of the thigh giving way is characteristic. One day the patient can scarcely walk, another day she feels nothing. No such variation is possible in pure osteoarthrosis.

If osteoarthrosis is complicated by a loose body, examination merely shows that the pain in the groin, thigh or front of the knee arises from the hip and that the capsular pattern is present. If by contrast a loose body is present in a hip-joint as yet normal, the examiner finds that a full range of movement is present, but passive lateral rotation hurts more than medial rotation—the exact opposite of the situation in early arthrosis.

Intention—To move the loose body to some other part of the joint whence it no longer gives rise to these momentary attacks of internal derangement.

Patient's Posture—The patient lies face upwards on a low couch, an assistant holding her pelvis, preventing her from being lifted off or pulled down the couch by the operator's traction. The physiotherapist holding the pelvis can often feel a click which the operator is too far away to perceive.

Technique—The manipulator stands with both feet on the end of the couch holding the patient's ankle. He raises her limb to about 80° straight-leg raise and leans well back pulling with all his body weight. His hands at the heel and dorsum of foot rotate the leg; he now gradually steps off the couch backwards. He uses the foot, held at a right-angle to the leg, as a lever and forces medial or lateral rotation during traction, with a sharp jerk at the extreme of range. As this is carried out, his body is moving downwards and backwards, slowly extending the joint at the same time. He examines the joint after each manoeuvre to find out the result and often concludes that one rotation is more effective than the other. Several repetitions are now carried out in the more favourable direction.

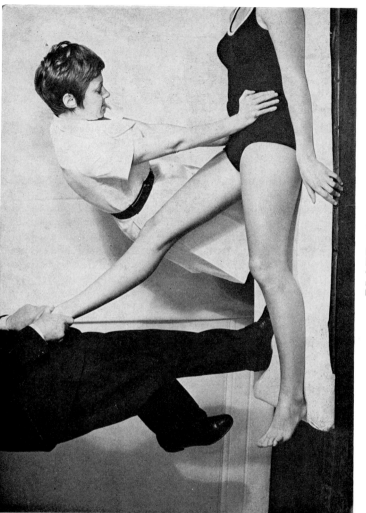

PLATE 96

HIP-JOINT: REDUCTION OF LOOSE BODY II

Indication—A subluxated loose body in the hip-joint for which the first manipulation has not sufficed. As a rule the last movements to stop hurting are full flexion and full lateral rotation. If the method of forcing shown in the previous plate does not render these two movements painless, this method is indicated, whereby stronger rotation using considerable leverage is carried out during traction.

Patient's Posture—The patient lies on her back on a low couch, and bends her hip and knee to a right-angle. Her pelvis is held down on the couch by an assistant applying her weight to the ilia at the anterior superior spines.

Technique—The operator puts one foot on the couch just beyond her buttock. He places the crook of her knee on his bent knee, holding it there with one hand and grasping her ankle with the other. He rotates the hip as far as it will go, in the direction that he found the more beneficial during the first manipulation. Holding her knee at a right-angle with the hand on her ankle, he plantiflexes his foot on the couch, thus raising her knee and with it her pelvis, where the assistant's counterforce is applied. During this traction, the femur is rotated smartly by means of the lever provided by the bent leg.

Result—Some two loose bodies out of three can be reduced and the patient walks out pain free. Some of the remainder are merely improved; occasionally the endeavour fails. Recurrence is common and has to be dealt with in the same way, since excision can be contemplated only when the loose body shows radiographically—most unusual.

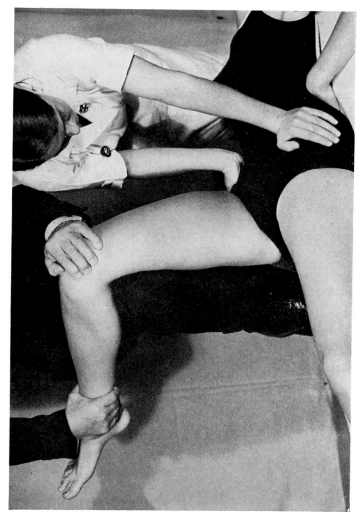

PLATE 97

HIP-JOINT

Intra-articular Injection

Lesion—Rheumatoid, spondylitic or traumatic arthritis at the hip—all respond well to intra-articular steroid suspension. Traumatic arthritis results from over-use, seldom one injury, and, if a few days in bed do not lead to recovery, should be treated by one infiltration with hydrocortisone. Caution should be exercised over repeated injections at short intervals for fear of a steroid arthropathy. The fibrous tissue lying at the back of the joint in pseudarthrosis due to an unreduced congenital dislocation is best treated by thorough infiltration with procaine; hydrocortisone has proved a failure.

Physical Signs—Limitation of movement in the capsular pattern. No radiographic change is to be expected in early rheumatoid or spondylitic arthritis.

Patient's Posture—The patient lies on his painless side. An assistant holds his foot and, if the upper edge of the trochanter proves difficult to find, abducts the limb. This relaxes the ilio-tibial fascia and simplifies palpation. The femur is moved to the neutral position (i.e. rotated medially to that point) so that the trochanter lies vertically above the acetabulum.

Technique—There is obviously more than one way to reach the hip-joint. The simplest is the lateral approach; for the upper surface of the greater trochanter is easily identified and there are no large nerves or blood vessels in the vicinity. A 5 ml syringe is filled with steroid suspension and a needle 10 cm long is fitted. A spot is chosen at mid-trochanter, just above its upper surface. If the thumb and long finger span the greater trochanter, identifying the anterior and posterior margins of the bone the index finger is free to identify the upper edge. The needle is inserted here and thrust vertically downwards until the resistance of the thick capsule is felt. Traversing this, the needle strikes bone at the neck of the femur close to, or at, its junction with the head. The injection is painful and for a minute or two quite severe aching is felt down the front of the thigh to the knee. It then abates, but some two hours later may recur and last several hours. If, therefore, the patient is not in hospital, he must arrange to get home by not later than two hours after the injection. A tablet of 50 mg pethedine is given to him to take home, in case this reaction follows.

Repeat Injection—If the patient remains comfortable for, say, six months, another injection can be given at this sort of interval indefinitely. Monthly injections, however, may provoke a steroid arthropathy and are not advisable.

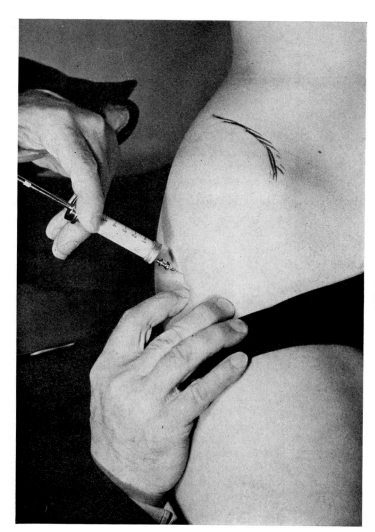

PLATE 98

HIP-JOINT

Injection of Silicone Oil

Indication—Osteoarthrosis at the hip.

Lubricant Liquid—The fluid is pure dimethyl polysiloxane of 12 000 centistoke viscosity, as recommended by Ongley.

Supplier—A sterile syringe filled with 20 ml Jointsil with a suitable needle is obtainable in a plastic pack from F. Fennell, 66 Old Pasture Road, Frimley, Camberley, Surrey. The empty syringe is returned by post and is recharged, sterilized and sent back within a week.

Anaesthesia—Though the oil is bland, it distends the joint, causing pain. A short-acting intravenous anaesthetic may be preferred by nervous patients. A painful reaction is apt to start some hours after the injection, hence the patient should be driven home at once after the injection, and the doctor warned that sedation may be required that evening.

Patient's Posture—The patient lies on her side, the affected hip uppermost. The physiotherapist supports her thigh in the greatest possible extension. The knee is bent to a right-angle and held horizontal, to ensure that a vertical insertion of the needle reaches the hip-joint.

Technique—Scrupulous sterility is observed throughout; for sepsis following a persistent foreign fluid would be a disaster.

The upper margin of the trochanter is identified and the skin in this region sterilized. Local anaesthesia is induced at a small area 1 cm above this line. The radiograph is now inspected to determine the angle that enables the needle just to clear the medial edge of the trochanter, aiming at the junction of the head with the neck of the femur. The needle, still in its plastic casing, is now held against the radiograph, and the length of needle projecting beyond the skin when its tip reaches bone is noted. The skin is now punctured at the anaesthetized point with a tenotomy knife, and the skin sterilized afresh. By this means the needle never traverses the skin.

The syringe has been lying nozzle upwards for some hours, so that any air in it has risen above the oil. The box is opened and the cap on the nozzle screwed off with sterile forceps. The needle is removed from its envelope and screwed on. The syringe is held vertical and the plunger is turned until all air has been expelled and a bead of oil appears at the tip of the needle. The way the bevel on the needle slopes is now noted. The needle is thrust through the tenotomy incision towards the femoral neck. At about 10 cm the leathery resistance of the capsule is felt and after another 1 cm bone is reached. The syringe is now rotated until the bevel of the needle lies facing the neck of the femur and parallel to its surface.

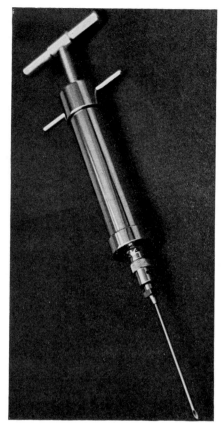

PLATE 99a

No vein exists on the periosteum large enough to take a needle of so wide a bore. The length of needle projecting beyond the skin is noted as correct. The piston is now screwed forwards until enough oil has been injected. Ninety half-twists (each of 180°) correspond to the expulsion of 20 ml of oil. The passage of the needle has been oblique, and the pressure of oil within the joint approximates the punctured surfaces on withdrawal of the needle, thus providing a valve hindering escape of the oil.

Twisting the piston is quite hard work and about ten minutes are required.

Reaction—For the first hour or two after the injection, little discomfort is experienced. Some hours later, quite a severe reaction may start, lasting from some hours to a week. If so, the patient should stay largely in bed and she should be warned of the possibility.

Results—These are not brilliant, but adequate, when the intractability of the disorder is borne in mind. One-third of the patients are very much better; one-third slightly better; one-third no better.

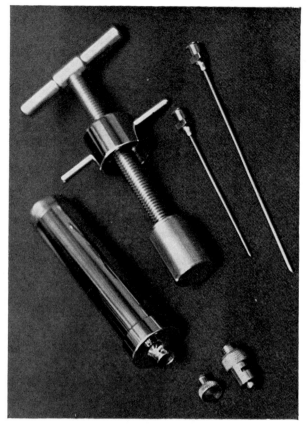

PLATE 99b

GLUTEAL BURSA

Injection I: Lateral Approach

Lesion—Gluteal bursitis comes on gradually for no apparent reason and can continue unchanged for years. It causes aching in the buttock and lateral aspect of the thigh. Since the radiograph of the hip shows nothing, it is usually mistaken for a disc lesion.

Physical Signs—The lumbar movements and testing the sacro-iliac joints provoke no pain. The symptoms are elicited at the extremes of passive range at the hip-joint but in a non-capsular pattern and with a non-capsular end-feel. As a rule full flexion and full lateral rotation bring the symptoms on; sometimes also full passive abduction, which squeezes the bursa against the blade of the ilium. Often resisted abduction hurts, since contraction of the gluteus medius muscle also squeezes the tender bursa.

Intention—The injection has a dual purpose. First, to confirm what is always an uncertain localization, since clear tenderness in the region of the bursa can seldom be established. Hence, after the local anaesthetic solution has been given time to take effect, the movements known to hurt are tested again. If they no longer hurt, the right place has been reached. If not, the search must be renewed.

Secondly, it so happens that what was originally intended as a purely diagnostic injection usually affords considerable lasting relief.

Patient's Posture—The patient lies prone and the operator identifies the upper edge of the greater trochanter. Tenderness is sought in the area lying between the trochanter and the iliac crest and the spot marked.

Injection Technique—A 50 ml syringe is filled with 1:200 procaine solution and fitted with a needle 10 cm long. A horizontal insertion is made just above the trochanter, the likely depth of the lesion is 5 to 8 cm from the skin. A 50 cm cubic area is infiltrated by a series of part withdrawals and reinsertions at a slightly different angle.

Result—The immediate result is diagnostic; the result a week later is a measure of the therapeutic effect. If the injection has helped, as is usual, it is repeated two or three times, until the patient is well. If the diagnosis is established but no lasting benefit accrues, 5 ml steroid suspension are injected in the same place. Between those two solutions, failure is exceptional.

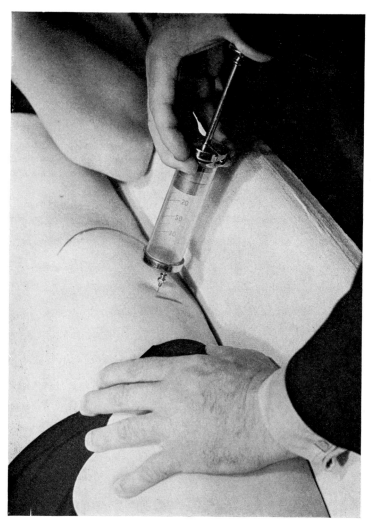

PLATE 100

GLUTEAL BURSA

Injection II: Vertical Approach

Patient's Posture—The patient lies prone on a high couch, her thigh hanging vertically downwards over the edge. Her bent knee rests on a chair. The upper surface of the greater trochanter can now be seen and felt as a horizontal plateau. This posture sometimes enables a tender spot lying close to the trochanter to be identified more accurately.

Injection Technique—A 50 ml syringe is filled with 1:200 procaine solution and fitted with a needle 6 cm long. The needle is inserted vertically downwards until the tip is felt to touch bone. It is then withdrawn about 1 cm and the area thereabouts infiltrated.

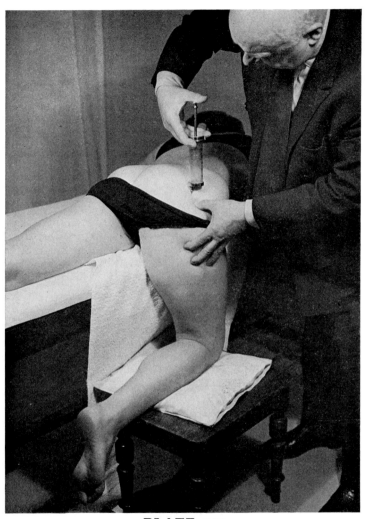

PLATE 101

PSOAS BURSA

Injection Technique

Lesion—Psoas bursitis is an uncommon cause of pain felt at front of the upper thigh. It appears gradually, for no apparent reason, and can go on for years causing pain near the groin on walking.

Physical Signs—These are difficult to interpret, since full passive flexion at the hip squeezes the tender bursa painfully, and full extension and lateral rotation stretch it. Medial rotation is free. The psoas muscle itself is exculpated when resisted flexion is found not to hurt. In gluteal bursitis the reference is to the outer side of the thigh. A loose body in the hip sets up twinges. Osteoarthrosis hurts on passive medial rotation, gives rise to a hard end-feel and shows radiologically.

Intention—The injection has a dual purpose. First, to confirm what must always be a tentative diagnosis. After local anaesthesia has been induced, the movements known to be painful are tested again. If they no longer hurt, the right spot has been reached. Secondly, the injection, though intended diagnostically, is often found therapeutic as well, affording lasting benefit.

Patient's Posture—The patient lies on the couch, his trunk well flexed, so as to relax the tissues at the groin. The anterior superior spine of the ilium is found; pulsation identifies the position of the femoral artery. The femoral nerve lies just lateral to the artery and both are avoided by choosing a point well lateral to the mid-point of the inguinal ligament and 5 cm below it.

Injection Technique—A 50 ml syringe is filled with 1:200 solution of procaine and fitted with a needle 8 cm long. The needle is inserted pointing upwards and medially until it strikes the bone near the junction of the head and the neck of the femur. The needle is withdrawn a few millimetres, until it lies outside the articular capsule. By a series of small withdrawals and reinsertions at a slightly different angle, the area between the hip-joint and the psoas muscle is infiltrated.

Result—If the movements that previously hurt no longer do so, the diagnosis is confirmed. A correctly placed injection often has a lasting therapeutic result, though two or three may be required for full relief. If the diagnosis is confirmed but no lasting improvement is afforded, 5 ml of steroid suspension are substituted.

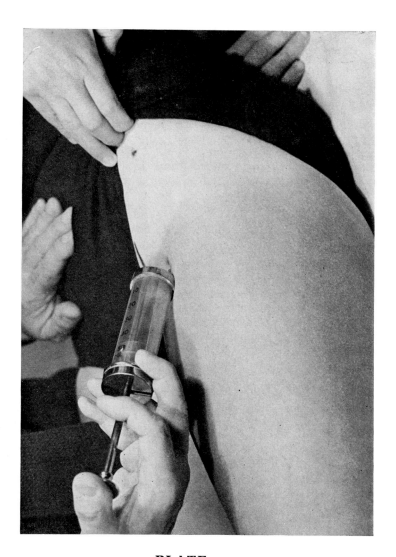

PLATE 102

RECTUS FEMORIS TENDON

Massage Technique

Lesion—This is usually a tendinitis due to over-use. Athletes are apt to develop strain here.

Physical Signs—Examination shows the pain in the groin to be brought on by resisted extension of the knee tested in the prone position. It may be elicited also by full passive flexion of the hip, which pinches the tender part, and/or by full passive rotation, which applies a localized stretch. Hence, a full range of movement is present at the hip-joint, but every extreme is not necessarily painless.

Patient's Posture—The patient sits well up on the couch, so that the hip-joint is held in 90° flexion, otherwise the tissues overlying the tendon are too taut to allow the physiotherapist's finger to penetrate deeply enough.

Technique—The physiotherapist sits at the patient's side facing his thigh. She identifies the anterior superior spine of the ilium and discovers the tendon some 8 cm below this point and in line with it. She places her index and middle fingers on the tendon, using her thumb, placed near the greater trochanter of the femur, for counter-pressure. She imparts her friction deeply, by alternately flexing and extending her wrist, together with a slight adduction–abduction movement at the shoulder.

Duration of Treatment—Twenty minutes twice a week suffice. Three or four weeks' treatment is usually needed.

Result—Uniformly good.

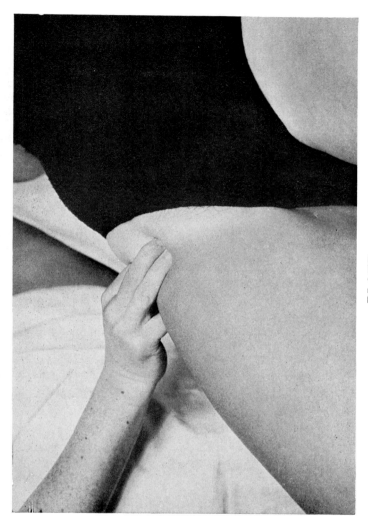

ADDUCTOR LONGUS MUSCLE: MUSCULO-TENDINOUS JUNCTION

Massage Technique

Lesion—This is traumatic and nearly always the result of a sudden over-contraction of the adductor muscles, such as occurs during riding, but nowadays chiefly during football. Ballet dancers may overstretch the muscle.

The lesion more often occurs at the teno-periosteal junction than the musculo-tendinous; occasionally the uppermost part of the belly suffers a minor rupture.

Physical Signs—There is a full range of passive movement at the hip-joint. Full passive abduction may hurt; resisted adduction is painful.

Tenderness is sought at the teno-periosteal junction, the musculo-tendinous junction and the uppermost part of the belly. In the first case massage or steroid is effective; in the second, only massage; in the third, massage or local anaesthesia.

Patient's Posture—The patient adopts the half-lying position on the couch, holding the affected thigh somewhat in abduction and lateral rotation.

Technique—That illustrated is for a lesion at the musculo-tendinous junction. The physiotherapist sits level with the patient's knees, facing him. Her hand grasps the affected area of muscle between her thumb and her index and middle fingers. She imparts the friction by drawing her hand medially.

Duration of Treatment—Twenty minutes twice a week are enough and three or four weeks' treatment may be required.

Results—In all recent and most chronic cases the results are good.

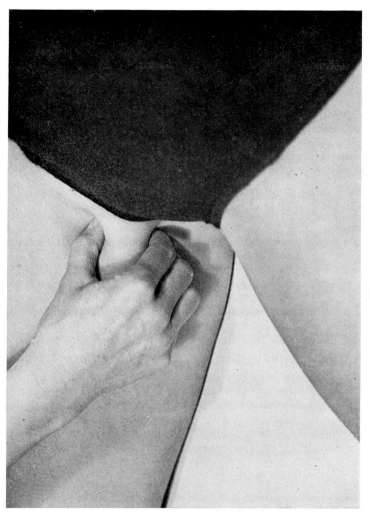

PLATE 104

HAMSTRINGS: BELLY

Massage Technique

Lesion—This is the common injury of sprinters and footballers. The athlete feels the muscle give way painfully at the back of the mid-thigh. Some hours later he is scarcely able to walk.

Physical Signs—Prone-lying resisted knee-flexion hurts. If the muscle tear is extensive, the muscle belly will not stretch fully and straight-leg raising is not only painful but slightly limited for the first few days. The tender area is identified, which may not be easy, since the lesion may lie deeply.

Patient's Posture—The patient lies prone, his knee held well flexed, his leg supported by a cushion. The muscle belly is now relaxed.

Technique—The physiotherapist sits facing his limb and puts both hands on his thigh at the correct level. She presses downwards until her fingers on one side, and her thumb on the other, grasp the belly of the muscle. She alternately flexes and extends her thumb and fingers; at the height of her flexion she draws her hands upwards by flexing her elbows a little so as to increase the transverse effect of her friction. This treatment is extremely tiring and five minutes' friction, five minutes' rest three times in the course of half an hour is about as much as is practicable. Ideally, patients should be treated daily for the first week and on alternate days after that.

After-treatment—The patient lies prone, a cushion under his thigh. His ankle is fixed against his buttock by a strap. Full extension at the hip and full flexion at the knee now so completely relax the hamstring muscles that their full contraction can not pull on the healing breach. Faradic stimulation is now administered for some ten minutes. The muscle is thus broadened out fully, without any strain falling on it. Mobility of the muscle-fibres between each other is maintained without any fear of recurrent rupture.

Duration of Treatment—The muscle is treated until resisted flexion at the knee no longer hurts. To make sure, since recurrence is so common, another week's treatment is given. The muscle, if strained again too hard too soon, is apt to give again; hence he must be warned against premature return to athletics. A minimum is three weeks.

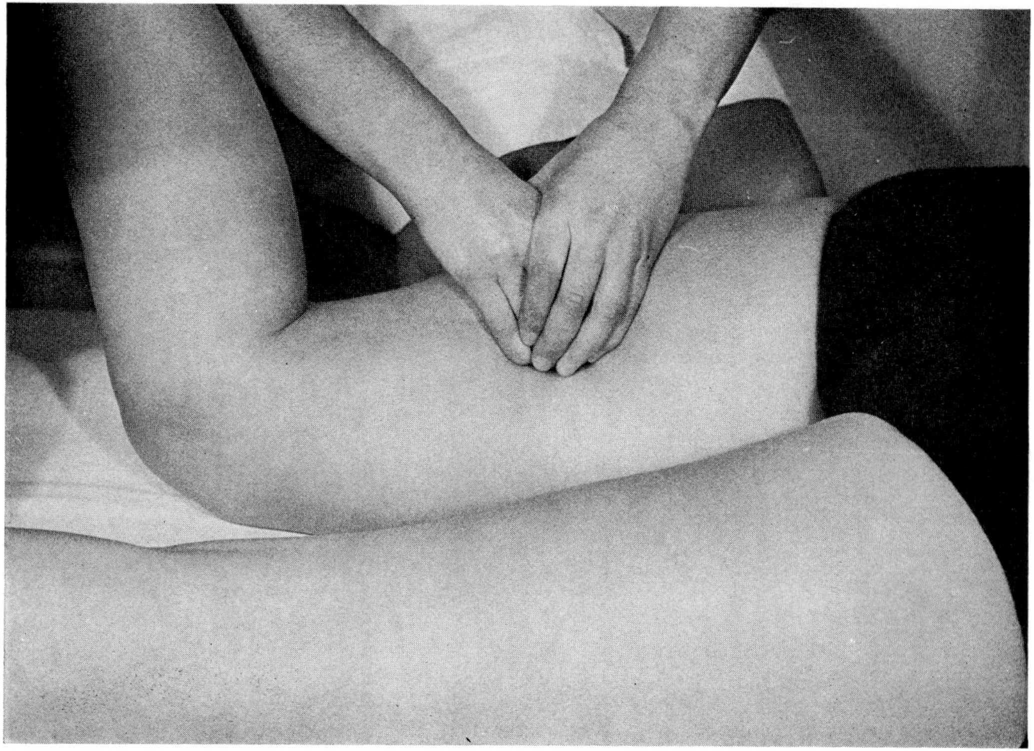

PLATE 105

HAMSTRING: ISCHIAL ORIGIN

Massage Technique

Lesion—Strain occurring at the insertion of the hamstring tendon at the ischium results from a flexion injury of the hip while the knee is held in extension. It is thus uncommon and confined to athletes and dancers.

The tendons are affected usually at the upper 5 cm of their extent.

Physical Signs—The pain in the thigh close to the gluteal fold is brought on by prone-lying resisted knee-flexion. Occasionally, the extreme of straight-leg raising is uncomfortable, since the tendon is then strongly stretched.

Patient's Posture—Unless the hamstring muscles are kept fairly stretched, the tendon lies too loose and deep to be properly palpable. Hence the massage must be given with the tendon fairly taut. To this end the patient lies face upwards with her hip well flexed. A suitable posture is afforded by a stool supporting the patient's calf horizontally, with the result that the thigh lies vertically.

Technique—The physiotherapist sits facing the patient's hip. She should apply two or three fingers to the tendons so as to cover their whole affected extent. Her thumb affords counter-pressure at the outer aspect of the thigh. Her fingers are moved across the tendon by an alternating abduction and adduction movement at the shoulder; there is a slight flexion–extension movement at the wrist as well.

Duration—Twenty minutes' treatment two or three times a week.

Results—In recent cases a fortnight's treatment usually suffices. In chronic cases, treatment may need to be continued for up to two months. Hence, infiltration with steroid suspension should be substituted.

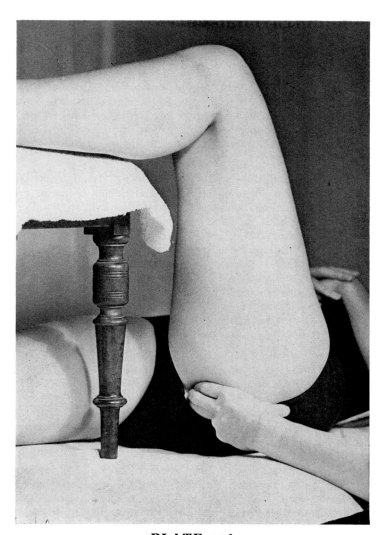

PLATE 106

KNEE-JOINT: TIBIAL COLLATERAL LIGAMENT

Massage in Extension

Lesion—In youngish patients this is nearly always traumatic; in middle age and later chronic strain at this ligament often complicates an impacted loose body at the knee. The lesion commonly lies at that part of the ligament overlying the joint-line and attached to the medial meniscus. A lesion at the femoral condyle is uncommon. Adhesions leading to chronic sprain are frequent. Less commonly a lesion of the lateral collateral ligament occurs, caused by a varus strain.

Physical Signs—Immediately after a severe sprain, the consequent acute traumatic arthritis overshadows the ligamentous lesion, rendering proper examination impossible. The patient, however, knows that he suffered a valgus strain at his knee and felt the ligament tear. Examination reveals a hot joint, full of fluid and extreme tenderness at some point along the medial ligament. When post-traumatic adhesions limit the mobility of the ligament, the knee is adequate for careful use, but hurts on the inner side and swells for a few days after strenuous activity. Examination now shows full passive extension hurting with 5° or 10° limitation of flexion. Considerable discomfort is elicited on passive valgus strain, with clear tenderness at the site of the ligamentous adhesions. The lateral ligament is less intimately connected to the knee joint and the swelling is less marked and the range of movement full. A varus strain hurts and the ligament is tender.

Indication for Massage—All lesions of the ligament without ossification. Immediately after the sprain, the intention is to maintain mobility of the ligament while it is healing. However, traumatic arthritis prevents the bones being moved under the ligament to full range. The alternative is to move the ligament to and fro on the bone. The ligament is moved in relation to the bone, in imitation of its normal behaviour, by the physiotherapist's finger applying transverse friction.

Adhesions require manipulative rupture (see Plates 122–7). Preliminary friction is then less important. However, if the lesion in the ligament lies at the femoral condyle—a part of the ligament that does not move on bone—the treatment remains massage or alternatively hydrocortisone, however long the trouble has lasted. Manipulation is useless at this site.

Contra-indication—Ossification in the ligament (Stieda-Pellegrini's disease). The radiographic finding of a small opaque node is unimportant.

Patient's Posture—The patient lies on the couch with his knee held in as full extension as possible. The ligament now lies at the anterior extreme of its range of movement and mobility is maintained here.

Technique—The physiotherapist sits by the patient's knee and places her fingers on the inner and her thumb on the outer side of the joint in such a

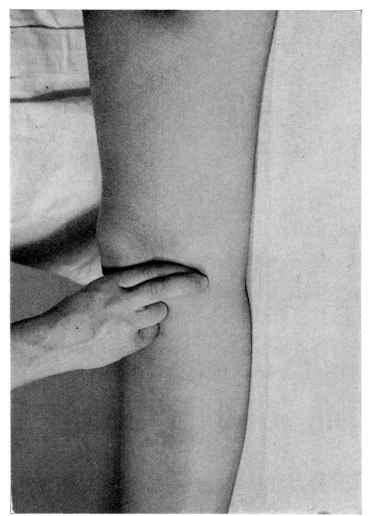

PLATE 107

way that the index finger covers the affected part of the ligament. The grip is strengthened by reinforcement with the middle finger. By alternately flexing and extending her wrist, she moves the forefinger to and fro over the ligament, keeping the thumb still to form the fulcrum. The ligament is thus moved over the bone at the anterior part of its range of movement. If the injury is very recent, great tenderness will be found necessitating a gradual beginning to the friction. Indeed, it may well take the physiotherapist a quarter of an hour of very gentle massage to prepare the spot for the one or two minutes' relatively deep friction that really moves the ligament. If the massage has been adequately given, a large increase in the range of flexion is immediately obtainable without pain; e.g. 90° limitation of flexion may give way to only 45° limitation by next morning. The technique for the lateral ligament is similar. The physiotherapist sits on the opposite side to apply the friction to the affected part of the ligament with the knee in extension. Stretching is seldom necessary.

After-treatment—During the first few days the massage provides the entire treatment. Then, as the range returns, gentle pressure towards extension and flexion follows the massage. When the arthritis is recovering (which is far quicker when massage to the ligament is given) stronger pressure is used, but not beyond the point of causing some discomfort.

KNEE-JOINT: TIBIAL COLLATERAL LIGAMENT

Massage in Flexion

Patient's Posture—The patient lies on the couch with his knee well bent up. Flexion draws the ligament towards the posterior extent of its range of movement and the physiotherapist's friction, by moving the ligament to and fro here, imitates its normal behaviour and maintains range.

Technique—The physiotherapist sits facing the knee, grasping it in such a way that her index finger lies at the central point of the medial aspect of the joint line. Here the ligament can be clearly felt. Keeping her finger-tip on the affected part of the ligament, she imparts the friction by alternately flexing and extending the wrist. By using the thumb as a fulcrum, her index finger is drawn backwards and forwards over the affected part of the ligament.

Massage here is tiring; it is therefore quite a good idea either to sit on the other side of the patient's knee and put the thumb on the ligament, using the finger-tip as fulcrum, or to use first the right hand for five minutes then the left.

Duration of Treatment—The physiotherapist should spend ten minutes on massage of the ligament in the extended position and another ten minutes on massage of the ligament in flexion. Gentle forcing of movement (see Plates 122–7) should immediately follow each of these massage periods, except during the first few days after the sprain.

Result—Massage to the site of the sprain followed by movement greatly diminishes the time required for full recovery after a recent sprain. Most patients get well in a fortnight instead of three months.

Caution—When the ligamentous strain is secondary to a loose body lying at the inner side of the joint, massage is useless. Only manipulative reduction is effective.

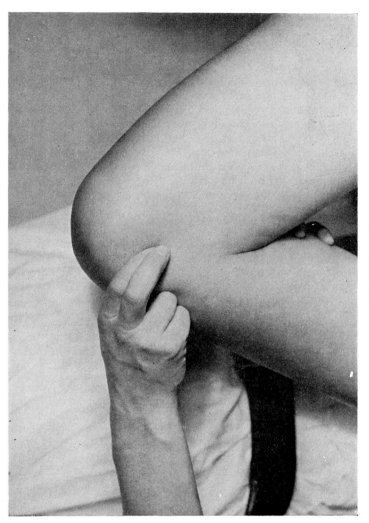

PLATE 108

KNEE-JOINT: TIBIAL COLLATERAL LIGAMENT

Injection Technique

Lesion—Recent sprain of the tibial collateral ligament results in quite severe local pain, considerable fluid in the joint and marked limitation of movement in the capsular pattern. During the first few days, extension is usually 10° restricted, and flexion 90°; after a week, the untreated case may still show 5° and 60° respectively. If massage to the ligament is adopted, the knee recovers in about a fortnight. Steroid suspension is equally effective. The traumatic inflammation at the healing breach is wholly inhibited and in about ten days the knee is practically normal. The scar in the ligament is not yet consolidated, however, and the knee should not be used fully for another week. In the long run, therefore, the two methods have almost identical results.

Contra-indications—
1. An adhesion holding the ligament abnormally adherent, for which massage and manipulation are indicated.
2. Stieda-Pellegrini's shadow, caused by raising up of periosteum.
3. Strain secondary to an impacted loose body at the inner side of the knee, for which manipulative reduction is required.

Physical Signs—The patient knows that his knee was subjected to strain in the valgus direction, and felt a sudden pain at the inner side of the joint. An acute traumatic arthritis is present and the central part of the medial ligament is very tender.

Technique—After examination, the patient is given a strong analgesic, e.g. pethedine, since the injection is very painful at the moment of infiltration and for several hours afterwards. A 2 ml syringe is filled with steroid suspension and fitted with a fine needle 2 cm long. The operator sits facing the inner side of the knee and thrusts the needle in horizontally. He has an area 1 cm square and 0·5 cm thick to infiltrate, and injects a series of droplets all over the affected area.

After-treatment—The patient lies in bed till next day. No further treatment of any sort is given. If the knee is still uncomfortable after a week, a second injection may be given or massage started. The patient can walk as from the morning after the injection, but must be careful of his knee for another two weeks, until the ends of the ligament have united.

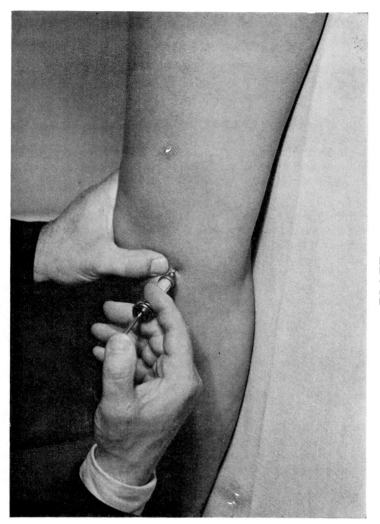

PLATE 109

KNEE-JOINT: CORONARY LIGAMENT

Massage Technique

Lesion—This is always traumatic and just as the meniscus is more often torn on the inner side of the knee so is the medial coronary ligament more often overstretched than the lateral. The cause is a rotation sprain; excessive medial rotation strains the outer coronary ligament, lateral rotation strains the inner. A considerable twist of the femur on the stationary tibia overstretches and sprains the coronary ligament holding the meniscus to the edge of the tibia. This is particularly apt to happen if the knee is slightly bent, since the menisci then move with the femur. If the twisting force continues, the meniscus tears as well.

Intention—To maintain or restore mobility to the coronary ligament. This cannot be done by moving the knee-joint, i.e. the tibia on the femur, for this is the wrong joint. It is at the tibio-meniscal joint that the passive movement must take place. There is only one way to secure such mobility: by means of the physiotherapist's finger. Hydrocortisone is of little avail on account of the thin line of tissue requiring infiltration; technically it is almost impossible. The treatment of coronary sprain, acute, subacute or chronic, is the same—deep friction to the ligament. It is extremely effective.

Physical Signs—The patient knows that his knee has suffered a rotation strain and that a sudden pain was felt at the inner or outer side of the knee. The traumatic arthritis is less severe than in collateral ligament sprain and the tenderness is at the edge of the tibial condyle not on the medial ligament.

Patient's Posture—The patient lies on the couch with his knee not quite fully flexed. In full flexion, even if it is obtainable, the capsule of the knee-joint tautens to the extent of holding the physiotherapist's finger off the ligament. By rotating the tibia on the femur the tibial condyle can be brought into greater prominence. External rotation will bring the medial coronary ligament within easier reach and internal rotation renders the lateral coronary ligament more accessible.

Technique—The physiotherapist sits level with the injured knee. If the medial coronary ligament is at fault, she sits on the same side of the patient as the damaged knee; if the lateral ligament, on the far side. She identifies the tibial condyle by coming down on it from above, and places her index finger on it. She reinforces with the middle finger. She presses her index finger towards the femur, so as to indent the superficial tissues and now presses downwards on to the ligament. Her *index finger-nail* lies *horizontally*, otherwise she cannot press downwards on to the shelf formed by the tibial condyle. Her finger is all but straight; very slight flexion is required to bring the tip on to the ligament. Her finger lies horizontally, in

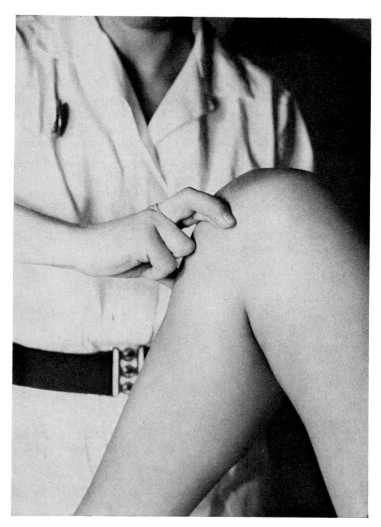

PLATE 110

line with the movement to be imparted. The thumb is used opposite the index to supply counter-pressure downwards; the pressure indenting the knee is maintained by the medial rotators of the shoulder. The movement to the ligament is imparted by her drawing her index finger-tip *horizontally* along the condyle by alternately flexing and extending her wrist.

Massage to the coronary ligament is often given the wrong way. The unwary physiotherapist may press her index medially against the femoral condyle, holding her finger-nail vertical. None of the friction then reaches the ligament, which is wasted on the articular cartilage of the femur. *The pressure must be exerted downwards*, where indeed the ligament lies.

Duration of Treatment—Ten or fifteen minutes daily the first week, on alternate days the second week. A coronary sprain usually gets well of itself in three months, but sometimes goes on indefinitely. A week or two's treatment is, in my experience, always successful, whether the patient is seen the day of the accident or many years later. There is no alternative. Hence, this is one of the most important frictional techniques that a physiotherapist needs to master.

PLATE III

KNEE-JOINT

Intra-articular Injection Technique

Lesion—Arthritis of the knee occurs in many diseases, rheumatoid arthritis or it may complicate, for example, ankylosing spondylitis, psoriasis, lupus erythematosus or non-specific urethritis.

Physical Signs—Warmth, fluid and capsular thickening at the joint. In the earliest stage, in spite of these local signs, the range of movement is full. Later restriction of movement in the capsular pattern supervenes. In advanced rheumatoid arthritis, crepitus and osteophyte formation may lead to a mistaken radiological diagnosis of osteoarthrosis.

Patient's Posture—The patient lies on the couch and consciously relaxes her quadriceps muscle. The operator places his thumb at the medial edge of the patella, lifting it off the femur by tilting it with his thumb.

Injection Technique—A 5 ml syringe is filled with steroid suspension and fitted with a thin needle 4 cm long. A point is chosen at the interval between the raised patella and the femoral condyle. The needle is thrust in horizontally and becomes intra-articular at about 2 cm. The injection is made here.

Result—Uniformly good except in Reiter's disease, for which steroids are useless.

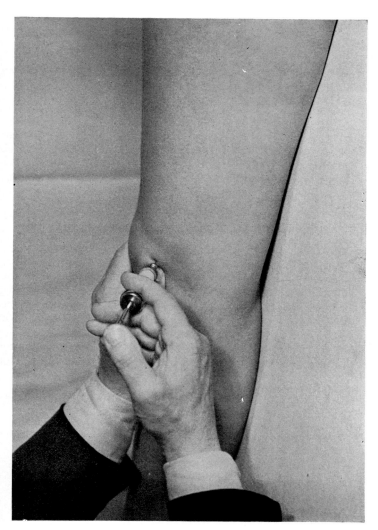

PLATE III

SUPRAPATELLAR TENDON

Massage Technique

Lesion—This is traumatic and lies at the insertion of the tendon into the patella. It is nearly always due to a sudden over-contraction of the quadriceps muscle. It also occurs as an over-use phenomenon in the one-legged.

Physical Signs—A full and painless passive range of movement is present at the knee. No warmth or fluid is detected. Resisted extension hurts at the front of the knee; resisted flexion does not. The tenderness is found at the insertion of the suprapatellar tendon into the bone. Infrapatellar tendinitis is commoner than suprapatellar.

Patient's Posture—The patient lies on the couch with the knee fully extended and the quadriceps muscle relaxed.

Technique—The physiotherapist sits facing the patient's knee. She presses downwards on the lower pole of the patella with the web of her thumb, her fingers to one and her thumb to the other side of the knee. This steadies the patella and at the same time tilts the upper pole forwards, thus bringing the lesion into a more accessible position. She places the middle finger of her other hand, reinforced by the index, against the upper pole of the patella. By pressing downwards and backwards she catches the tendinous fibres of insertion against the bone. The friction is imparted by a to-and-fro movement of her whole forearm and hand. It is very tiring to the physiotherapist.

Duration of Treatment—Twenty minutes two or three times a week. More than a month's treatment is seldom needed.

Results—Good, as long as the friction is given long enough and really hard over the entire extent of teno-periosteal junction affected.

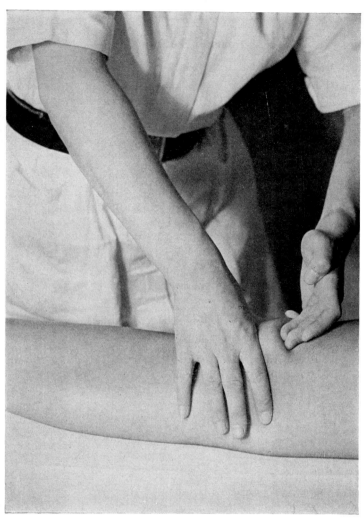

PLATE 112

SUPRAPATELLAR TENDON

Injection Technique

Lesion—See page 360.

Patient's Posture—The patient lies on the couch with the knee extended and the quadriceps muscle relaxed. The operator's left hand presses on the lower pole of the patella, so as to tilt the upper border forwards. This edge is now identified and the tender area singled out. It is from 1 to 2 cm long. A spot is now chosen about 1·5 cm above the centre of the affected region of tendon.

Injection Technique—A 2 ml syringe is filled with steroid suspension and fitted with a thin needle 2 cm long. It is inserted at the spot marked and a series of fanwise insertions made moving the tip along the affected area of the teno-periosteal junction. Nothing is injected until at each shift of the needle the tip is felt to touch bone. Accuracy is ensured by the tilting of the patella, whose upper edge projects.

After-treatment—There is considerable soreness for one or two days. The patient treats his knee as gently as possible for a week. He then tries it out and is seen again at the end of ten days.

Results—Two or three injections are often required, since a small spot may be omitted as the needle is moved along the edge of the bone.

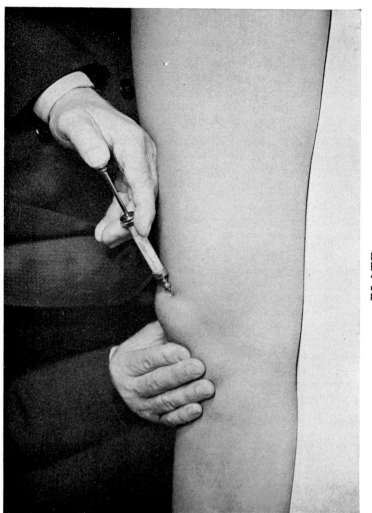

PLATE 113

QUADRICEPS EXPANSION

Massage Technique

Lesion—This is usually the result of over-use, but a direct blow is occasionally the cause. Footballers and the one-legged are prone to strain here. The inner or outer expansion may be affected, but the two lesions appear not to occur together. Recurrent dislocation of the patella strains the expansion on the inner side each time.

Physical Signs—There is a full and painless range of passive movement at the knee-joint. No warmth or fluid is present. The pain at the front of the knee is elicited by resisted extension; resisted flexion is painless. The tenderness is found at the insertion of the expansion at one or other side of the patella.

Patient's Posture—The patient lies with the knee extended and the quadriceps muscle fully relaxed.

Technique—The physiotherapist sits facing the patient's knee. One hand grasps the leg in such a way as to enable the thumb to push the patella well over towards the affected side. The ring finger of her other hand, reinforced by the middle finger, is placed behind the now projecting edge of the patella. This finger, by pressing forwards, catches the expansion against the bone. The friction is imparted by a horizontal movement of the physiotherapist's forearm and hand.

This treatment is often wrongly given. The physiotherapist must not use her finger with the nail vertical exerting pressure against the femur. Her nail is horizontal and her pressure against the back of the projecting edge of the patella.

Duration of Treatment—Twenty minutes' friction suffices.

Results—Recent sprains usually clear up after two or three sessions in the course of a week. In long-standing cases, two or three weeks' treatment may be required. Full lasting relief has always been attained in my experience. Steroid suspension is not effective.

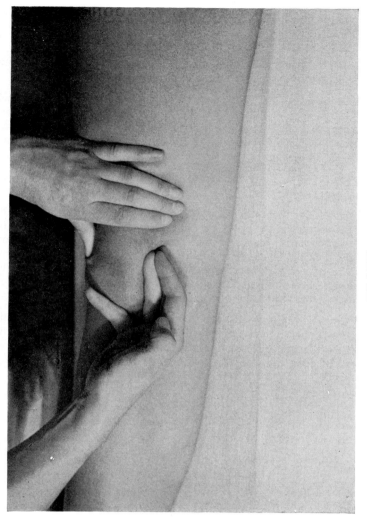

PLATE 114

INFRAPATELLAR TENDON

Massage Technique

Lesion—This is nearly always caused by over-use. Occasionally one sudden over-contraction of the quadriceps muscle is responsible.

Physical Signs—A full and painless range of movement exists at the knee. Warmth and fluid are absent. Resisted extension hurts at the front of the knee; resisted flexion does not. Tenderness is found at the lower pole of the patella at an area about 1·5 cm long. In my experience the tibial extremity of the tendon is never at fault.

Patient's Posture—The patient lies with the knee fully extended and the quadriceps muscle relaxed.

Technique—The physiotherapist sits facing his mid-thigh and places the web of her thumb on the upper part of the patella. Pressure here tilts the lower pole forwards, rendering the teno-periosteal junction prominent. She places the ring finger of her other hand on this line, pressing upwards against the edge of the bone. She reinforces with the long finger. The pressure is applied by adducting the arm strongly. The friction is imparted by alternate flexion and extension movements at elbow and shoulder.

Duration of Treatment—Twenty minutes suffice and are about as long as a physiotherapist can manage. Even long-standing lesions here usually clear up with friction given two or three times weekly for from two to six weeks. Recent injuries seldom need more than two or three weeks' treatment.

Results—Permanent relief is the rule.

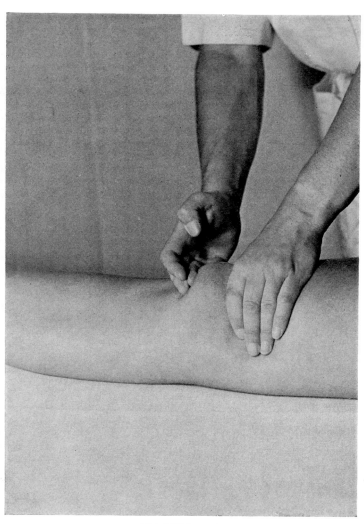

PLATE 115

INFRAPATELLAR TENDON

Injection Technique

Lesion—See page 366.

Patient's Posture—The patient lies face upwards on the couch, the knee extended and the quadriceps muscle relaxed. The operator's left thumb is pressed against the upper part of the patella so as to tilt the lower pole forwards. The exact extent of the tender aera at the teno-periosteal junction is identified. A spot is chosen 1·5 cm inferior to the mid-point of this area.

Injection Technique—A 2 ml syringe is fitted with a thin needle 2·5 cm long and filled with a steroid suspension. The patella is held tilted and the needle inserted at the point chosen, pointing directly superiorly. A series of droplets is injected along the line by a series of fanwise small withdrawals and reinsertions. The injections are given only when the tip of the needle is felt to touch bone. The bevel of the needle then ensures that the teno-periosteal junction is infiltrated.

After-treatment—Considerable soreness lasts one to two days. The patient uses his knee as little as possible for a week.

Result—Uniformly good, but two or three injections may be required since it is easy to omit a small extent of the lesion as the needle is moved along.

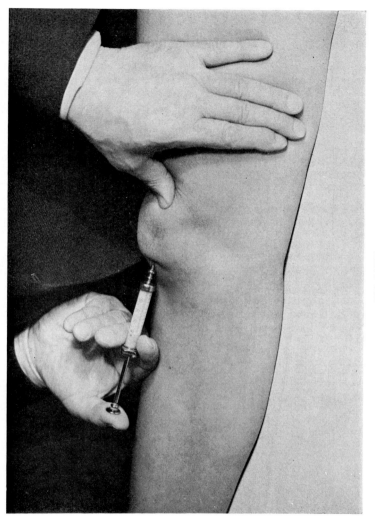

PLATE 116

BICEPS TENDON AT KNEE

Massage Technique

Lesion—Tendinitis here is nearly always due to over-use, and may result from the prolonged maintenance of active flexion at the knee, e.g. in driving a car whose seat is too low or too close to the foot controls. The lesion nearly always occurs at the fibres of insertion into the head of the fibula.

Physical Signs—The pain is felt at the outer side of the knee and is not elicited by any passive movement at the joint. However, resisted flexion and lateral rotation both bring the pain on and tenderness is found at the fibular insertion.

Patient's Posture—It matters very little if the patient lies prone or supine so long as his knee is extended; the illustration shows him lying face downwards.

Technique—The physiotherapist sits level with the patient's foot, facing his head. She can identify the head of the fibula most easily by coming up on to it from below. She then places her thumb on the tendon of the biceps muscle and grasps the patient's leg so that her fingers supply counter-pressure. By keeping her fingers still and giving small alternate pronation and supination movements to her forearm, she draws her thumb to and fro over the tendon.

Duration of Treatment—Twenty minutes twice a week are adequate. Three to six weeks' treatment may be required.

Results—Uniformly good.

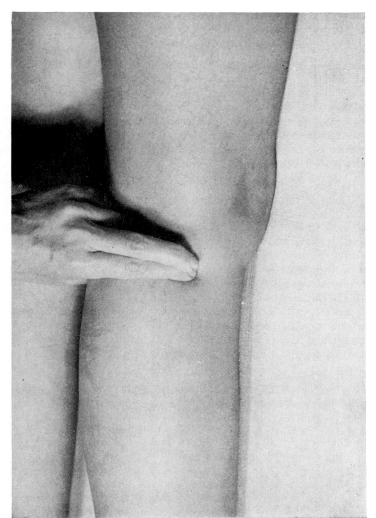

PLATE 117

ANTERIOR CRUCIATE LIGAMENT: ANTERIOR END

Injection Technique

Lesion—A hyperextension strain of the knee may overstretch the anterior cruciate ligament; so may a sudden jerk forcing the tibia forwards on the femur when the knee is held bent. In my experience, the lesion always lies at the ligamento-periosteal junction, but the physician has small means of knowing whether it is at the anterior attachment at the tibial spine or the posterior attachment to the medial surface of the lateral condyle of the femur. Other tissues may have been sprained too and require separate treatment.

Physical Signs—The patient sprains the knee, but describes pain felt within the joint. A minor degree of traumatic arthritis follows, and search for collateral and coronary tenderness shows that none of these four ligaments is involved. When the tibia is held at a right-angle to the femur and pulled sharply forwards, the pain within the knee is elicited. Excessive antero-posterior range shows the ligament to have become elongated. If the patient complains of pain, not instability, removal of the former restores full function. If the joint is unsound, though the infiltration will stop the pain, the knee will remain unstable.

The decision of which end of the ligament to infiltrate is hard to make; it can be only a guess. Examination determines which ligament; whereabouts the pain is felt is the only guide to which end. Usually there is no knowing. If so, one end is injected; then, if no benefit has acc ued by a week later, the other end.

Patient's Posture—The patient lies on the couch, the knee bent to a right-angle. The lower pole of the patella is identified.

Injection Technique—The injection is given the same day as the patient is seen; a duration of hours or years make no difference. A 2 ml syringe is filled with steroid suspension and a thin needle 5 cm long is fitted. Piercing the skin so as just to clear the patella, the needle is thrust downwards and backwards at an angle of 45°, aimed at the spine of the tibia. If it hits bone directly, the tip does not lie within the ligament. If the needle is felt to traverse a resistant tissue before touching bone, the tip lies at the ligamento-periosteal junction. By means of a series of small withdrawals and reinsertions, an area about a centimetre square is infiltrated.

Results—Whether the sprain is of a few days' or even years' standing, recovery is complete within at most ten days, provided that the entire area of the lesion has been adequately infiltrated. More than two injections are seldom required.

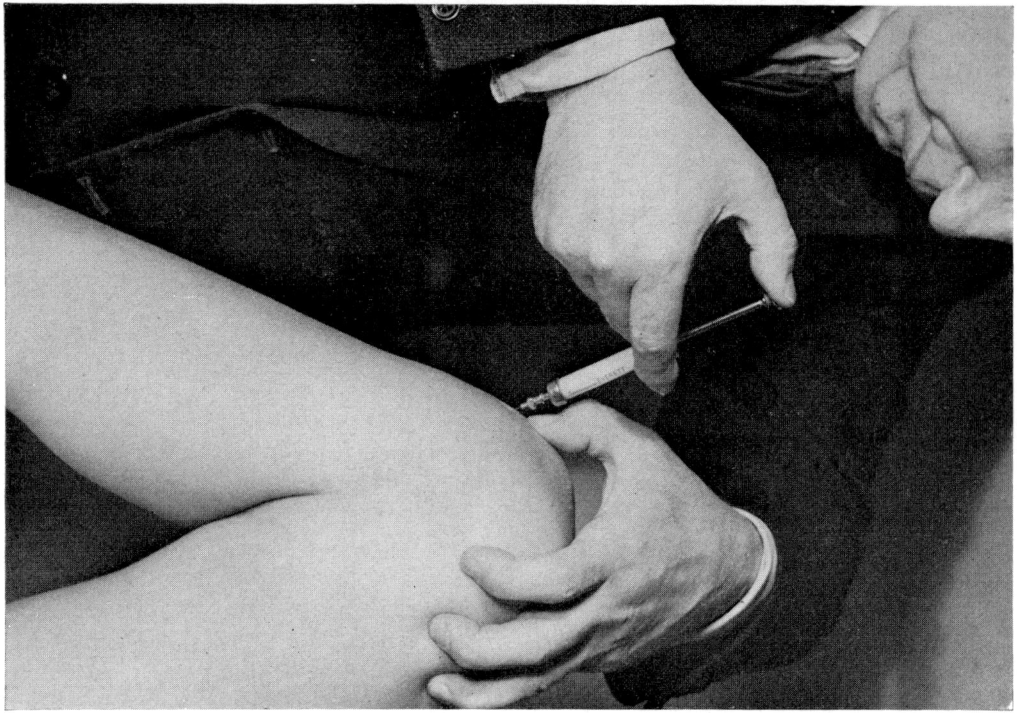

PLATE 118

ANTERIOR CRUCIATE LIGAMENT: POSTERIOR END

Injection Technique

Lesion—See page 372.

Patient's Posture—The patient lies prone, the knee extended. The projections formed by the two femoral condyles are identified. A spot is marked at the apex of the medial condyle.

Injection Technique—A 2 ml syringe is filled with steroid suspension and a thin needle 6 cm long is fitted. It is inserted at the marked spot and aimed at the medial surface of the lateral condyle, i.e. transversely and at an angle of 30° with the horizontal, thus passing well posterior to the popliteal vessels. If the tip strikes bone, the correct spot has not been reached. If the needle is felt to pierce a resistant structure and then to touch bone, the tip lies within the ligament. At each small withdrawal and reinsertion, this sensation must be sought afresh, so as to ensure that the multiple injections are all intra-ligamentous.

Result—The traumatic arthritis consequent upon a strained cruciate ligament ordinarily subsides in six to twelve months. After accurate infiltration, the knee should be fit for normal use in two weeks (including football). Pain is abolished, but instability caused by material lengthening is not altered. Slight lengthening, once the pain has ceased, often proves no disability.

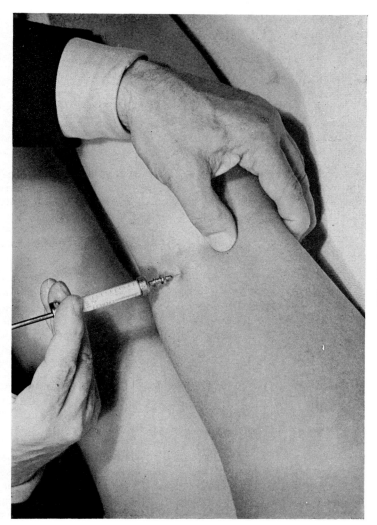

PLATE 119

POSTERIOR CRUCIATE LIGAMENT: POSTERIOR END

Injection Technique

Lesion—If the tibia is forced backwards on the femur while the knee is held bent, the posterior cruciate ligament can be overstretched, e.g. a dashboard injury. In my experience, the lesion always lies at the attachment of ligament to bone, but it is scarcely possible to determined at which end. However, the posterior end of the ligament is much more often affected than the anterior; hence this should be infiltrated first.

Physical Signs—The patient reports the nature of the sprain, and describes pain felt within the joint. A minor degree of traumatic arthritis supervenes, but search along the collateral and coronary ligaments reveals no tenderness. When the tibia is held at a right-angle to the femur and pushed backwards, the central pain is evoked. Excessive range shows that the ligament has become overstretched; this is permanent. The injection relieves pain but cannot alter instability.

Patient's Posture—The patient lies prone, the knee extended. The level of the upper surface of the tibia is identified by palpation at the antero-lateral side of the joint, where the interval between tibia and femur is most easily felt. The posterior end of the posterior cruciate ligament lies at the exact mid-point of the tibia, at this level. A spot is marked at the apex of the lateral condyle of the femur, some 3 cm above the level of the tibial surface.

Injection Technique—A 2 ml syringe is filled with steroid suspension and fitted with a thin needle 5 cm long. At the marked spot the needle is inserted, aiming at the centre of the posterior tibial edge. It is directed slightly inferiorly and at 60° to the horizontal. This lateral approach avoids the popliteal vessels. By means of a number of small withdrawals and reinsertions, the posterior aspect of the tibia is found. The direction of the needle is then progressively altered, until resistance ceases, the needle passing without obstruction into the knee-joint. This is just too far, and the needle is directed back to the previous point. The area here is infiltrated, the tip being felt to penetrate ligament before touching bone each time it is shifted a little.

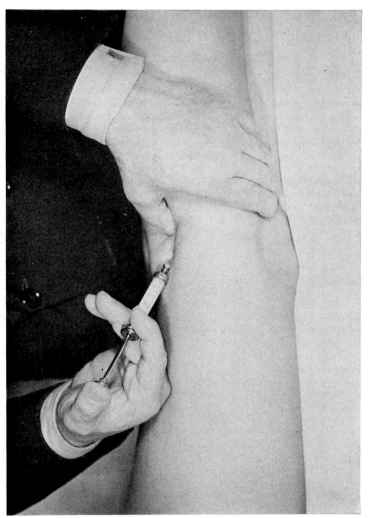

PLATE 120

POSTERIOR CRUCIATE LIGAMENT:
ANTERIOR END

Injection Technique

Lesion—See page 376.

Patient's Posture—The patient lies supine, the knee straight. The midpoint of the outer border of the patella is identified. A spot is chosen here just beyond the patellar margin. The operator applies the thumb of his left hand under the upper part of the lateral patellar edge and tilts it so that the surface of the patella is lifted off the femoral condyle.

Injection Technique—A 2 ml syringe filled with steroid suspension is fitted with a thin needle 6 cm long. At the marked spot, the needle is inserted parallel to the articular surface of the patella and pushed on until the tip meets the lateral aspect of the medial surface of the femoral condyle. It must then be moved, little by little, until the resistance of the ligament is felt before bone is touched. A number of small injections is made here.

Result—Many months of traumatic arthritis and pain are obviated. Within two weeks a patient with a recent sprain is fit for football again; a chronic sprain may have ceased in a week. Instability is unaffected, but slight permanent lengthening may not matter, once pain ceases. Material elongation naturally goes on causing symptoms.

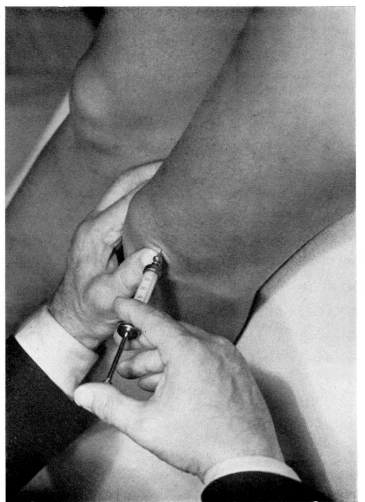

PLATE 121

KNEE-JOINT

Forced Extension

Lesion—Adhesions form about the medial collateral ligament if the knee is not moved adequately during healing from a sprain. The scar develops abnormal adherence to bone and the ligament is no longer fully mobile. Hence recovery is never complete, the knee hurting at the inner side for several days after any exertion.

Physical Signs—The pain is at the inner side of the knee. Full passive extension hurts there; flexion is 5° or 10° limited. Medial rotation is painless; lateral rotation hurts at the extreme. Applying valgus strain to the knee also hurts and the mid-part of the ligament is tender.

Indication—Abnormal adherence to the medial ligament to the femur.

Contra-indications—Recent strain of the ligament. Stieda-Pellegrini's periosteal elevation of the ligament.

Patient's Posture—The patient lies supine on the couch and extends the knee as much as he can.

Technique—The physiotherapist stands by the patient's side, level with his leg. She lifts his heel off the couch with one hand and presses down on his knee, just above the patella with her other palm. Since an adhesion is to be broken, the movement should be a quick jerk.

After-treatment—For a few days afterwards the patient repeats this movement actively at frequent intervals, so as to maintain the increased range.

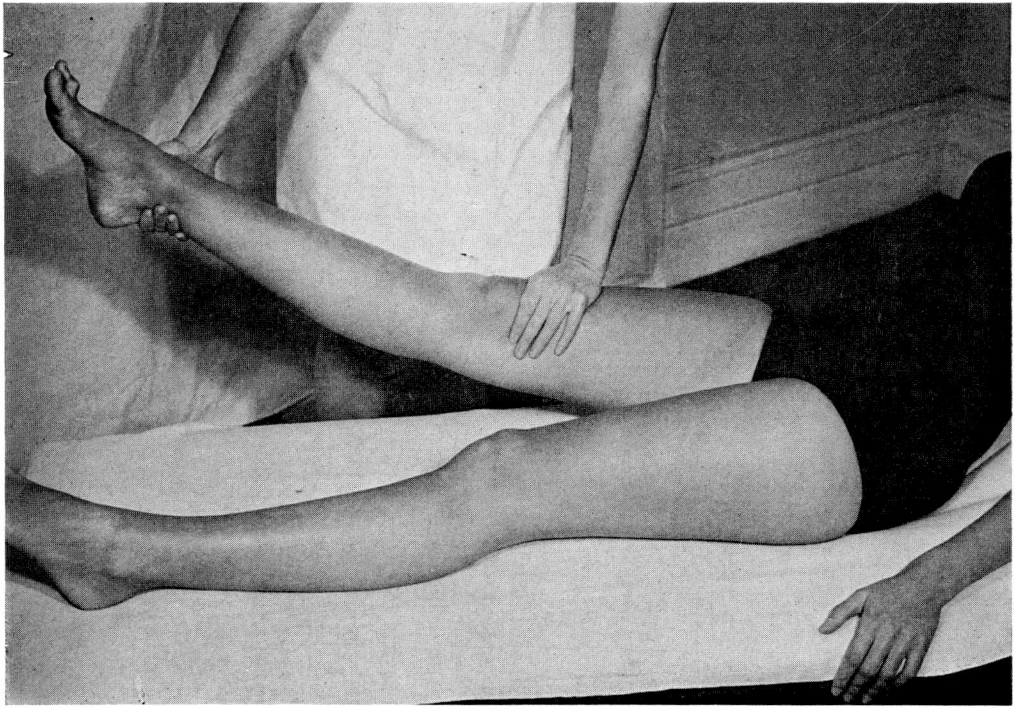

PLATE 122

KNEE-JOINT

Forced Flexion I

Indications—Limitation of flexion due to adhesions about the medial collateral ligament.

Contra-indications—As for forced extension (see page 380).

Patient's Posture—The patient adopts the half-lying position on the couch. The back of the couch should not be tilted too high, since the patient's trunk then interferes with the preliminary achievement of the necessary considerable flexion at the hip-joint.

Technique—The physiotherapist stands level with the patient's other knee. She flexes his thigh at the hip as far as it will comfortably go; unless this is done, she has very little control when flexion is forced at the knee. She places one hand at this knee, thus steadying it and maintaining flexion at the hip. She then places her other hand on his ankle and forces the patient's heel towards his thigh with a smart jerk. The movement ends when the heel hits the upper thigh. The adhesion parts with a tiny snap, scarcely enough to convince the manipulator that his work is done.

After-treatment—For the next few days, the patient squats every few hours, thereby using his body weight to ensure full passive flexion at the knee. The added range is thus maintained.

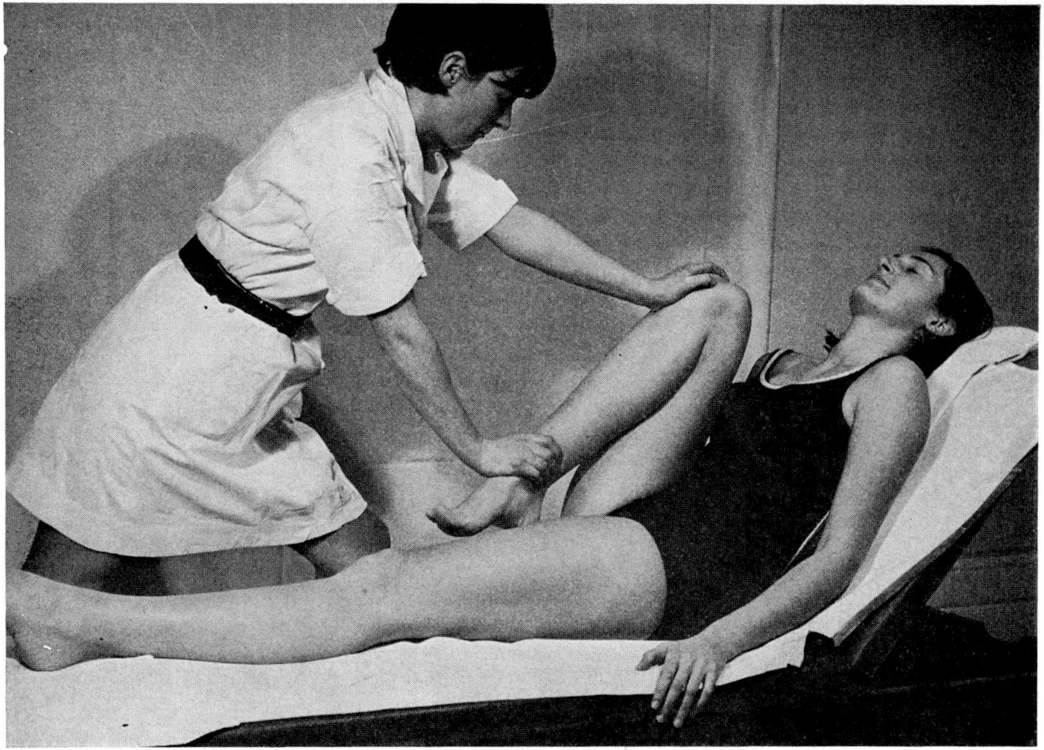

PLATE 123

KNEE-JOINT

Forced Flexion II

Lesion—A curious condition exists at the knee when, some weeks after an operation or an injury to the inner femoral condyle, increasing limitation of flexion sets in without any corresponding restriction of extension or rotation. The joint appears normal otherwise; it is not warm and no fluid is present.

Gentle forcing does not prevent flexion becoming increasingly restricted.

Physical Signs—The knee will not flex beyond 90°; no other sign is present. The nature of the lesion becomes clear only during the manipulation, when a loud sound resembling the tearing of a piece of silk is heard. Where such a gross adhesion lies is a mystery to me.

Patient's Posture—The patient lies prone on a high couch, and flexes his knee as much as he can.

Technique—The operator stands facing the patient's knee and crooks her elbow about the front of his ankle; she presses with her other forearm against the back of his knee. She then clasps her hands. By maintaining this position of her forearm and tilting her body towards the patient's head, she keeps his knee on the couch while the knee-joint is forcibly flexed. Great power is obtained in this way.

After-treatment—Next day, the knee is warm, full of fluid and considerably more painful than before the manipulation. A 10 kg weight is attached by a rope passing over a pulley to the patient's leg by means of an ankle-strap. The pull on the cord is horizontal and towards his head. He is told to extend the knee actively and then to relax, letting the weight swing his leg back towards flexion at the knee. When the limitation of flexion has fallen to 45°, weight-bearing knee-flexion exercises restore the full range in about a month.

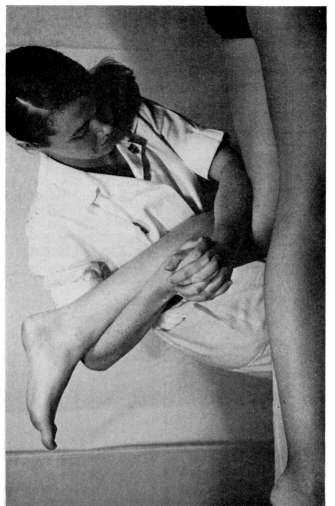

PLATE 124

KNEE-JOINT

Forced Lateral Rotation

Lesion—Adherence of the medial collateral ligament to bone causes pain on full lateral rotation of the knee. This movement must therefore be forced.

Physical Signs—See page 380.

Patient's Posture—The patient adopts the half-lying position on the couch, and flexes his thigh at the hip-joint.

Technique—Since the rotation range at the knee is at its greatest when the joint is well flexed, the physiotherapist must hold the hip and knee in considerable flexion by pressing one hand on the patient's knee. She then hooks the fingers of her other hand round the back and outer side of the patient's heel, applying her forearm to the inner border of his foot. The greatest pressure is taken by the distal part of his first metatarsal bone. She now forces lateral rotation of the tibia on the femur, using his foot, held at right-angles to his leg, as a lever. When an adhesion requires rupture, the movement is an abrupt adduction of the physiotherapist's elbow.

After-treatment—The patient stands and bends his knee about 45°. He then twists his body round away from the affected knee. This turns his femur inwards on the stationary tibia, thus forcing lateral rotation.

He does this exercise each few hours for a few days, ceasing when the movement is free and quite painless.

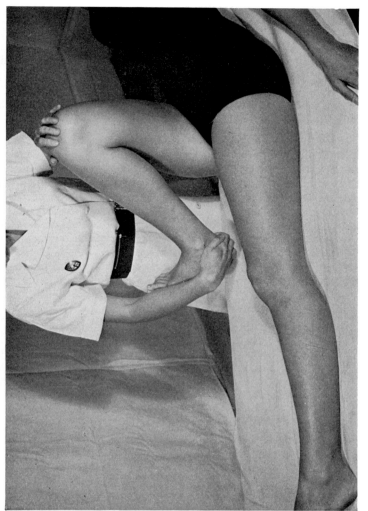

PLATE 125

KNEE-JOINT

Forced Medial Rotation

Lesion—Adhesions limiting mobility of the medial collateral ligament.

Physical Signs—See page 380.

Patient's Posture—The patient adopts the half-lying position on the couch and flexes his thigh at the hip-joint.

Technique—The reverse of the method illustrated on Plate 125 cannot be used, since it is easy to sprain the patient's ankle in this way. Only the heel can safely be used as a lever when medial rotation of the leg is forced.

The physiotherapist stands at the patient's side level with his thigh. She clasps her hands tightly about his heel and holds the knee and hip flexed. By a combined movement of both wrists, she twists his heel strongly, thereby forcing medial rotation at the knee-joint. As long as her hand on the outer side of his ankle does not exert pressure beyond the calcaneo-cuboid joint line, the fibular collateral ligament of the ankle joint is safe.

Some physiotherapists find it easier to pass the forearm belonging to the hand which grasps the inner side of his heel in front of rather than behind the patient's leg.

After-treatment—As for forced lateral rotation, but the body is turned towards the painful side.

N.B.—Lateral and antero-posterior mobility at the knee-joint are undesirable movements that never require increasing. Thus it is no part of the restoration of range at the knee-joint to attempt to overstretch the collateral or cruciate ligaments.

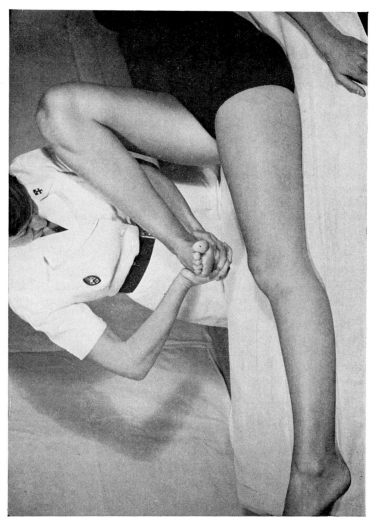

PLATE 126

KNEE-JOINT: REDUCTION OF SUBLUXATED MENISCUS

Lesion—Displacement of the loose portion of the intra-articular meniscus is the result of a rotation sprain. This first overstretches the coronary ligament, then ruptures the meniscus. A rim of cartilage attached to the ligament remains in place; the body of the meniscus slips over the dome of the femoral condyle to lie towards the centre of the joint. The medial meniscus is more often ruptured than the lateral; hence the manipulation illustrated is that for the former lesion.

Physical Signs—The history describes a rotation sprain followed by such severe pain at one side of the joint that the patient falls to the ground. When he tries to get up, he finds the knee locked in flexion.

There is a springly block limiting extension at the knee by 10°. Traumatic arthritis limits flexion by perhaps 30°—the non-capsular pattern. The coronary ligament on the affected side is very tender.

Anaesthesia—General anaesthesia is often required, especially on the first occasion.

Patient's Posture—The patient lies face upwards on the couch and flexes both hip and knee to a right-angle. She relaxes her thigh muscle as best she can.

Technique—The manipulator has, in the case of the medial meniscus, to move the cartilaginous fragment medially, since it lies displaced towards the centre of the joint. He must therefore apply strong valgus strain on the joint so as to open the inner aspect and encourage reduction in that direction. At the same time he must gradually extend the knee while rotating it to and fro rapidly. His one hand is therefore placed at the outer side of the knee and presses medially and towards the floor; the other hand at the foot rotates the leg and pulls it laterally, also holding it up so that the pressure of his first hand on the knee causes the joint to extend.

As the full range of extension is reached, reduction is signalled by a small click, whereupon extension at the knee is immediately felt to become free. The manipulation may have to be repeated several times before it succeeds.

When the lateral meniscus is at fault, the manipulator must apply varus strain to the knee-joint; hence his one hand must be placed at the inner side of the joint and his other hand at the ankle must press the leg medially (not illustrated). Otherwise the movement is the same.

Should skilled manipulation under anaesthesia fail to secure reduction—a rarity—the whole meniscus should be removed at operation as soon as possible.

After-treatment—If reduction is carried out shortly after a recurrent displacement no after-treatment is required. Otherwise it is as for sprain of

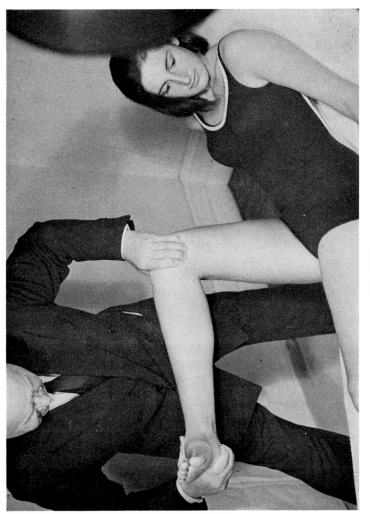

PLATE 127

the coronary ligament (see page 354) which, especially on the first occasion of the meniscal rupture, is painfully strained. A second attack of internal derangement calls for excision of the entire meniscus.

A cyst of the lateral meniscus requires puncture of its cartilaginous wall. Several punctures should be carried out since it may be loculated. The aperture remains patent lastingly, since an avascular structure cannot heal; cure therefore results. If the cyst has led to rupture the entire meniscus requires removal.

KNEE-JOINT: REDUCTION OF IMPACTED LOOSE BODY I

Lesion—Middle-aged people are apt suddenly to develop causeless pain at, usually, the inner side of the knee. Twinges make the patient apprehensive walking downstairs. The cause is sudden non-traumatic impaction of a loose body at the inner side of the joint. It is nearly always a cartilaginous fragment, and so does not show radiologically. In consequence, a diagnosis of osteoarthrosis is often made. But osteoarthrosis does not come on suddenly, at one side of the joint only, and cause twinges.

Physical Signs—The signs of an active lesion are usually present—warmth and fluid. The movements indicate sprain of the medial collateral ligament; full extension and full lateral rotation hurt at the inner side of the joint; flexion is painful and 5°, perhaps 10°, limited. Valgus strain hurts and the central part of the medial collateral ligament is tender. Clearly the ligament is sprained, but there has been no sprain by extrinsic force. It is therefore intrinsic, from within the knee, i.e. a space-occupying lesion at the medial side. The diagnostic principle is simple: sprain of the medial ligament in a patient who has not sprained it.

The loose bodies which form in young patients as the result of osteochondrosis dissecans or chondromalacia patellae possess a bony nucleus. They show up radiologically and require removal.

Intention—The intention behind this manipulation is to move the loose body from its position between the articulating surfaces towards a neutral situation within the joint, i.e. posteriorly, where it no longer engages. To this end the tibia and femur must be distracted so as to give the fragment room to move.

Anaesthesia—As this method is practically painless, general anaesthesia is not required. Apprehensive patients should be told that the examination of the knee after each manoeuvre cannot be carried out in the unconscious patient, and the likelihood of success is correspondingly diminished.

Patient's Posture—The patient lies prone on the couch and flexes her knee to a right-angle. An assistant holds her lower thigh down on to the couch, pressing with her whole weight.

Technique—The operator stands level with the patient's knee, his one hand grasping the dorsum of her foot and the other her ankle. The web of his thumb catches under her heel, thus holding the foot in dorsiflexion; this gives a good purchase for his other hand. He now lifts the patient's thigh off the couch by hooking her foot on to his far thigh, his foot on the couch. The assistant now presses downwards as hard as she can, her hands applied to the back of the thigh close above the knee (Plate 128). This position is now maintained until the operator feels the quadriceps muscle relax and the tibia and femur come apart. He then removes his thigh

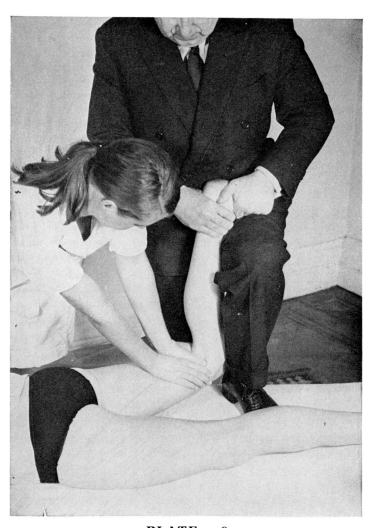

PLATE 128

supporting her foot and, during strong traction, fully rotates the foot
rapidly each way several times while he moves sideways towards the end
of the couch. The knee is thus rotated and extended during distraction of
the joint surfaces. The assistant holding the knee down feels the click, the
operator does not. After each manipulation the knee is examined again.
When nearly well, it may be only while walking or going downstairs that
the patient feels anything. This manoeuvre is painless and can be repeated
up to a dozen times during any one session. One or two sessions should
suffice for full relief even if the disorder has been present for many months.
If the operator is working single-handed, he can take his shoe off and
apply his foot to the back of the patient's knee for counter-pressure.

If this manipulation reduces an impacted loose body incompletely, those
illustrated in Plates 129 and 130 should be tried.

After-treatment—The patient must be warned that he has a loose body
inside the joint and that recurrence is not unlikely within a year or two. He
should not bend his knee more than he can help when he sits, and ought
not to kneel. He must come for treatment at once if the symptoms recur.

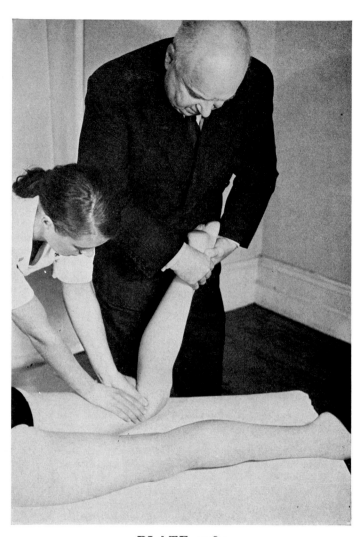

PLATE 128a

KNEE-JOINT: REDUCTION OF IMPACTED LOOSE BODY II

Indication—If the first manipulation has been repeated several times without affording full reduction and a small loose fragment of cartilage impacted at the inner side of the joint is still causing pain on full extension.

Patient's Posture—The patient adopts the half-lying position on the couch and co-operates actively. Since the operator's hands, when so placed as to exert pressure calculated to adduct the leg on the thigh (i.e. towards varus), are not suitably placed to force extension at the knee, this movement must be performed actively by the patient.

Technique—The operator rotates the patient's hip laterally and bends her knee to a right-angle. He applies one hand to the inner side of the knee and the other to the outer side of the ankle, and exerts varus pressure. He now asks her to extend the knee slowly while this stress is strongly maintained. At the moment of almost full extension, a slight jerk is given encouraging full extension, the varus strain being fully maintained.

This manipulation may have to be repeated several times. Examination after each manoeuvre indicates whether or not the click that is often heard and felt was significant.

After-treatment—The patient should sit cross-legged on the floor, the leg on the affected side in front of the other, and press strongly on the inner side of her knee, at the same time actively extending it. The floor exerts the counter-pressure at the ankle.

Result—Full extension at the knee can usually be rendered painless.

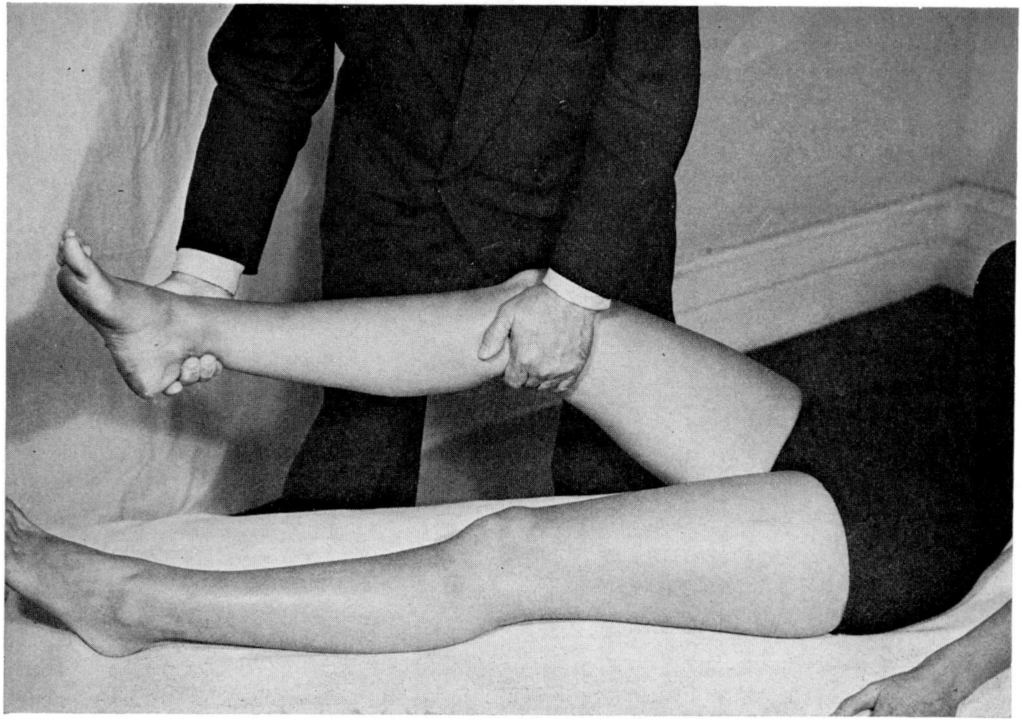

PLATE 129

KNEE-JOINT: REDUCTION OF IMPACTED LOOSE BODY III

Indication—If the previous manoeuvres have not restored a full and painless range of flexion to the knee-joint, this method of rocking the tibia on the femur during flexion should be employed.

Patient's Posture—The patient lies face upwards on the couch, bending her knee as far as she can, and relaxing her quadriceps muscles.

Technique—The operator inserts his wrist at the back of the patient's bent knee, so that it is squeezed between her femur and tibia. His other hand at her ankle jerks the tibia towards flexion and suddenly lets go, thus rocking the tibia forwards than back on the femur. A click may be felt, flexion suddenly becoming free. Should this manipulation fail, it may be repeated during rotation. An assistant places her wrist at the back of the patient's knee; the operator, holding the patient's foot and ankle in both hands, simultaneously forces flexion and rotation (see Plate 130a).

Caution—After each attempt at manipulation during flexion, the range of extension at the knee-joint should be tested. If, as the range of flexion gradually increases, that of extension is found to diminish, manipulation towards flexion must cease; for the preservation of a full range of extension at the knee-joint is always paramount.

After-treatment—The patient must be careful to avoid redisplacement of the loose fragment. This occurs most often when the knee is kept flexed for a long time; hence, he should not sit with the knee more bent than he can help, nor should he kneel.

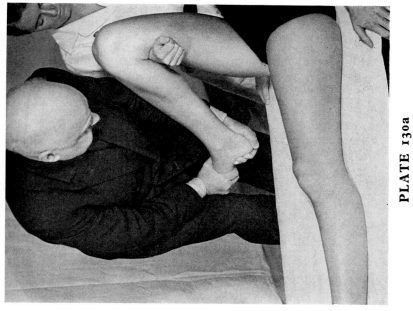

PLATE 130a

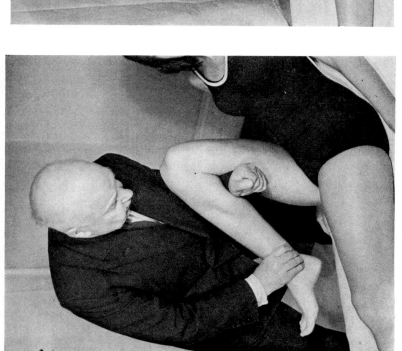

PLATE 130

GASTROCNEMIUS MUSCLE

Massage Technique

Lesion—Rupture of a few fibres of the gastrocnemius muscle so often occurs during a game of tennis that the condition is also known as 'tennis leg'. The so-called 'rupture of the plantaris tendon' has always proved in my experience to be caused by the lesion of the gastrocnemius muscle.

Physical Signs—In the recent case the patient walks in using the affected leg on tiptoe and complains of a sudden severe twinge at mid-calf with pain on walking ever since. Examination shows limitation of dorsiflexion of the foot because of pain in the calf. The gastrocnemius has gone into spasm about the breach; it is thus too short to allow the patient to get his heel to the ground. Rising on tiptoe is possible, with pain, since the upper and lower parts of the muscle are intact and working. Tenderness is found at the inner part of the muscle belly, at or just below its mid-point.

Patient's Posture—The patient lies face downwards on the couch, his foot resting in full equinus so as to relax the calf-muscles.

Technique—The physiotherapist sits at the level of the patient's leg facing towards it. She places three fingers on the affected area of muscle. The transverse friction is imparted by the physiotherapist drawing her hand to and fro horizontally.

Additional Treatment—The heel of the shoe must be raised at once, enough to allow painless weight-bearing. It is lowered daily, the criterion being the least height that enables the patient to stand painlessly. Local anaesthesia should be induced at the inception of treatment, but in recent cases the patient should rest for an hour and a half after the injection, in order not to overstrain the healing breach again. Friction is begun the next day. The patient should sit down and practise off-weight plantiflexion and dorsiflexion exercises as often as possible during the day.

Duration of Treatment—Massage should be given for twenty minutes daily for, say, three sessions, then three times a week.

Results—Patients seen the day after the injury, treated by local anaesthesia, then massage, raising the heel and constantly repeated active off-weight exercises, may expect to be back on the courts in two weeks. In chronic cases, full relief usually takes a month of treatment on alternate days.

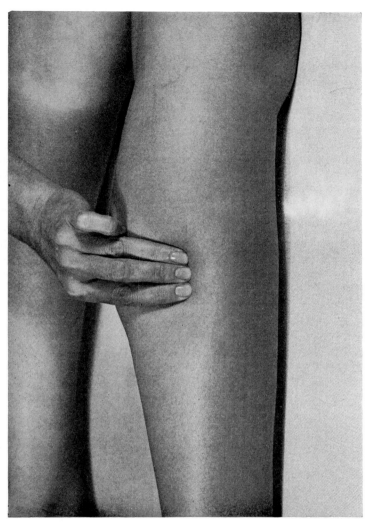

PLATE 131

PERONEAL TENDONS: UPPER PART

Massage Technique

Lesion—Tendinitis here usually follows a varus sprain of the tarsus, but may appear as an over-use phenomenon as the result, for example, of unaccustomed exercise on uneven ground.

Physical Signs—The patient is often an athlete complaining of 'shin soreness'. The pain is at the lower half of the leg on the lateral side. No passive movement at the ankle or other tarsal joints hurts, but resisted lateral rotation of the foot elicits the pain above the ankle. Tenderness of the peroneal tendons must be sought anywhere from the musculo-tendinous junction downwards.

Patient's Posture—The patient lies with his lower limb held medially rotated so that its lateral surface lies uppermost.

Technique—The physiotherapist sits facing the patient's foot, which she holds in inversion so as to stretch the tendons. She places the tips of two or three fingers, held slightly flexed, on the tendons, thereby pressing these against the shaft of the fibula. The friction is imparted by a to-and-fro movement of the forearm, which makes her fingers ride over the tendons.

Duration of Treatment—Twenty to thirty minutes' friction are usually required, since a stretch of two or three inches of tendon may have to be treated. The duration of treatment is very variable; two to four weeks of massage given two or three times a week may be needed. The patient should avoid such exercise as results in pain until he is well.

Result—Uniformly good.

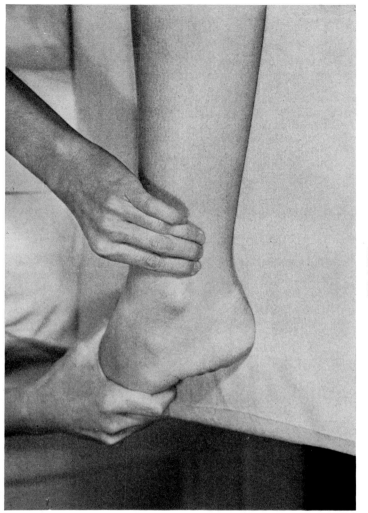

PLATE 132

PERONEAL TENDONS: LOWER PART

Massage Technique

Lesion—Strain of the tendons here usually follows a varus sprain of the ankle, but may be caused by over-use.

Physical Signs—The only painful movement is resisted eversion of the foot and is felt at the ankle. Tenderness is sought along the tendons, at the back of the lateral malleolus and at the calcaneus.

Patient's Posture—The patient lies with his lower limb held medially rotated so that the outer edge of his foot faces upwards.

Technique—The physiotherapist sits facing the patient's foot, holding it in inversion and adduction so as to stretch the tendons. The tender length of tendon is identified and the physiotherapist puts her middle and ring finger-tips on it. She gives the friction by moving her forearm to and fro, so that her fingers ride over the tendons.

Duration of Treatment—Two to four weeks' treatment two or three times weekly may be required. The patient should not walk farther than strictly necessary until he is well.

Results—In my experience no case has failed to yield to treatment by deep friction, though a few long-standing cases have taken a good month to clear up.

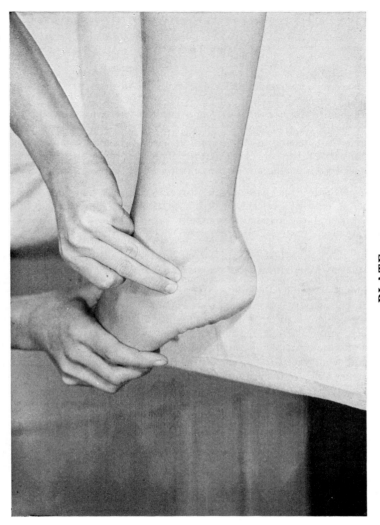

PLATE 133

POSTERIOR TIBIAL TENDON: UPPER PART

Massage Technique

Lesion—Strain here is the result of over-use, either owing to unaccustomed exercises or secondary to a pes planus deformity. It is sometimes called 'shin soreness'.

Standing with the heel held in valgus and the forefoot abducted puts a constant strain on the posterior tibial tendon and sets up particularly intractable pain starting usually in middle age. In these cases a mid-tarsal support must be fitted, otherwise continued over-use of the muscle prevents the massage from having any lasting effect.

Physical Signs—The pain is felt just above, or at, the ankle, and is brought on only by resisted inversion of the foot. The other resisted movements and the passive movements prove painless. Tenderness is sought along the posterior tibial tendon.

Patient's Posture—The patient lies on the couch with his leg held laterally so that its inner surface faces upwards.

Technique—The physiotherapist sits by the patient's foot, facing it. She holds his leg laterally rotated and his foot at about a right-angle by grasping the inner side of his forefoot. She lays her middle finger, reinforced by the index, flat on the affected length of tendon in the sulcus between the tendo Achillis and the tibia. She imparts the friction by rotating her forearm, and the operative finger with it, by alternating full pronation and full supination movements. Unless this technique is used, her finger slides from the tibia to the tendo Achillis, missing the posterior tibial tendon altogether.

Duration of Treatment—Tendinitis here usually clears up with twenty minutes' treatment twice a week for a month or less. When the lesion is secondary to a pes planus deformity, it is no use starting the massage until the valgus support has been supplied. Until well, the patient should stand and walk as little as possible.

Result—Uniformly good.

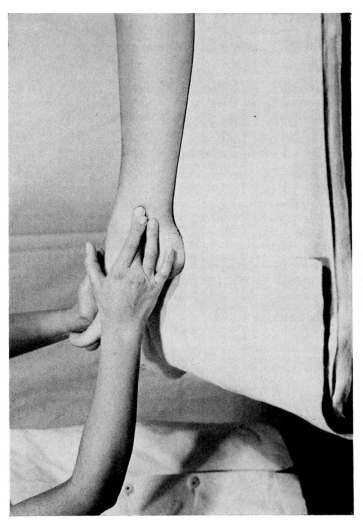

PLATE 134

POSTERIOR TIBIAL TENDON: LOWER PART

Massage Technique

Lesion—See page 408.

Physical Signs—The pain is felt at the inner side of the hind foot and is evoked only by resisted inversion of the foot. The tenderness of the posterior tibial tendon is found at the calcanean extent.

Patient's Posture—The patient lies on the couch with his leg laterally rotated so that the inner border of the foot faces upwards.

Technique—The physiotherapist stands by the side of the patient's leg. She holds his foot at right-angles and the leg in lateral rotation by grasping the inner side of his forefoot. She places the tips of her ring and middle fingers on the affected length of tendon and imparts the friction by a flexion–extension movement at her wrist using her thumb as fulcrum. She feels her fingers ride over the tendon at each stroke.

Duration of Treatment—Twenty minutes' treatment twice a week for a few weeks is usually enough. The patient should not walk more than he need until he is well. A support is required (see page 408).

Results—Uniformly good.

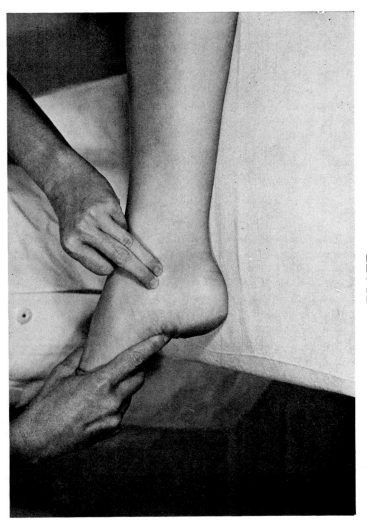

PLATE 135

TENDO ACHILLIS

Massage Techniques

Lesion—This is a tendinitis due to over-use and is thus common in athletes.

Physical Signs—The patient feels a pain at the back of his heel on rising on tiptoe. Nothing else produces any pain. The patient has almost always made a correct diagnosis himself. Tenderness is sought along the tendon; it is never found on the posterior aspect of the tendon, often on both sides, and often on the anterior surface. This is an important point; for massage cures tendinitis only if the correct area is treated. Hence the patient will not improve if treatment to the anterior aspect of the tendon is omitted when part of the lesion lies there. Occasionally the lesion lies only at the tendinous insertion at the upper border of the calcaneus.

Contra-indications—Multiple xanthomata, rheumatoid or gonorrhoeal tendinitis, or that due to gout or chondrocalcinosis. Structural change in the tendon itself naturally cannot be reversed by massage, hence partial rupture with an enlarged area of chronic fibrosis is not suitable.

Patient's Posture—The patient lies face downwards on the couch.

Techniques—

1. The patient's foot projects just beyond the edge of a low couch. The physiotherapist sits at his foot and puts her knee against the patient's sole, thus maintaining dorsiflexion to a right-angle. She grasps the tendon between her finger and thumb. She imparts the friction by drawing her hand backwards until her digits slip from the side towards the posterior aspect of the tendon (Plate 136).

2. The anterior aspect of the tendon may be affected (usually in addition to each side). The patient moves farther up the couch, in order that his foot shall lie fully plantiflexed. This relaxes the tendon enough to give it good lateral mobility. With one thumb, she pushes the tendon sideways as far as it will go. She can now reach the anterior aspect of the tendon with the tip of her ring finger, which is strongly applied there by her flexing her elbow. The transverse friction is carried out by alternating supination and pronation movements of the forearm, which rotates the finger on the tendon. The finger, hand and forearm are held in a straight line (see Plate 137).

3. The lesion may lie at the lowest part of the tendon level with the upper surface of the calcaneus. The tendon must again be relaxed, so that it can be indented enough to allow access to the fibres adjacent to its insertion. Using both hands, the physiotherapist makes a ring round his heel, her thumbs at its plantar surface, one index finger-tip reinforced by the other at the lesion. She presses hard, and draws her finger across this area by moving her forearm to and fro (see Plate 138).

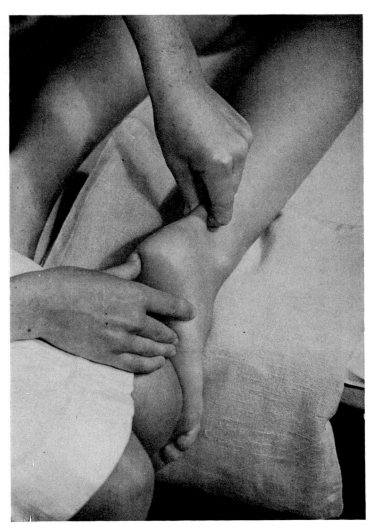

PLATE 136

Duration of Treatment—A quarter of an hour's friction every other day for a week or two is usually required. Until well, the patient should not walk farther than necessary.

Results—Uniformly good. The only failures are the cases of nodular scarring about an old partial rupture.

Complete Rupture

Complete rupture of the tendo Achillis must be treated by immediate operative suture, otherwise some lasting disability always remains. If a patient is seen too late for operation, deep massage to the thickened tendon, twice a week for a couple of months, and to the swollen areas to either side of it anteriorly, markedly diminishes symptoms. Cure is not obtainable.

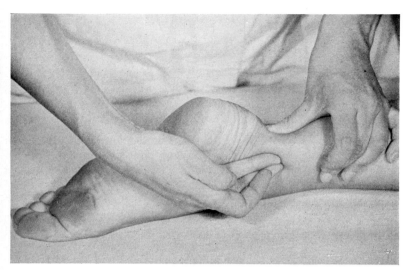

PLATE 137

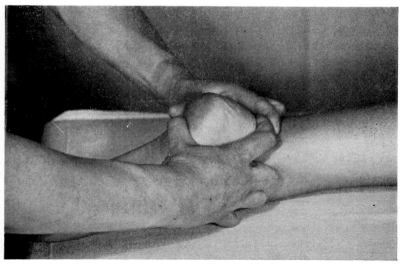

PLATE 138

TENDO ACHILLIS

Injection Technique

Indication—Tendinitis resulting from over-use.

Contra-indication—A palpable swelling indicates an area of localized scarring within the substance of the tendon, left over from a minor rupture. Such a structural alteration implies that conservative treatment will fail.

Patient's Posture—The patient lies prone on a high couch with his foot held in dorsiflexion by an assistant. The tendon is thus stretched so that the affected area can be accurately mapped out and also so as to provide a stiff flat surface along which to run the needle. If a large area of tendon is at fault it is often best to get rid of all but the most resistant spot by massage first.

Injection Technique—A 2 ml syringe is filled with steroid and fitted with a thin needle 5 cm long. Since the linear surface of the tendon is likely to need infiltration, the needle should be introduced some 3 cm away from the lesion. It is pushed forwards parallel to the tendon until the tip reaches the far edge of the lesion. The injection is given while the needle is being drawn back again as far as the near edge of the affected area. As the needle travels along the surface of the tendon, constant pressure on the plunger maintains a flow of the suspension. This is repeated a little to one side of the previous line three or four times using 0·5 ml at each infiltration.

After-treatment—The patient avoids running for a week.

Results—Uniformly good.

Caution—The steroid should not be injected into the substance of the tendon; rupture has resulted later.

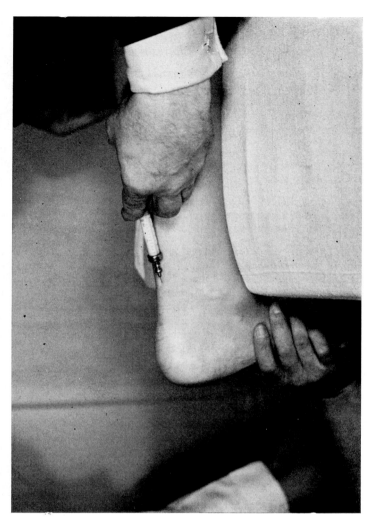

PLATE 139

DANCER'S HEEL

Injection Technique

Lesion—Dancers provoke a traumatic periostitis at the posterior articular margin of the tibia by pressure there from the upper surface of the calcaneus. It results from overpointing, i.e. plantar-flexion beyond the 180° position when she is *sur les pointes*. Since the pain is at the heel, it is mistakenly ascribed to a lesion of the tendo Achillis.

Physical Signs—Full passive plantiflexion of the foot sets up the pain at the back of the heel, i.e. something is pinched. Rising on tiptoe is painless, thus exculpating the tendo Achillis.

Patient's Posture—The patient lies prone on the couch with the foot in the neutral position. The posterior articular margin of the tibia is identified, 2 cm superior to a line joining the tips of the malleoli.

Injection Technique—A 2 ml syringe is filled with steroid suspension and fitted with a fine needle 4 cm long. The suspension must be injected along the bruised edge. It is identified by thrusting the needle vertically downwards and feeling for the point at which bone (tibia) gives way to articular cartilage (talus). The tip is now moved a millimetre or so superiorly, to rest on the tibial edge. A line of little droplets is now injected all along this horizontal line. Pressure on the piston is applied only when the tip is felt to lie in contact with periosteum.

After-treatment—The dancer must not rise *sur les pointes* for a week, but can carry out ordinary exercise as soon as she likes. She must avoid overpointing permanently.

Result—Uniformly good.

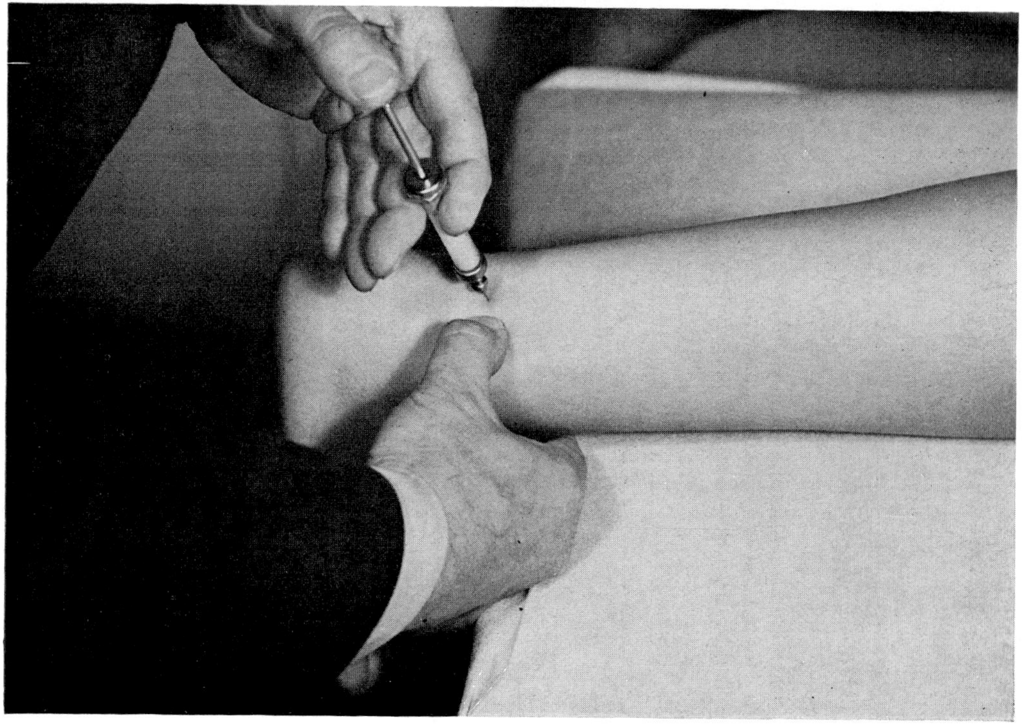

PLATE 140

SPRAINED ANKLE: FIBULAR COLLATERAL LIGAMENT

Massage Technique

Lesion—This is always traumatic and the commonest result of a sprained ankle. The usual place for some fibres of the ligament to part is at their origin from the fibula.

Intention—To move the injured fibres of ligament to and fro over bone in imitation of their normal behaviour. In recent sprain this is best secured by friction with the physiotherapist's finger.

Physical Signs—In a recent varus sprain of the ankle, bruising and oedema prevent the arrival at a diagnosis by palpation for tenderness, for the swelling and tenderness are diffuse. The diagnosis must therefore be made by study of which movements hurt. The examination involves testing:

1. Inversion in plantiflexion which stretches the fibular collateral ligament.
2. Inversion in dorsiflexion which stretches the fibulo-calcanean ligament.
3. Rotation of the forefoot on the hind foot which stretches the calcaneo-cuboid ligament.
4. Resisted eversion which tests the peroneal tendons.

Patient's Posture—The patient lies on the couch with his limb medially rotated so that the outer border of the foot faces upwards.

Technique—The physiotherapist sits at the medial aspect of the patient's foot. She stretches the ligament by holding the foot in as much inversion and plantiflexion as is comfortable. She places her middle finger, reinforced by the index, on the site of the lesion. If this lies at the fibular origin, her forearm is fully pronated so that her finger presses upwards as well as inwards; if it lies at the talar extent of the ligament, her pressure is directed medially only (not illustrated). She imparts the friction by drawing her hand and forearm to and fro.

If the sprain is very recent, the friction is not vigorous, being only deep enough adequately to move the ligament on the subjacent bone; for there are as yet no adhesions to rupture. It is preceded by effleurage to diminish the oedema and followed by passive, then active, movements. Finally the patient is taught how to walk slowly with a heel-and-toe gait, without limping.

Duration of Treatment—In recent sprains the patient should be treated daily; in such cases a few minutes' deepish friction is ample. More than two weeks' attendance is seldom needed. In chronic cases friction followed by manipulation should not be necessary on more than two or three occasions.

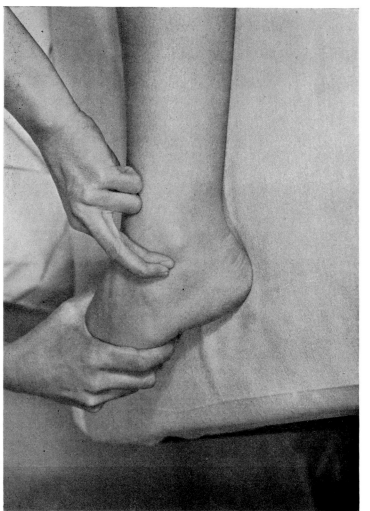

PLATE 141

Results—In recent cases, uniformly good; in chronic cases, nearly always good. If a long-standing sprain here does not recover quickly the question of mistaken diagnosis arises. If this is clearly correct, mobilization under anaesthesia is called for.

Deltoid Ligament at Ankle

This ligament behaves quite differently from its fellow at the lateral aspect. Massage is useless and manipulation harmful.

The fact that the sprain took the unusual direction should lead to examination of the whole foot. A marked valgus deformity may be detected, for which a support designed to take excessive strain off the inner side of the ankle is required. In these cases the ligament is apt to be overstretched anew at each step the patient takes; a varus support relieves the repeated stresses that maintain the chronic sprain.

Full relief is much hastened if, once the support has been fitted, steroid suspension is injected (see page 430).

SPRAINED ANKLE: FIBULAR COLLATERAL LIGAMENT

Injection Technique

Lesion—The commonest lesion in a sprained ankle occurs at the fibular origin of the anterior fasciculus of the collateral ligament.

Physical Signs—Stretching the ligament by passive plantiflexion and rotating the foot medially is painful. This movement also stretches the peroneal tendons but tendinitis here is excluded when resisted eversion is found not to hurt.

Indication—Only in recent sprain, the sooner after the accident the better. Once adhesions have formed they require rupture; by then hydrocortisone is no longer any help.

Patient's Posture—The patient lies on a high couch, his limb in medial rotation, to bring the outer side of the foot uppermost. An assistant holds the foot in as much plantar flexion and inversion as is comfortable. The line of tenderness at the lateral malleolus is defined from end to end.

Injection Technique—A 2 ml syringe is filled with steroid suspension and fitted with a thin needle 3 cm long. A spot is chosen 2 cm away from the mid-point of the ligamentous origin at the edge of the fibula and the needle thrust in almost horizontally until it meets bone. A series of droplets is injected fanwise from one end to the other of the ligamentous attachment to bone.

After-treatment—The pain is quite considerable for two days, and an analgesic may well be required that night. Rapid improvement then ensues and in a few days the patient is well. The normally slow resolution of post-traumatic inflammation is greatly hastened, but at the expense of increased symptoms for two days. Unless, therefore, the patient can take it quietly for these two days, treatment by massage is to be preferred.

Result—Uniformly good.

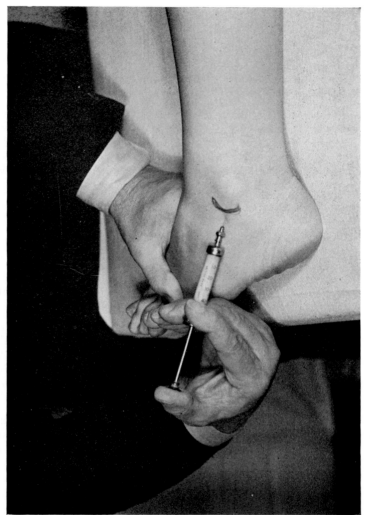

PLATE 142

SPRAINED ANKLE: CALCANEO-CUBOID JOINT

Massage Technique

Lesion—This is always traumatic. The medial rotation and adduction force exerted when the ankle is sprained tears some fibres of the ligament lying at the outer side of the calcaneo-cuboid joint.

Physical Signs—The calcaneo-cuboid ligament is usually sprained with the talo-fibular ligament. Testing the calcaneo-cuboid ligament in isolation involves holding the foot in dorsiflexion and valgus via the heel. The talo-fibular ligament is thus fully relaxed. The forefoot is now fully rotated on the motionless heel. Pain felt at the outer side of the mid-foot must arise from the calcaneo-cuboid joint.

Caution—Peroneal tendinitis following a sprained ankle is often mistaken for adhesions and treated in vain by manipulation. It is important therefore to test eversion against resistance in these cases.

Intention—To move the ligament manually to and fro over the bone in imitation of its normal behaviour.

Patient's Posture—The patient lies with his lower limb extended and medially rotated so that the outer border of the foot faces upwards.

Technique—The physiotherapist sits facing the foot, approaching it from the medial aspect. She steadies the forefoot with one hand and holds it adducted, thereby bringing the calcaneo-cuboid joint into prominence. She lays the middle finger of the other hand, reinforced by the index, on the joint line. Friction is given by a vertical movement of her finger, imparted by moving the whole forearm.

Duration of Treatment—In recent sprains, a week or two's treatment suffices. The massage is followed by gentle passive movements and instruction in gait. In chronic sprain, the adhesions require manipulative rupture, not massage (see page 434).

Results—Uniformly good.

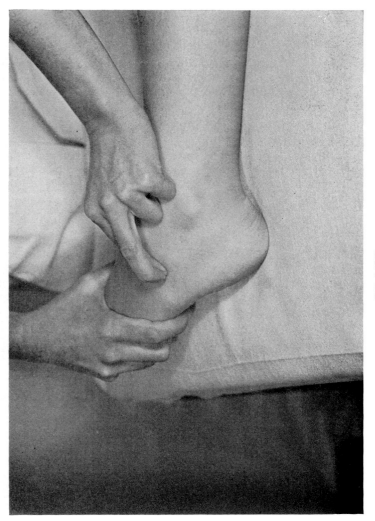

PLATE 143

SPRAINED ANKLE: CALCANEO-CUBOID JOINT

Injection Technique

Lesion—If a considerable medial rotation and adduction strain of the forefoot on the hind foot is included in the force spraining the ankle, the calcaneo-cuboid joint suffers as well as the fibular collateral ligament. It is seldom sprained alone.

Physical Signs—The heel is held and drawn downwards so as to dorsiflex the ankle. With his other hand the examiner rotates the forefoot, while keeping the heel still, thus obviating tension on the fibulo-talar and fibulo-calcaneal ligaments. If rotation and/or adduction hurt, the lateral calcaneo-cuboid ligament is strained. Tenderness along a 2 cm extent of the joint line is found.

Patient's Posture—The patient lies on a high couch, his limb in full medial rotation, so as to bring the outer border of the foot uppermost.

Injection Technique—A 2 ml syringe is filled with steroid suspension and fitted with a fine needle 2 cm long. The needle is thrust in at the lowest extent of the joint-line at an angle of 45° and a droplet of suspension injected. It is then slightly withdrawn and pushed on to a point just superior to the previous infiltration, and so on until the whole area has been dealt with.

Results—Uniformly good, but the patient is very sore for a few days and will have increased difficulty in walking during that time.

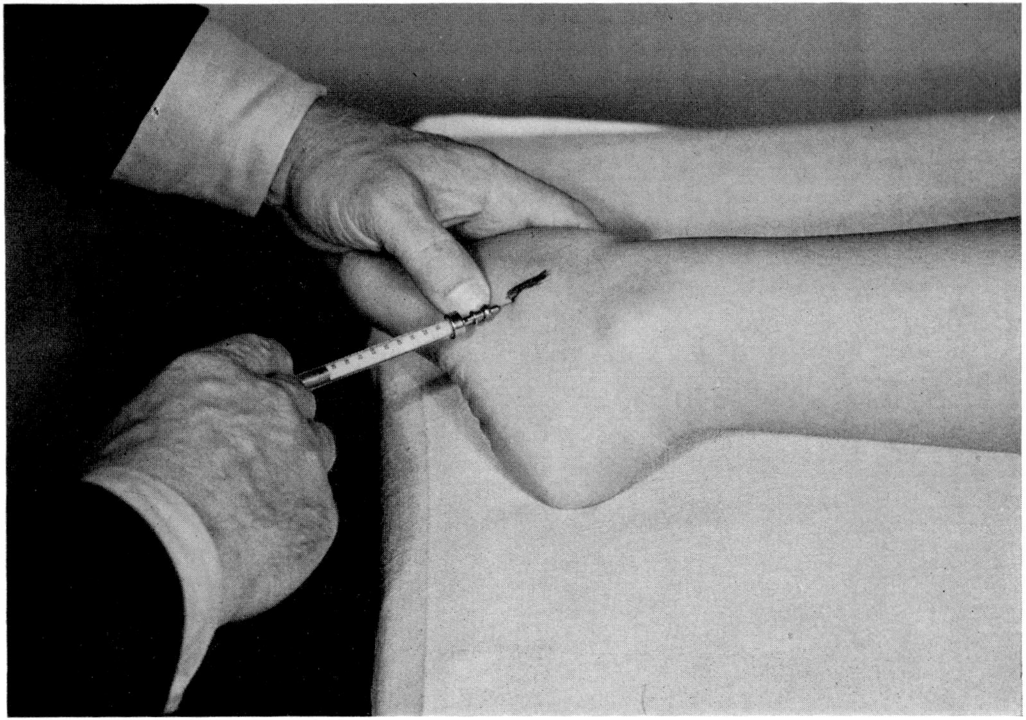

PLATE 144

SPRAINED ANKLE: DELTOID LIGAMENT

Injection Technique

Lesion—This is post-traumatic or, more often, the result of chronic strain in a patient with a valgus foot. After an eversion sprain of the ankle, pain at the inner side may persist indefinitely, sometimes for years. Every step hurts, because the traumatic lesion has never had the chance to subside, being maintained by repeated traction each time the foot bears weight and is forced again into valgus at the heel and abduction at the forefoot.

Physical Signs—Stretching the deltoid ligament by full passive eversion and plantiflexion of the foot is painful. Resisted inversion is not; this finding exculpates the posterior tibial tendon. Tenderness is present at the tibial origin of the ligament.

Caution—Since the lesion is caused by repeated traction, the worst possible treatment is further overstretching, i.e. manipulation. Analogy with the fibular collateral ligament is entirely misleading. Treatment therefore consists in relief from tension. Massage is useless.

Support—A support 1 to 2 cm thick is fitted under the inner mid-tarsal area; this obviates the repeated stretch at each step.

Injection of Steroid Suspension—This serves to allay the persistent post-traumatic inflammation. The precise extent of the painful scar is determined. An assistant holds the foot in eversion, thus rendering the medial malleolus prominent. A 2 ml syringe is filled with steroid suspension and fitted with a thin needle 3 cm long. A point is chosen 2 cm below and in front of the tender line of ligament and the needle inserted there. It is directed at the inferior aspect of the tibia and, by a series of partial withdrawals and fanwise reinsertions beads of fluid are injected all along the affected extent of the ligamento-osseous junction.

The ankle is painful for twenty-four hours.

After-treatment—The patient bears weight on that foot as little as possible for a few days, and goes on wearing the support for some months.

Results—Uniformly good.

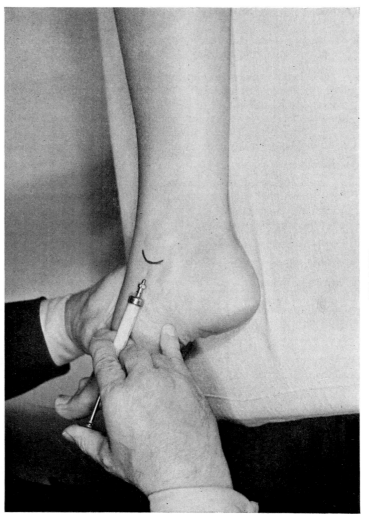

PLATE 145

POSTERIOR TIBIO-TALAR LIGAMENT

This treatment was devised by Mr F. Harris, M.C.S.P., of Solihull who kindly supplied the text and the photograph.

Lesion—This is post-traumatic, secondary to a sprain of the ankle. If a sprain of this ligament has been allowed to heal in the absence of adequate movement adhesions form, binding it abnormally to bone.

After a few weeks the patient reports that he can walk normally and that the sprain has largely recovered, but when again attempting certain movements, like kicking a football, severe twinges are experienced around the inner malleolus.

Physical Signs—All resisted movements are painless; this finding exculpates the posterior tibial tendon. Pain is felt only on a forced plantar flexion movement, suggesting that some lesion is being pinched at the extreme of range, at the posterior aspect of the inner malleolus.

Patient's Posture—The patient lies prone on a high couch with the knee flexed to a right angle.

Technique—The operator stands facing the foot, supporting it with the left hand, and applying deep friction to the site of the lesion, with the middle finger of the other hand reinforced by the index finger. The friction is imparted by drawing the hand and forearm to and fro.

Duration of Treatment—However chronic these adhesions have become, response to treatment is very quick. Deep transverse friction on three or four occasions is usually sufficient.

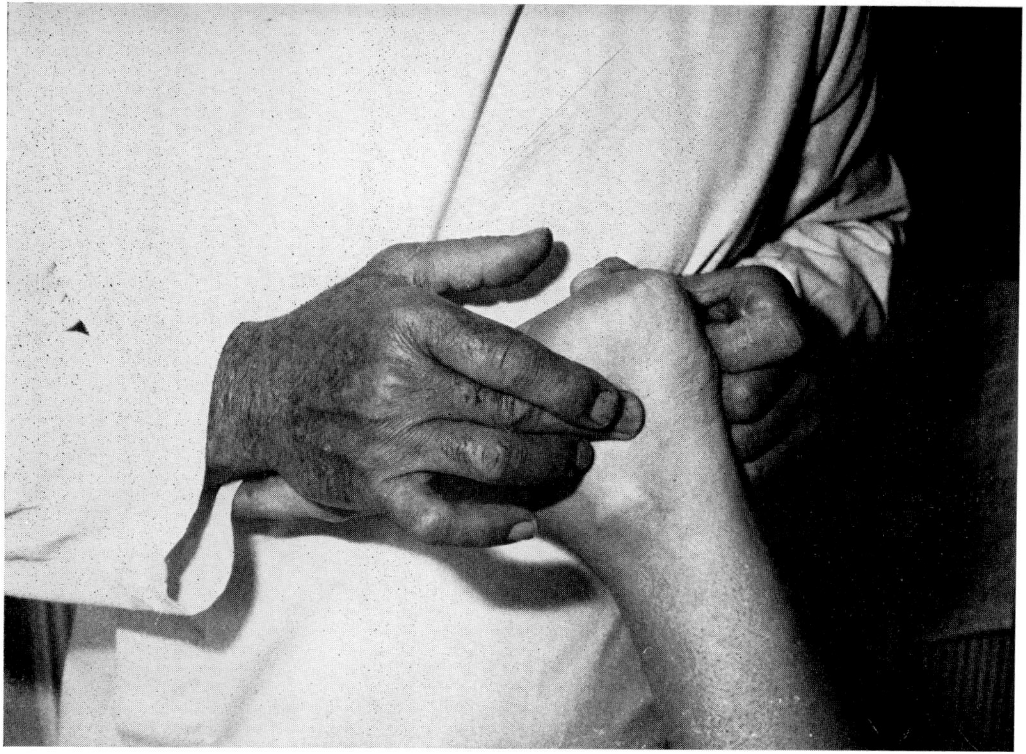

PLATE 146

SPRAINED ANKLE: MANIPULATION

Lesion—If sprain of the anterior fasciculus of the fibular collateral ligament or of the calcaneo-cuboid ligament has been allowed to heal in the absence of adequate movement, adhesions form binding them abnormally to bone. The patient reports after a few months that the sprain has largely recovered, but that the ankle hurts and swells at the outer side for some days after strenuous use.

Physical Signs—Pain felt at the outer side of the ankle on full inversion of the foot during plantiflexion (talo-fibular ligament). Pain felt on full rotation at the mid-tarsal joint (calcaneo-cuboid ligament). No pain when the resisted movements are tested; this finding exculpates the peroneal tendons.

Intention—This manoeuvre simultaneously ruptures adhesions at the outer side of both the ankle and the calcaneo-cuboid joints.

Indication—Adhesions remaining after a varus sprain of the ankle and tarsal joints.

Contra-indications—If a varus sprain has resulted in peroneal tendinitis, no advantage accrues from manipulation of the joint. Forced movement is, of course, unsuited to the treatment of a recent sprain.

Patient's Posture—The patient lies supine on a high couch.

Technique—The operator stands at the patient's foot, holding it away from him at arm's length and facing him. If the left ankle is to be manipulated, he adducts his left arm across his chest and grasps the patient's heel, which he forces into full varus as it rests on the couch. He places the right hand downwards on the dorsum of her forefoot, curling his fingers round the shaft of the first metatarsal bone. He employs his other hand to do three things at once (*a*) plantiflex the foot, (*b*) medially rotate the forefoot on the hindfoot, and (*c*) adduct the forefoot. This triple movement is carried out by pressing his hand towards the floor, with the greater pressure exerted by the heel of his hand on the outer border of the foot. For the simultaneous forcing of adduction he uses his fingers on the inner side of her forefoot as a fulcrum and draws his elbow sharply towards his side. Unless the operator holds his right elbow well away from his body, little force can be exerted at the final moment.

Results—Good. Only an occasional case needs this manoeuvre carried out under anaesthesia.

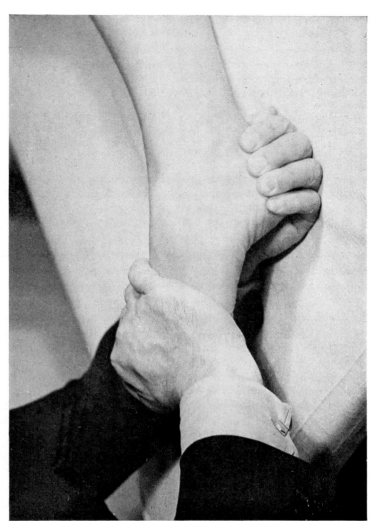

PLATE 147

ANKLE-JOINT: REDUCTION OF LOOSE BODY

Lesion—After a sprain, a small fragment of cartilage may become loose within the joint, usually anteriorly. In consequence the patient complains of sudden erratic twinges on plantiflexion the foot, usually as she walks downstairs. There may be several in a day, then none for weeks.

Physical Signs—The subluxation is momentary and spontaneous reduction the rule. Hence, when the patient attends, her ankle is normal. The only other condition that leads to similar symptoms at the ankle-joint is a sprung mortice and, when this is tested, it is found intact.

Intention—To shift the loose body to another part of the joint whence it will no longer subluxate. But the operator has no means of knowing at the time of the manipulation whether this has been achieved or not. The best that can be done is to perform the manoeuvres, whereupon the patient reports the result some days later.

Patient's Posture—The patient lies supine on the couch, her heel exactly level with its edge. An assistant at the other end grasps her upstretched hands for counter-pressure.

Technique—The operator grasps the patient's heel with his left hand, his finger protected from the hard edge of the couch by a thick foam-rubber pad. This hand does not pull; it provides the fulcrum. He grasps the dorsum of her foot with his right hand and leans back, pulling as hard as he can. He is now using the lever extending from the posterior surface of the calcaneus to the metatarsal area for distracting the talus from its mortice. Now, he carries out a strong circumduction movement several times.

If this method fails he passes on to that required for a loose body in the talo-calcanean joint, since strong varus and valgus strains there also reach the ankle joint (see page 442).

Result—About half of all cases are relieved. The remainder have to put up with the disorder, unless, rarely, the loose body contains an osseous nucleus and shows radiologically. If so, it can be removed.

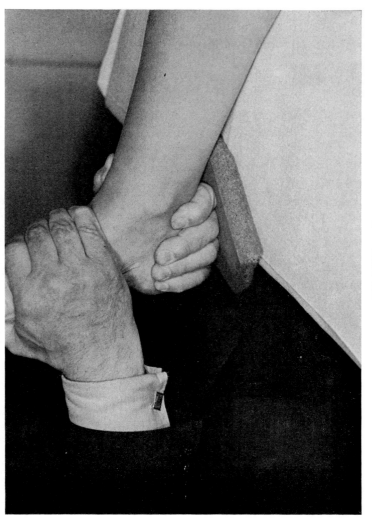

PLATE 148

TALO-CALCANEAN JOINT

Injection Technique

Lesion—Rheumatoid arthritis is common at the two talo-calcanean joints, leading to increasing limitation of varus movement. Finally fixation in full valgus results.

Contra-indications—Steroids are of no help in the osteoarthrosis that follows fracture involving the articular surface of the calcaneus, nor in spasmodic pes planus.

Patient's Posture—The patient lies on his side on a high couch, the inner side of his heel uppermost.

Injection Technique—Since the joint is fixed in valgus, there is more room to approach from the medial aspect. The sustentaculum tali is identified. A 2 ml syringe is filled with steroid suspension and fitted with a thin needle 2 cm long. A point is chosen close to the tip of the sustentaculum and the needle thrust in just above it, parallel to the joint surface. If it meets bone at about 1 cm from the skin, the needle is manoeuvred about until it is felt to slip in further without resistance. The tip now lies within the anterior joint and 1 ml is injected. It is then partly withdrawn and reinserted 45° posteriorly and the remaining 1 ml injected into the posterior joint.

Result—In advanced cases, one or two intra-articular injections may not restore much movement, but pain ceases for months, even years.

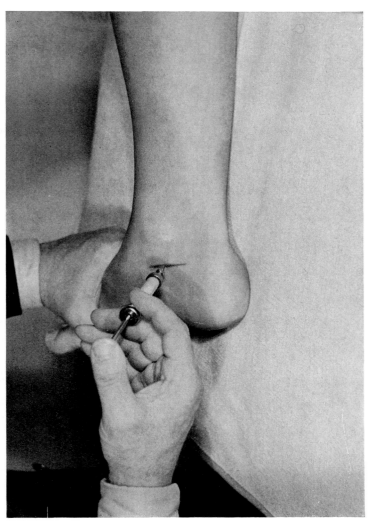

PLATE 149

TALO-CALCANEAN JOINT: MOBILIZATION

Lesion—Limited movement after immobilization in plaster for tibio-fibular fractures. The joint is fixed in the mid-position, whereas in arthritis it fixes in full valgus.

Physical Signs—Immobilization with subsequent restricted varus and valgus range at the talo-calcanean joint.

Contra-indications—Osteoarthrosis following fracture of the articular surface of the calcaneus, spasmodic pen planus, subacute traumatic or rheumatoid arthritis.

Patient's Posture—The patient lies face upwards on the couch.

Technique—It is very difficult to obtain any leverage at this joint, whether manually or even with a Thomas's wrench. The physiotherapist sits at the patient's foot and clasps her fingers behind his heel, compressing the calcaneus as strongly as she can with each palm. By swinging one elbow away from the other towards herself, she imparts a varus or valgus movement to the talo-calcanean joint. This forcing must be repeated with the utmost vigour a great many times at each session.

Results—If only half the normal range can be restored, the patient may lose all the symptoms arising at this joint. Several months of treatment are usually required.

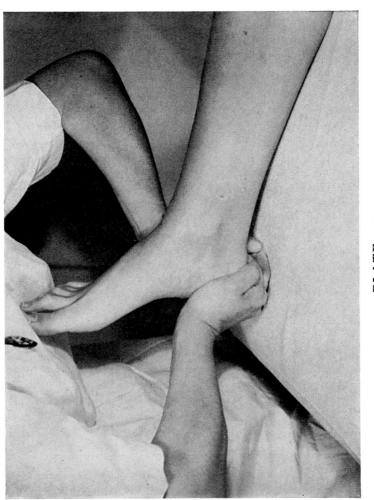

TALO-CALCANEAN JOINT: REDUCTION OF LOOSE BODY

Lesion—A loose body in the joint causes either sudden twinges or attacks of sudden fixation in valgus.

Physical Signs—During an attack of internal derangement, the joint is fixed in valgus, but the short history of recurrent attacks indicates that the cause is not arthritis. Between attacks the joint appears normal clinically. The loose body consists of cartilage and thus does not show radiographically.

Patient's Posture—He lies prone on the couch holding on to the edge with his hands. He pulls himself up the couch until the dorsum of the affected foot is strongly applied to the lower edge of the couch, and maintains this pressure during the manipulation.

Technique—The operator locks his two hands round the patient's heel, his crossed thumbs engaged against the upper posterior edge of the calcaneus. He keeps his fingers against the edge of the couch, protected by a thick foam-rubber mat. His feet are steadied against the legs of the couch and he hangs backwards, exerting the utmost possible traction on the bone. He now flexes at one wrist and extends at the other; then he reverses the movement. As a result, varus then valgus movement is forced at the joint during strong traction.

Results—Fixation in valgus is seldom difficult to overcome, but to get the loose body to a position whence it no longer subluxates is more difficult. Several attempts may be necessary at a few days' interval.

This manipulation often succeeds when a loose body is present within the ankle joint.

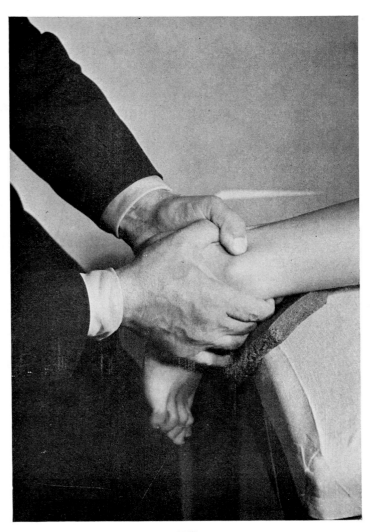

PLATE 151

MID-TARSAL JOINT: FORCING LATERAL ROTATION

Indications—Limitation of movement due to ligamentous adhesions, to early osteoarthrosis, or to the capsular contracture that maintains a congenital inversion deformity of the fore foot on the hind foot. Adhesions may form after a sprained ankle or in the course of the immobilization necessitated by the treatment of tibio-fibular fractures.

Patient's Posture—The patient lies face upwards on the couch.

Technique—The operator sits at the patient's foot, facing him.

In adults, great strength is required to achieve an adequate movement. Thus the operator's hands should be clasped about the outer aspect of the forefoot. The heel of his dorsally placed hand presses chiefly on the first metatarsal bone; that of his other hand acts mostly against the plantar surface of the fifth metatarsal bone. The rotation is imparted to the forefoot by the operator swinging his elbows, one towards, the other away from, himself. This movement is repeated scores of times at each session, since an increase in the range is difficult to attain.

In children, even at the age of two or three, a surprising degree of vigour is necessary. If the operator's strength is adequate he can grasp the child's heel with one hand, his thenar eminence lying at the outer side of his heel and his fingers at the inner side. The fingers of his other hand are hooked about the outer side of his fore foot, his palm lying dorsally. By a simultaneous movement of both hands his heel is forced towards varus and the forefoot laterally rotated again and again (not illustrated).

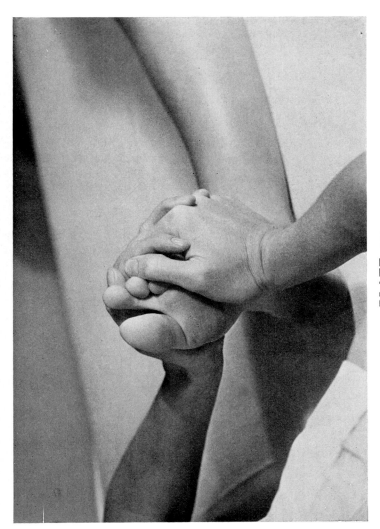

PLATE 152

DORSAL INTEROSSEOUS MUSCLE OF FOOT

Massage Technique

Lesion—This may be traumatic, and is then secondary to direct injury or to a marching fracture. Alternatively the cause may be overstrain. In either case, chronic pain may ensue, lasting for years.

Patient's Posture—The patient lies supine on the couch.

Technique—The physiotherapist sits facing the patient's foot. With one hand she flexes the patient's toes so as to relax the muscle. She places the middle finger of the other hand, reinforced by the index, in the groove between the two metacarpal bones. She imparts a transverse friction by rotating her finger by alternate pronation and supination movements of her forearm.

Duration of Treatment—Ten or fifteen minutes' friction thrice weekly for two to four weeks usually suffices. After the massage, faradic and resisted flexor exercises are given to the toes.

Results—Full relief is nearly always attained. Local anaesthesia is diagnostic, not curative. There is really no other treatment for this condition but deep friction, hence many patients suffer indefinitely. The result of this treatment is excellent.

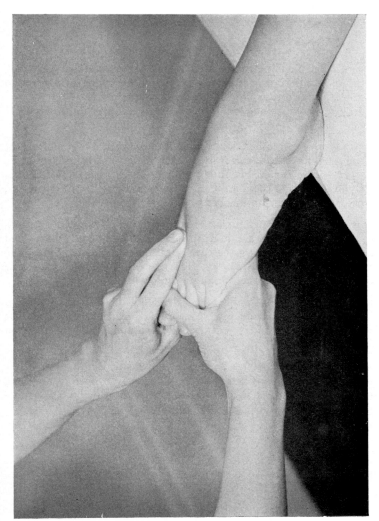

PLATE 153

METATARSO-PHALANGEAL JOINT

Injection Technique

Lesion—At the first metatarso-phalangeal joint, rheumatoid arthritis, osteoarthrosis or a traumatic arthritis alone or superimposed on an hitherto symptomless osteoarthrosis are all frequently encountered.

At the other four joints, only rheumatoid or traumatic arthritis is common.

Physical Signs—At the first joint, limitation of extension is marked, of flexion slight. At the others, curiously enough, the reverse pattern indicates arthritis—restricted flexion but little limitation of extension. The pain is accurately localized and the joint tender. Resisted flexion proves painless, thus exculpating the sesamo-metatarsal joint.

Patient's Posture—The patient lies on a high couch, an assistant grasping the big toe and distracting the joint surfaces. The joint-line is identified with her help, for by rotating the toe she renders the lower edge of the proximal phalanx easier to identify. This presents no difficulty at the hallux but is quite hard at the other four joints.

Injection Technique—A 1 ml syringe is filled with steroid suspension and fitted with a thin needle 2 cm long. The assistant pulls hard; the needle is passed into the space between the two bones and the injection given.

Result—It is remarkable that traumatic arthritis in the finger-joints is not improved by steroids, whereas at the metatarso-phalangeal joints the patient is lastingly pain-free within twenty-four hours. Rheumatoid arthritis responds equally well, of course, at hand or foot.

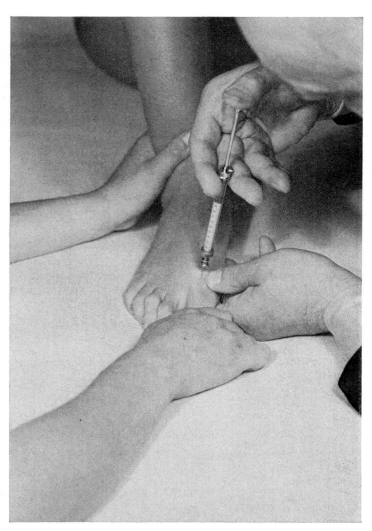

PLATE 154

HALLUX

Traction

Lesion—A minor degree of osteorathrosis or of traumatic arthritis at the first metatarso-phalangeal joint, particularly in a ballet dancer, is suitable for traction.

Physical Signs—Painful limitation of extension, with full flexion causing some discomfort.

Apparatus—This is shaped like a box and carries a foot-piece with straps to hold the patient's foot motionless. The handle at the back screws out the forward projection, increasing tension. This is applied by a spring, housed in the projecting cylinder and distracting up to 10 kg. A handle at the side alters the position of the cylinder in relation to the patient's foot, enabling pull at any desired angle to be achieved.

Patient's Posture—The patient sits and places his foot on the box. The straps are tightened and one layer of thin sponge rubber is wound round the big toe. A Japanese fingerstall is then put on and the loop at its end hooked on to the spring. The angle of traction is adjusted. The posterior handle is now turned until satisfactory traction is secured.

Duration of Treatment—Five to ten kg of traction retained for twenty minutes are usually required.

Result—Some immediate relief is to be expected and two or three treatments should suffice.

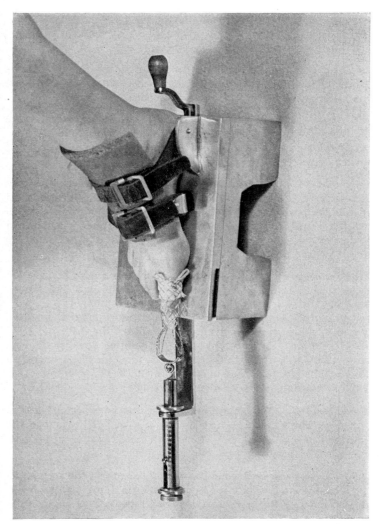

PLATE 155

PLANTAR FASCIA

Injection Technique

Lesion—The usual cause is prolonged strain during standing by patients with an over-arched foot. If periosteum is raised from the bone by such tension, a calcanean spur results, visible radiologically.

Physical Signs—The pain is felt at the inner side of the heel and is severe on taking the first few steps after sitting. Examination of the joints, ligaments and tendons reveals no lesion. The tender spot is easily identified at the medial edge of the calcaneo-fascial origin.

Patient's Posture—The patient lies prone on a high couch, his knee flexed to a right-angle. The operator stands at his toes, with his left hand encircling the heel, pressing hard on the lesion with his index finger, which he uses to feel, as the injection proceeds, where each droplet is placed. An assistant dorsiflexes the foot so as to render the plantar fascia taut and easy to identify when the needle touches it.

Injection Technique—The plantar skin overlying the tender point is too thick to be sterilized; hence an oblique approach through thin skin is necessary. This makes it more difficult to reach the right spot.

A 2 ml syringe is filled with steroid suspension and fitted with a needle 5 cm long. A spot is chosen, along the medial side of the foot, 3 to 4 cm anterior to the lesion. The needle is thrust in pointing downwards from the horizontal and advanced until it traverses resistant fascia and then touches bone. The affected area is now infiltrated all over by minor withdrawals and reinsertions of the needle.

After-treatment—Severe pain lasting two days is to be expected, and the patient must be warned that he may not be able to put his foot to the ground during this reaction. The injection is therefore best carried out on a Friday evening and a strong analgesic prescribed.

Prevention of Recurrence—Raising the heel of the shoe while keeping its upper surface horizontal enables the forefoot to drop down slightly, relaxing the fascia. Faradic foot baths and short flexor exercises strengthen the muscles that maintain the arch of the foot.

Results—Good.

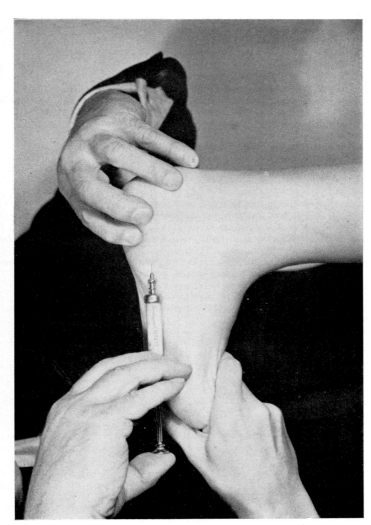

PLATE 156

References

BAYLIS, P. (1966) Some legal aspects of private practice. *Physiotherapy*, **52**, 303.
BRODIN, H., BANG, J., BECHGAARD, P., KALTENBORN, F., & SCHOITZ, E. (1966) *Manipulation av Ryggraden*. Stockholm: Scandinavian University Books.
BROWN, T. (1828) Irritation of the spinal nerves. *Glasg. med. J.*, 158.
COLDHAM, M. (1975) Chiropractic. *Canad. med. J.*, **112**, 929.
CYRIAX, J. (1945) Lumbago: The mechanism of dural pain. *Lancet*, **ii**, 427.
———— (1948) Fibrositis. *Brit. med. J.*, **ii**, 251.
———— (1950) Treatment of lumbar disc lesions. *Brit. med. J.*, **ii**, 1434.
———— & TROISIER, O. (1953) Hydrocortisone and soft-tissue lesions. *Brit. med. J.*, **ii**, 966.
GOWERS, W. R. (1904) Lumbago. *Brit. med. J.*, **i**, 117.
GRIFFIN, J. E. & TOUCHSTONE, J. S. (1963) Ultrasonic movement of cortisol into pig tissues. *Amer. J. phys. Med.*, **43**, 77.
HARRISON, E. (1920) Effect of spinal distortion on sanguineous circulation. *London med. phys. J.*, **44**, 373.
HIRSHFELD, P. F. (1962) Die konservative Behandlung des lumbalen Bandscheiben-vorvalls nach der Methode Cyriax. *Dt. med. Wschr.*, **9**, 299.
HUNERFAUTH (1887) *Handbuch der Massage*, p. 113.
KALTENBORN, F. (1967) *Frigjoring av Ryggraden*. Oslo: Universitets Forlaget.
KLEINKORT, J. A. & WOOD, F. (1975) Phonophoresis with 1 % versus 10 % hydro-cortisone. *Phys. Ther.*, **55**, 1321.
MAITLAND, G. D. (1964) *Vertebral Manipulation*. London: Butterworths.
MIXTER, W. J. & BARR, J. S. (1934) Rupture of intervertebral disc with involve-ment of spinal canal. *New Engl. J. Med.*, **211**, 210.
PRINGLE, B. (1956) Approach to intervertebral disc lesions. *Trans. Ass. indust. med. Offrs*, **5**, 127.
RIADORE, J. E. (1843) *Irritation of Spinal Nerves*. London: Churchill.
SEGUIN, (1838) Torticollis guéri par extension, massage et percussion candencée. *Rev. med. franc.*, **75**, 2.
TROISIER, O. (1973) *Les Algies Discales et Ligamentaires du Rachis*. Paris: Masson.
WILSON, D. G. (1962) Manipulative treatment in general practice. *Lancet*, **i**, 1013.
YOUNG, B. K. (1969) *The Observer*, Sunday 12 October.

Index

Index